CHILDREN'S COSTUME 1860-1920

Darlings of Dress

Norma Shephard

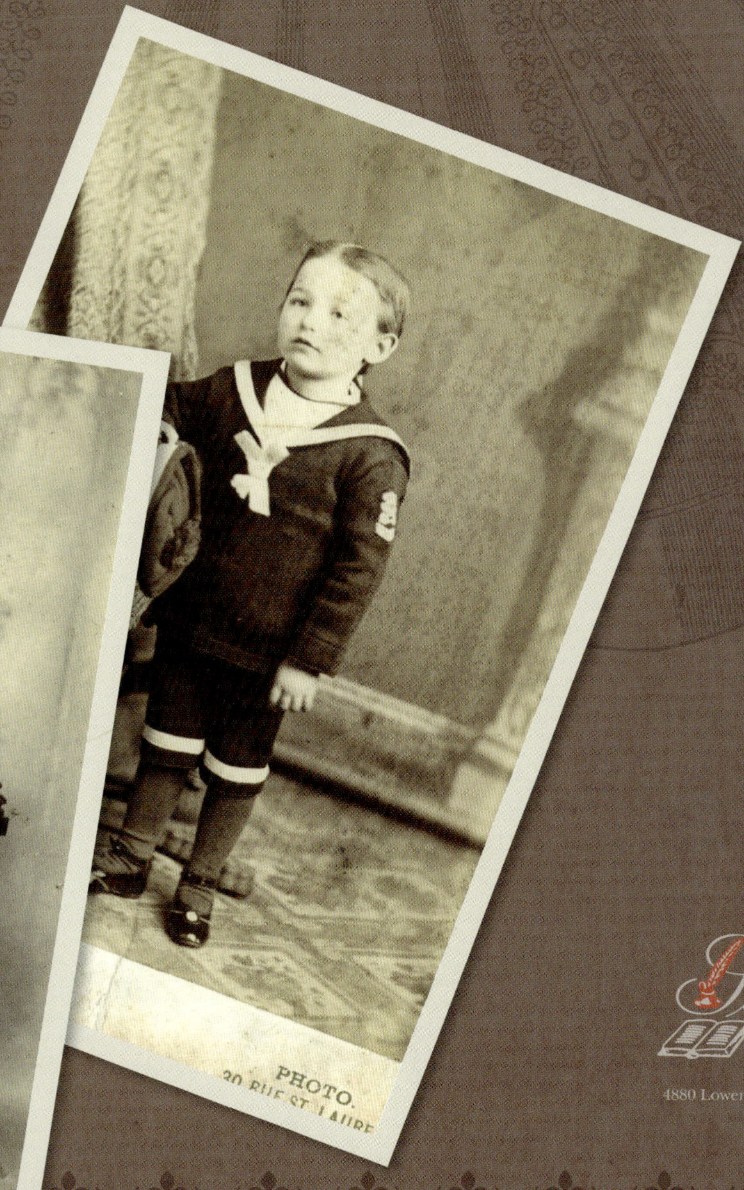

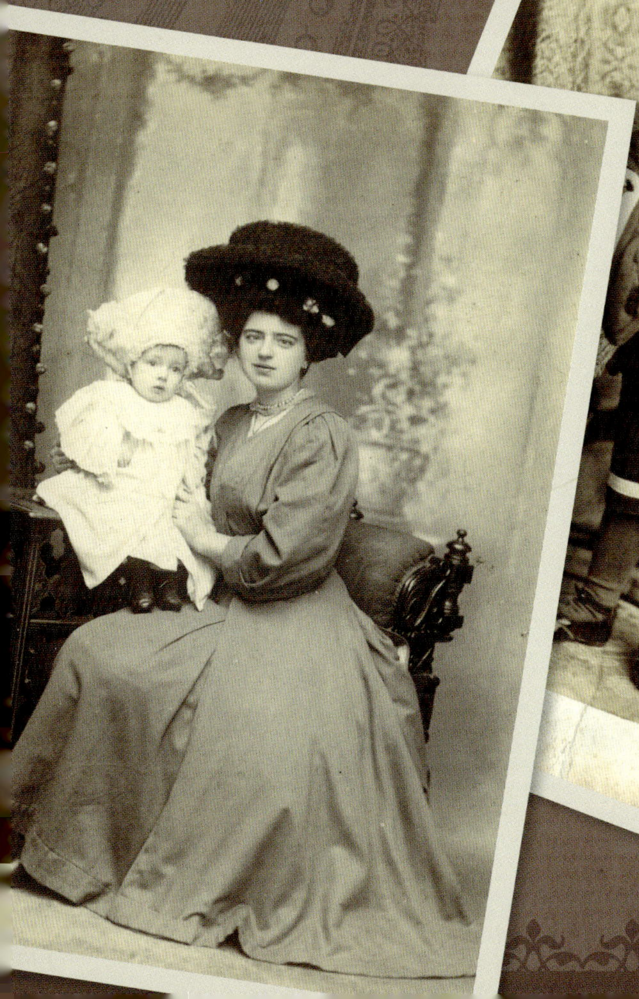

Schiffer Publishing Ltd
4880 Lower Valley Road • Atglen, PA 19310

Other Schiffer Books by Norma Shephard:

Accessorizing the Bride: Vintage Wedding Finery through the Decades, ISBN 978-0-7643-2185-6

In Step with Fashion: 200 Years of Shoe Styles, ISBN 978-0-7643-2817-6

Lingerie: Two Centuries of Luscious Design, ISBN 978-0-7643-2818-3

Library of Congress Control Number: 2017940409

Designed by Molly Shields
Cover design by Brenda McCallum
Type set in Egregio Script/Adobe Caslon Pro

ISBN: 978-0-7643-4939-3
Printed in China

Published by Schiffer Publishing, Ltd.
4880 Lower Valley Road
Atglen, PA 19310
Phone: (610) 593-1777; Fax: (610) 593-2002
E-mail: Info@schifferbooks.com
Web: www.schifferbooks.com

For Abigail Corinne Kramer, Sidney Patricia Shephard, and James Conor Shephard: within these pages you will find many of your foremothers and forefathers as they appeared in childhood.

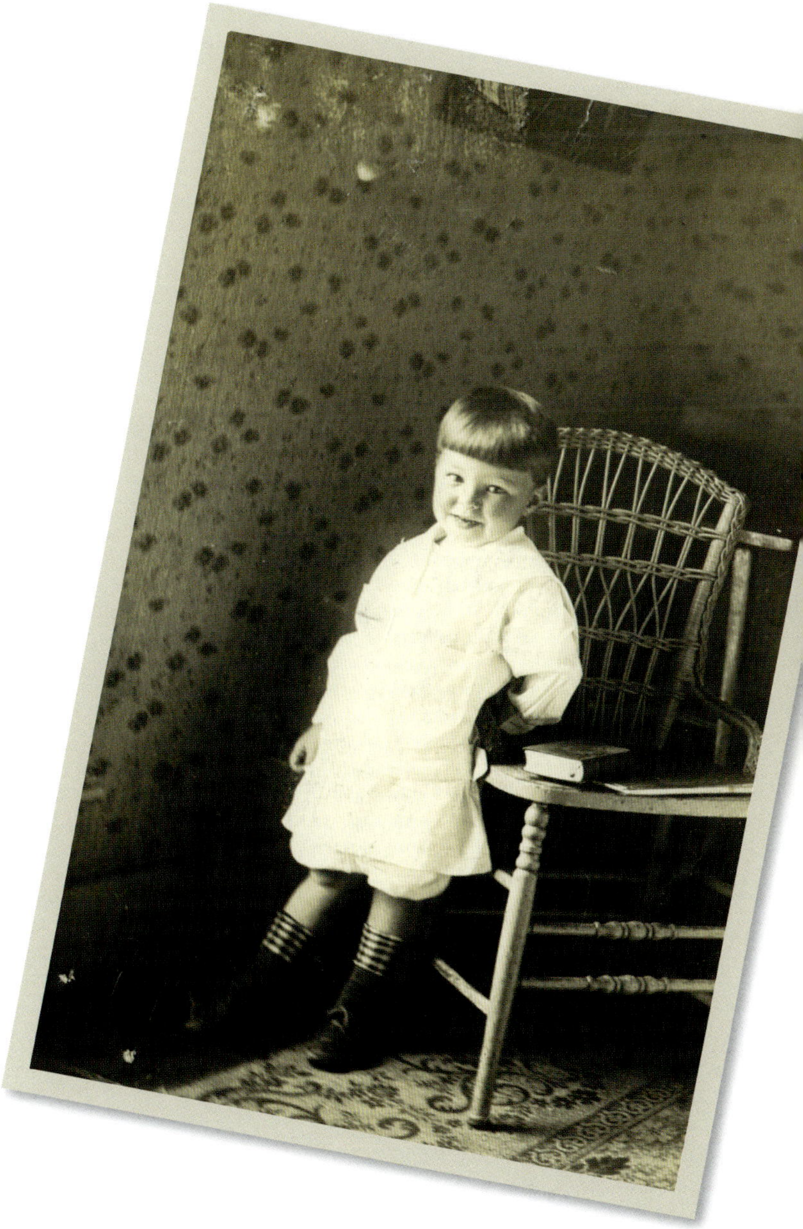

Contents

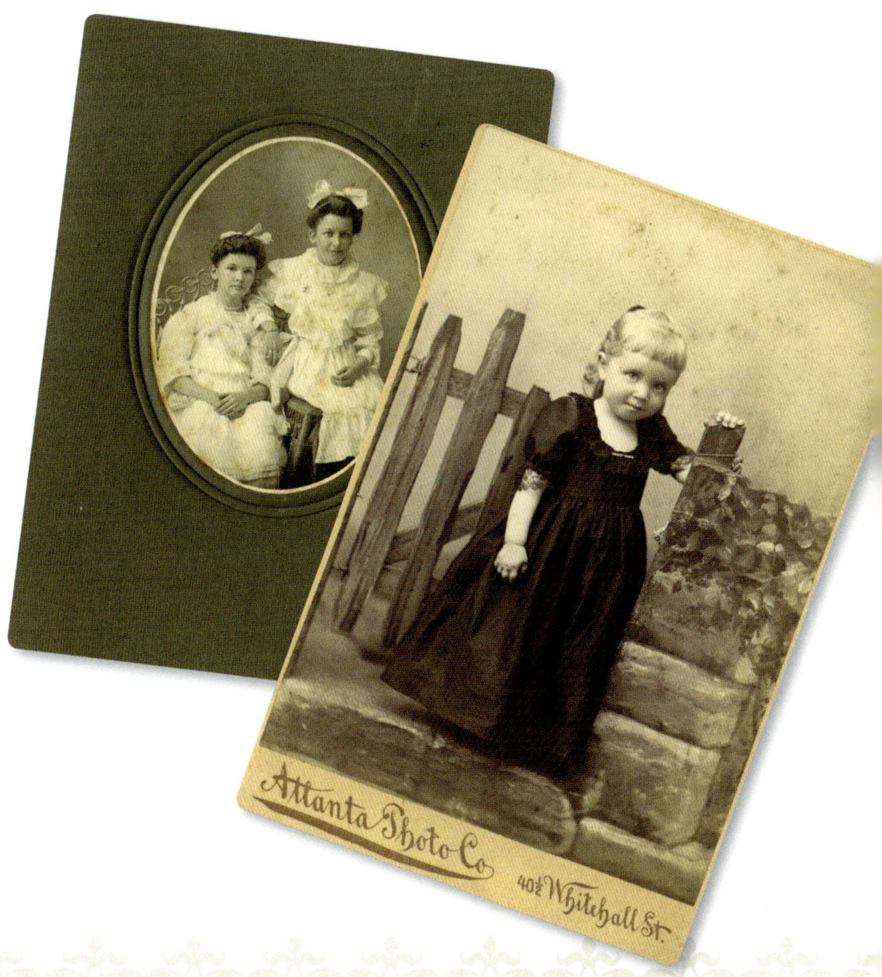

Acknowledgments

Many an archivist will admit there is a fine line between conservation and hoarding. In this age of consumerism it is often difficult when editing our possessions to have an eye for what future historians will find of interest.

I am grateful for parents and grandparents who honored their family history enough to preserve letters, portraits, and scores of artifacts, making space for them through many moves. And to other families of like mind, whose children's clothing, family portraits, periodicals, and catalogs they tucked dutifully away and then released for me to find at antique shops, thrift stores, and flea market stalls. I would not be able to do that were it not for the wonderful vintage clothing shopkeepers and dealers I have met along the way, chief among them Connie Bulagic, Jentine Gootges, Jill Silverstone, and Laura Skrovonek.

On a more personal level, I wish to thank my brother, Bruce Hillyer, for keeping me sane through that damp spring weekend of sorting through over one hundred years of documents at the old Brigham homestead.

Thanks also to the many friends and family of the Mobile Millinery Museum and Costume Archive who supplied additional images and artifacts, particularly Kathy Crow, Jean Burbidge, Ron Minaker, and Nancy Rasmussen.

As always, I owe a debt of gratitude to my husband and fellow author, Jim Shephard, for overlooking—and only occasionally commenting on—my ever-growing hoard of period photographs, documents, and costume artifacts. Jim is also the co-founder of Northshore Wordsmiths, a writers' group whose members—Anne Gwaza, Bobbie Smith, Elsie Thorn, Diana Walsh, and John Wilkinson—were always ready to offer enthusiastic support and insightful critique. Thanks as well to the encouragement and insight of fellow writers Jean Burbidge and Kathy Crow. I'm also grateful to my editor, Cheryl Weber, and the team at Schiffer Publishing.

Finally, to readers of my previous fashion history books, and to the vintage costume enthusiasts who attend my many annual exhibits and installations, thank you for sharing stories of your own treasures and for posing the questions that keep me seeking answers to the who, what, when, where, why, and how of vintage and antique costume.

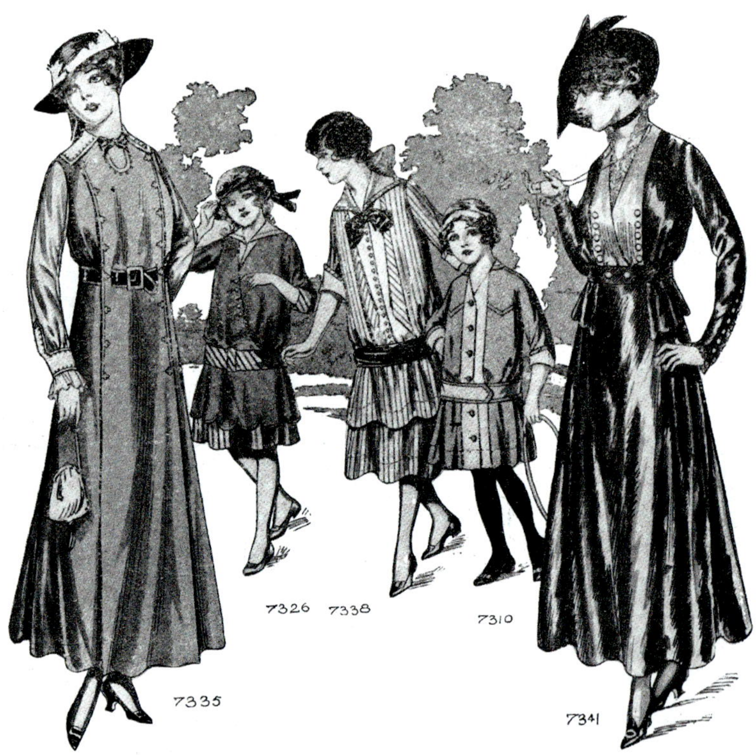

Introduction

Oh, Baby!

> "We may say that many, if not all, of the personality traits that we have called masculine or feminine are as likely linked to sex as are the clothing, the manners, and the form of headdress that a society at a given period assigns to either sex."—Margaret Mead, cultural anthropologist

One of my favorite things to do at Christmas is to attend a matinee performance of the *Nutcracker*. I always plan to arrive early to people-watch. For the attendees with kids in tow it is an extra special occasion for which the children are suitably and often lavishly attired.

While there is no official dress code for attending the ballet, most people prepare for the magical experience by dressing up in something special and/or holiday inspired. The aspiring ballerinas are easy to spot in their red velvet coats and taffeta dresses or crinolined tutu-like skirts. Some dress in long gowns and even the boys get into the act.

At times undervalued or trivialized, fashion is an integral component of our recollection of historical events. Costume helps shape individual and collective identity while providing very real physical defenses against the elements. Costume is more intimately connected to the human experience than any other artifact; indeed, period garments bear witness to the personal daily existence of those who have gone before.

Over the past dozen years I have presented a number of costume exhibits and museum installations throughout Ontario, the most popular of which has been "Unsinkable Fashion: Costume From the Titanic Era." At each of these presentations, the artifacts that received the most attention were those made for and worn by children.

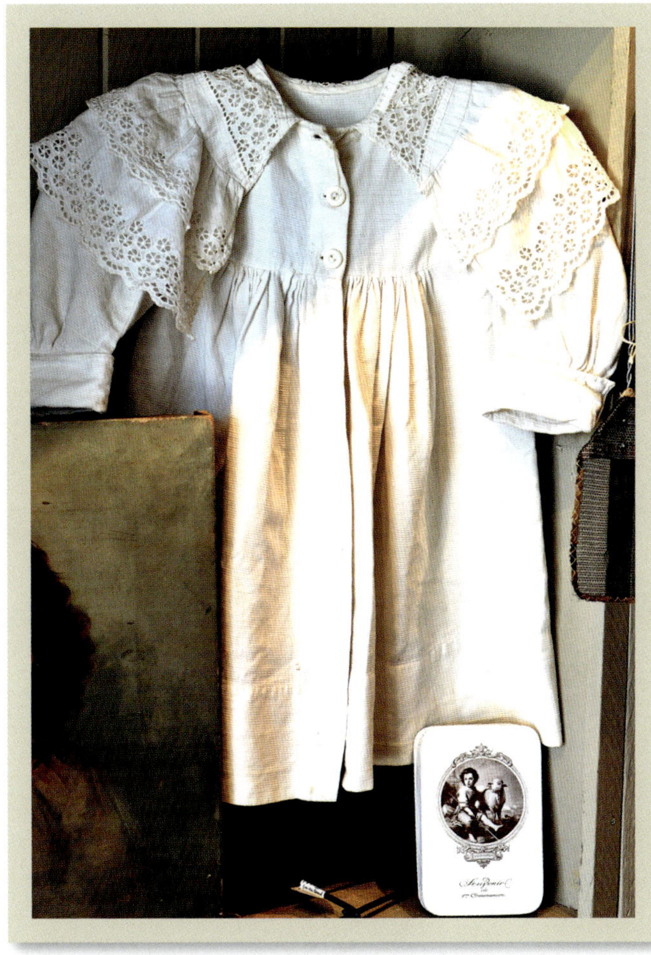

A sepia-toned Victorian vignette featuring a young child's cotton coat with layered cutwork collar.

Sleuthing for Historic Costume

> "Vintage, to me, means that the clothing is at least thirty years old and wearable; antique clothing, to me, is a piece that predates the 1940s."—Karen Augusta, Augusta Auctions

Who doesn't love a mystery? Certainly, I do. As a girl, I devoured Nancy Drew books and their Hardy Boys equivalents, trekking to the library for the next volume practically before finishing the last. I went into nursing to satisfy my curiosity about how the body works, and when my husband hung up his shingle as a private investigator, I was only too happy to assist with his cases. We once found a runaway teen girl after I suggested staking out the local laundromats. Even then, my thoughts ran to fashion.

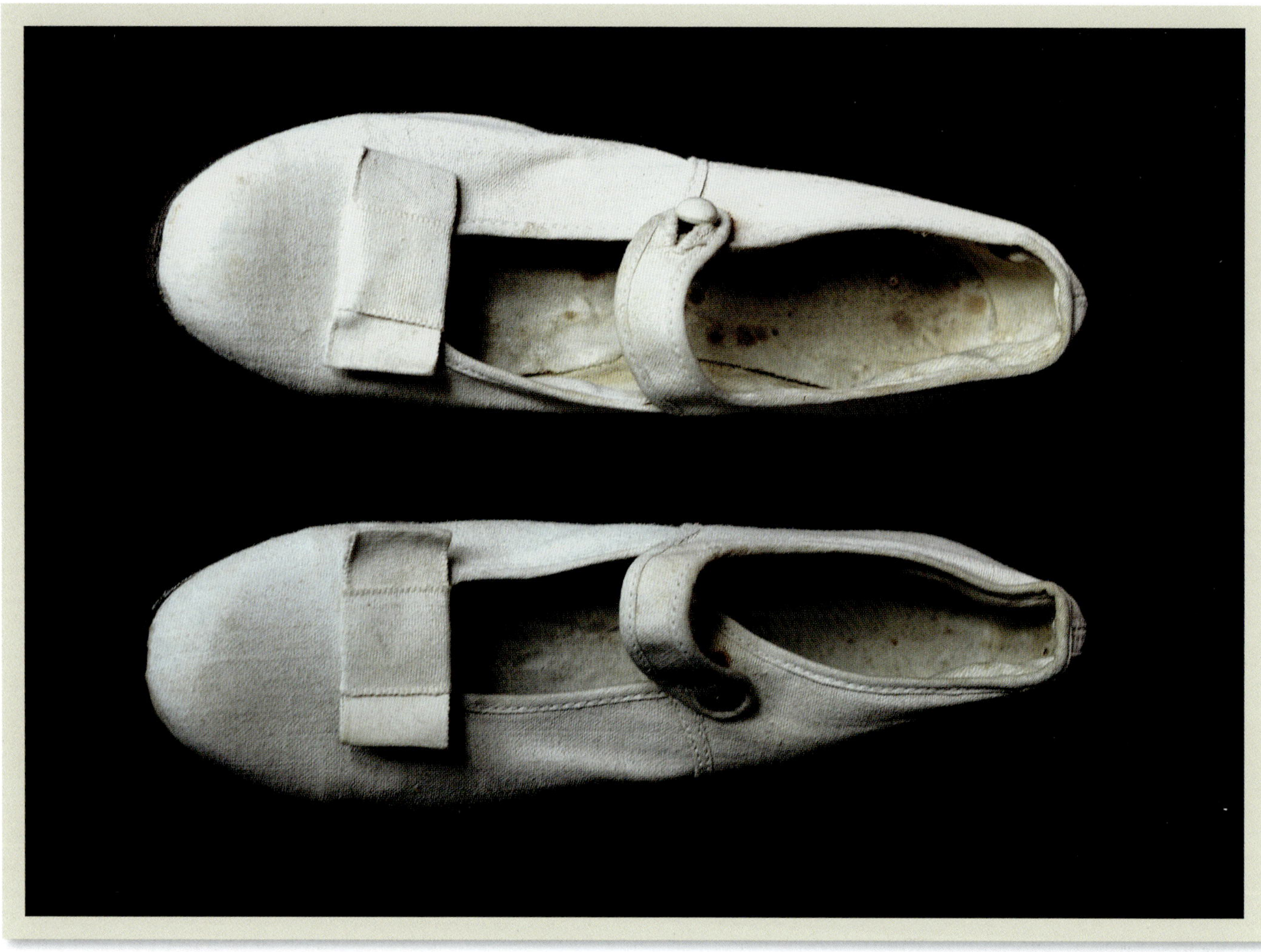

Girl's white canvas shoes with button closure.

It wasn't until I founded the Mobile Millinery Museum—a textile archive that now houses close to 3,000 hats and hundreds of period costume goodies—that I was able to combine my love of fashion with my penchant for puzzle solving. In 2004, after amassing a selection of period wedding gowns, I wrote and photographed *Accessorizing the Bride: Vintage Wedding Finery through the Decades*, a project that required me to research each of the pieces, matching them to their place in social history.

1,000 Hats followed in 2006, then *In Step with Fashion: 200 Years of Shoe Styles* and *Lingerie: Two Centuries of Luscious Design* (my husband's favorite), in 2008. Along the way, I became fascinated with the study of children's dress and joined the throng of museum buyers, decorators, costumers, and photographers in search of nineteenth- and twentieth-century children's clothing, accessories, embroidery transfers, luggage, portraits, and sewing patterns.

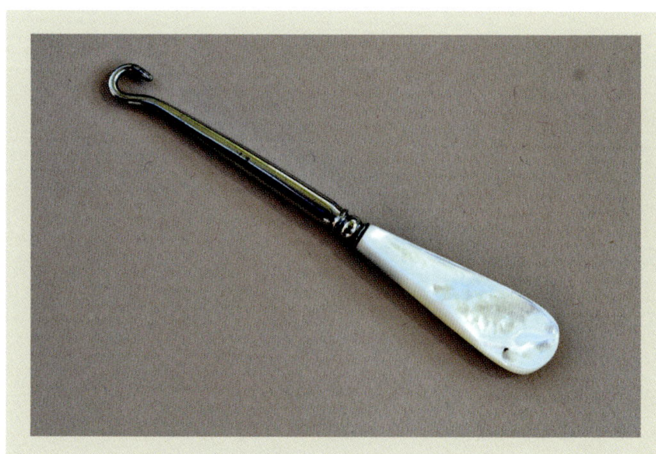

Child's mother-of-pearl button hook.

Part of the appeal of vintage and antique costume is the outstanding quality and uniqueness of the pieces available for

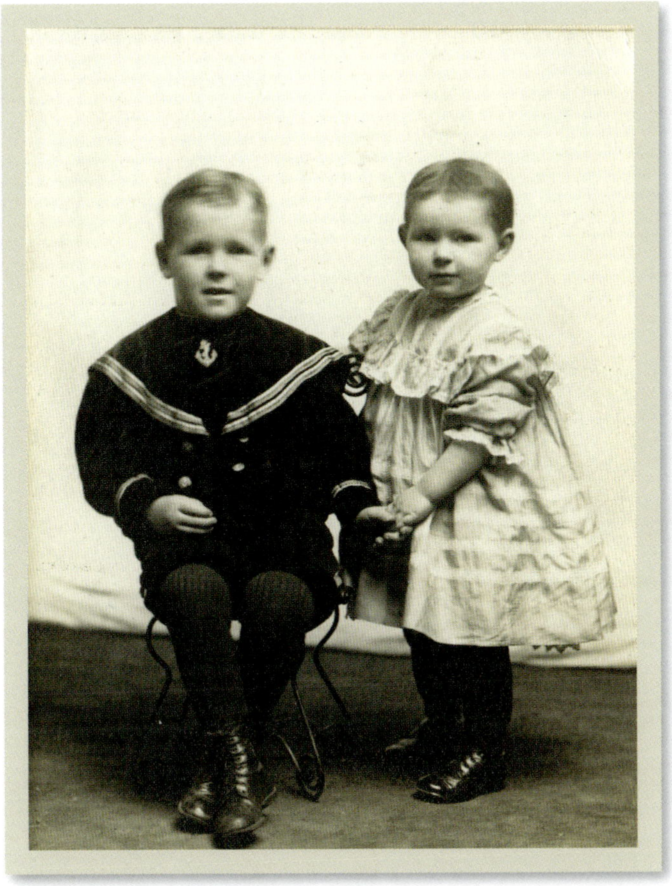

Siblings dressed in gender-specific attire.

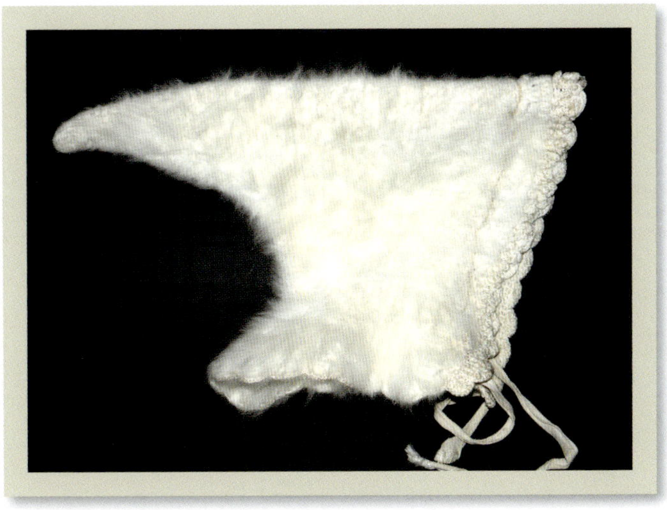

A child's white angora pixie hat with hand worked crochet trim, discovered in the children's corner of Vintage Soul Geek in Hamilton, Ontario.

sale, many of which speak distinctly of their times. Discerning enthusiasts search for delightful designs fashioned from one of the many tantalizing textiles of ages past. Those in the know employ various strategies for finding that next great treasure, some choosing to make regular forays into their local vintage store or charity shop. Stopping in for a quick raid on the way home from work will not result in a great find on every visit, but this shopping style ensures the occasional successful plunder.

Those with a fondness for online auction sites such as eBay and Etsy enjoy the quality and variety of items listed. Passwords and a PayPal account at the ready, this group shops from home at any hour of the day or night.

Still others take a festival approach to their vintage clothing searches, saving up for a weekend of extended browsing at special vintage clothing shows like the three held in Sturbridge, Massachusetts, each year. Like big game hunters, they prefer the jungle atmosphere of bustling crowds, long lineups, and competitive buyers.

For ready-to-wear, carefully curated vintage pieces from the 1920s to the 1970s, my favorite shop is Vintage Soul Geek in Hamilton, Ontario, but when I'm in the mood for a good dig, I like to visit The Little Shop on Ogilvy Street in Montreal. This textile treasure trove has anything and everything, including a festive atmosphere and an owner who will serve you tea. Closer to my home is Laura Skrovonek's stall at Aberfoyle, Canada's oldest antique market.

Many vintage shops keep limited hours, and some only accept cash, so check details before heading out.

Christening Gowns

The most collectible of all vintage children's garments is the christening gown. This religious vestment was traditionally worn within the first few weeks or months following the infant's birth when the child received the sacrament of baptism. In Victorian times the gown might be handmade by the mother, at times using fabric from her own wedding dress. Tradition being what it is, the gown was put away for use by subsequent children and was even handed down through the generations.

Christening gown style and workmanship varied little from 1860 to 1900. The dresses were generally made of white cotton, silk, or flannel and embroidered with rosettes and/or ribbon work. These opened at the back and were fitted across the shoulders, but fell in long swoops that would drape over the arms of the officiant's black robes when he held the child, eliciting oohs and aahs even from a distance. Depending upon the season, the ensemble might include a matching cloak, but bonnet and booties were a must. For sentimental reasons, a daughter's bonnet might be fashioned from her mother's lacy bridal hanky, then unstitched years later to be used for its original purpose.

By 1900, fashion dictated a lighter aesthetic, and gowns of this nature were primarily fashioned of white cotton or

INFANT'S CHRISTENING ROBE.

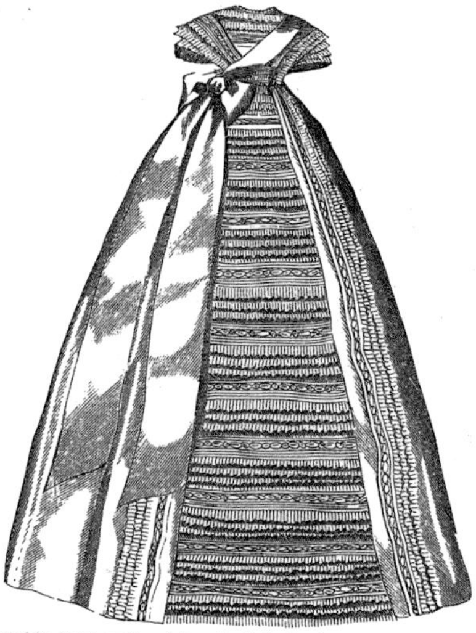

MADE of fine French muslin, and trimmed with fluted ruffles and inserting. The sash is of very broad white ribbon.

A formal christening robe set with insertion lace and sashed with ribbon. *Godey's Lady's Book and Magazine*, July to December 1861.

INFANT'S CHRISTENING ROBE.

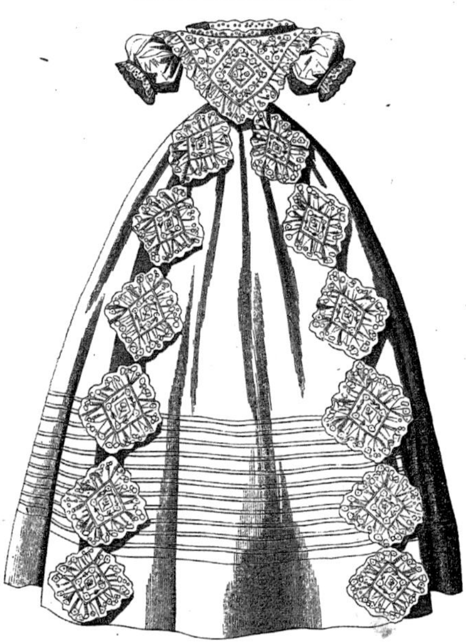

Rosettes made of flouncing decorate this 1860s illustration of a fashionable christening robe. *Godey's Lady's Book and Magazine*, January to June 1861.

NOVELTIES FOR MARCH.

JUVENILE FASHIONS.

Fig. 1.

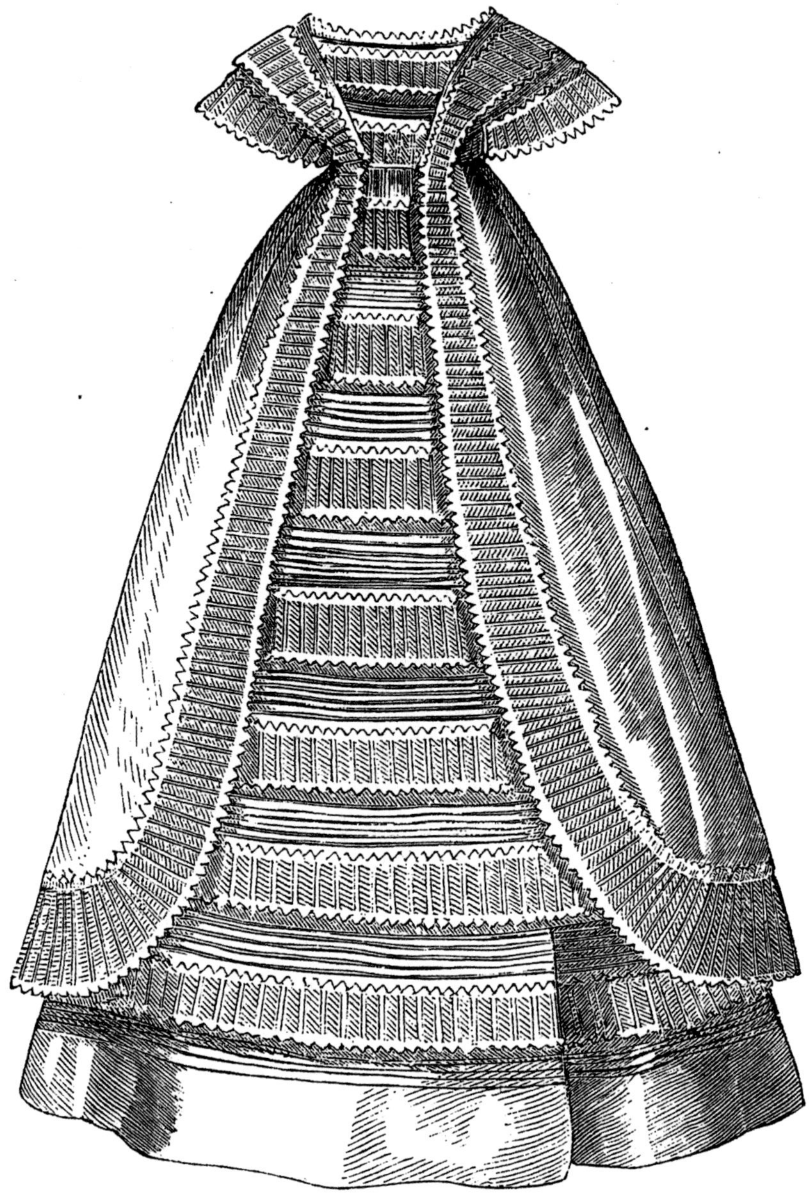

Illustration of the latest in christening robes in March 1861; a ruffled and pin-tucked gown with vertical and horizontal embellishment. *Godey's Lady's Book and Magazine*, January to June 1861.

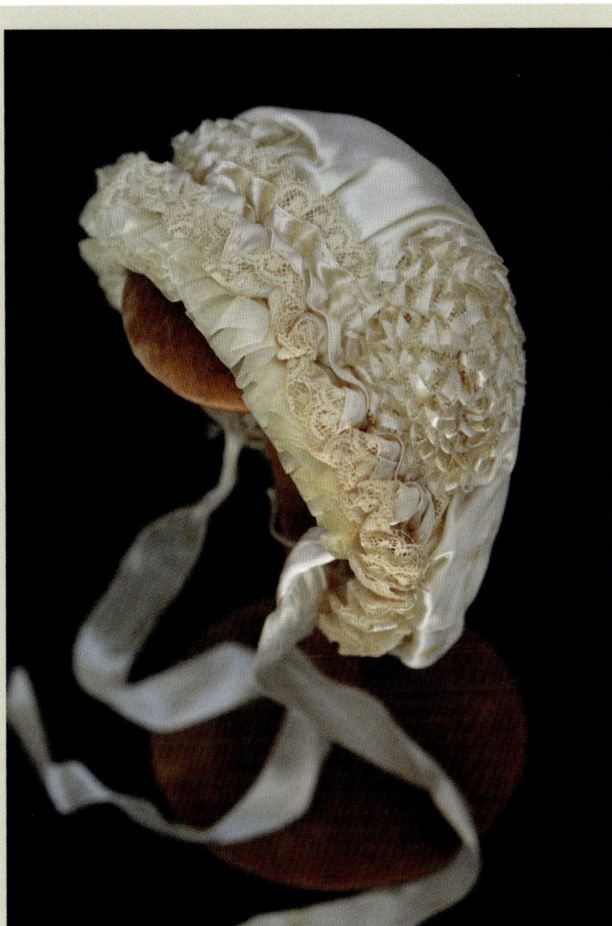

Silk satin christening cap with padding and ribbon ties, c. 1915.

dotted Swiss. Embellishment was easily achieved through machine-stitched pin tucks, lace insertions, cutwork, or through the purchase of pre-embroidered fabric. By the teens, it was perfectly acceptable to purchase ready-made christening gowns from a department store or mail order catalog.

Forensics of Costume Collecting

> "Children's clothes were definitely remade over and over to accommodate a growing body. A lot of the time, they were re-purposed for younger siblings as well."—Anna-Marie Hand, Maryland Historical Society

Often a collector starts out as someone who simply happens upon an aged but particularly interesting or tantalizing textile; a piece of handmade lace perhaps, or an exquisite silk christening gown, maybe even a pair of gold leather high-button boots or a beaded bag. Something falls into our hands that causes us to marvel at the design, workmanship, or embellishment. We wonder who wore it and when. Where and how was it made? What was its original cost, its present value?

If we are lucky, the object comes with an eyewitness, someone who can tell us the object's history. There may be an accompanying photograph or letter, even a sales receipt. We discover the wonders of provenance. But even if the object of our delight was snagged at a rummage sale or unearthed from a bag of discards destined for the local thrift shop, we can tell at a glance that it is old, out-dated, and special.

Just as fingerprints can be lifted from a piece of glass with the correct equipment and techniques, so too can perspiration and other stains be lifted from aged textiles, adding to the wearability of an antique or vintage article of clothing. But much of the antique children's clothing available to buyers today is too fragile to be worn, and serves instead as a study piece or decorative accent.

Antique and vintage children's clothing, like any other category of aged textile, is a finite commodity, one often overlooked by vintage costume buyers, most of whom are looking for wearable adult fashions, iconic of their times.

Age-Specific Cuteness and Era-Specific Appeal

> "Culture and fashion have an interlacing relationship."—Cece Scriver, vintage clothing dealer

What is it about children's clothing that draws the oohs and aahs from audience members and causes us to pack away outfits that our own offspring have outgrown months and even years before? Rory Evans, former editor of *Martha Stewart Living*, expressed it thus: "Some of my daughter's outgrown dresses are so inextricably linked to my memories of her age-specific cuteness, the thought of putting them away physically pains me." Evans encourages readers to frame such items and decorate with them.

Framing is certainly one way of living with our children's cherished clothing from years gone by, but placing such items under glass eliminates the possibility of being able to appreciate their tactile beauty or turn them inside out to gaze at the label or examine their construction.

Evans' theory of age-specific cuteness can be expanded to encompass era-specific appeal, as a study of children's costume through the decades reveals fashions, fads, and trends that ebb and flow with the changing social times.

Children's clothing has changed over the decades, and while it is the children themselves who put the darling in dress, parents have always enjoyed dressing their children up, whether it be the middle-class Victorian family who outfitted their offspring to echo their social status and reflect well on the family, or the 1950s mom who as a child spent hours at play dressing her dolls, and now can't wait to place her infant in the prettiest or handsomest attire money will buy.

Clothing has gone through a number of incarnations throughout the nineteenth and twentieth centuries with changes not only in style but in textile fabrication and clothing manufacture as well, thanks to innovations brought about after the industrial revolution. Throughout the sixty-year period covered by this book, the appearance, composition, and manufacture of children's clothing was further influenced by such diverse factors as war, literature, technology, music, transportation, agriculture, geography, chemistry, religious mores, commerce, and sometimes pure chance.

Precious Pigments

> "All who can, should grow their patches of flax and cotton. All who can should have sheep, if but a few. Our forests furnish dyes as various and as bright as the tints that make their foliage as glorious at 'the turn of the leaf.' With these materials, there is no reason why our ladies should not be clad in beautiful apparel, the product of their own industry and taste; while they also may clothe their husbands and sons."—*Clarke County Journal*, February 4, 1864

Much has been written about the discovery of aniline dyes and its boon to the textile industry, enabling it to produce dyes with exact shades. But there was magic in many of the organic pigments commonly used to color fabric prior to William Henry Perkins' accidental discovery of mauveine in 1856.

Nineteenth-century manufacturers and home economists alike developed their own recipes for dying woolens and cotton yarns using everything from walnut root to red oak, and hickory bark to moss. Sassafras (a root used to flavor root beer), poke berries, and the bark of wild plum root were also valued for their coloration properties. The processes were labor intensive and might involve the use of alum, vinegar, rusty pots or nails, cream of tartar, writing ink, or suet. The "animalizing" process might further require the use of urine, blood, milk, or even dung. Many recipes were carefully guarded, but the effects of the Civil War—factory fires, blockades, inflated prices, and the devaluation of the Confederate dollar—necessitated the public sharing of these home recipes and a return to the spinning wheel for many women, particularly in the South.

The widespread use of chemical dyes developed over time as more tints were developed.

It is no accident that the artist Henri de Toulouse-Lautrec became a master of pastels, coming as he did from the region of Lautrec, famous for its pigment known as pastel blue. This "perfect blue" is harvested from the *Isatis tinctoria* leaves, which when ground and dried produce a pigment that boasts a ten-year resistance to fading from sun and/or water exposure. Pastel blue was also valued for its antimicrobial properties.

Eventually, indigo, which produced a deeper intensity of color, brought about the decline of pastel, as it could be produced at one-sixth the cost and could also be adulterated to produce a range of tints.

Garments colored with this natural dye are still being produced today.

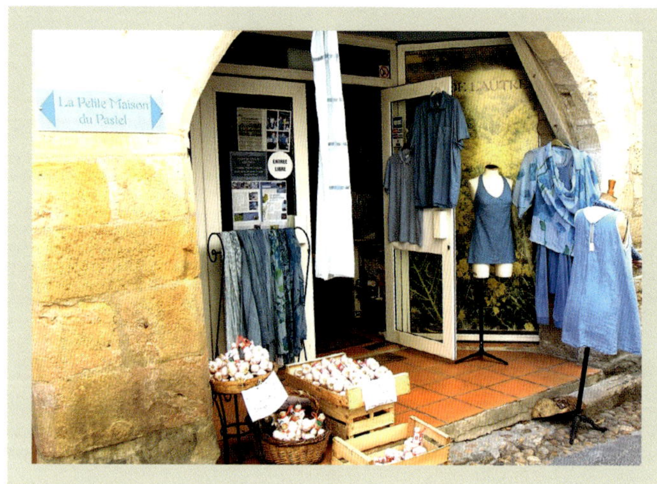

La Petite Maison du Pastel, a treasure trove of authentic pastel blue textiles and other handmade products.

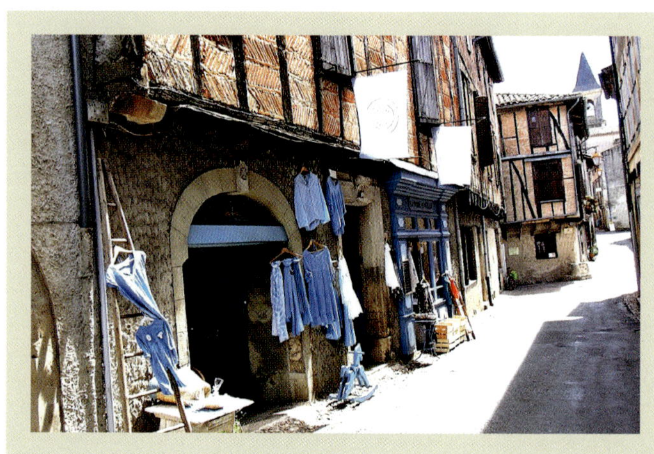

This shop selling pastel blue textiles is on the Rue du Mercadial in Lautrec.

The Influence of Literature on Children's Clothing Design

> "There is really nothing in the world that can be compared to red shoes!"—From "The Red Shoes" by Hans Christian Andersen

In children's literature, footwear, more than any other item of apparel, is used to convey allegory—"The Red Shoes," *Little Goodie Two Shoes*, *The Wizard of Oz*, "The Shoemaker and the Elves"—to name just a few. Often the shoes possess magical powers and at times are used to teach virtue or warn against misdeeds.

Clear plastic novelty heels, based on the Cinderella tale, have long delighted children and are a staple in any serious dress-up box. But illustrations of popular fictional characters as diverse as Alice in Wonderland, Little Lord Fontleroy, Buster Brown, and Davy Crockett have had a powerful influence on children's everyday wear as well.

The decision of a firm in Victorian London to initiate a children's clothing line based on Kate Greenaway's work proved lucrative, with followers of the arts and crafts movement choosing to dress their little girls in pantaloons, pinafores, and sublimely pictorial bonnets.

When Frances Hodgson Burnett's book, *Little Lord Fauntleroy*, was published in 1886, Burnett submitted a photograph of her son, Vivian, to the publishers as a guide for the illustrations. What they saw was a boy whose velvet tunic was lavishly trimmed with a lace collar and cuffs. A feather-trimmed floppy velvet hat topped his coif of fringe and curls—described as lovelocks by the author—and a low-slung satin belt presided over knee-length velvet pants.

The look was interpreted by illustrator Reginald Birch, whose pen and ink drawings of the boy so inspired American mothers that they clamored to dress their sons in the style of the little aristocrat they saw pictured in the pages of Burnett's book. Supply of the velvet suits, lace-trimmed blouses, and leggings soon met demand with multiple variations of the style made available. The story was later developed into a film starring Mary Pickford, which revived the popularity of the look in the 1920s.

General Observations

> "The use of a shoeing horn in putting on the children's low shoes saves the heels of the stockings."—Elizabeth Robinson Scovil, *Ladies' Home Journal*, April 1898

Before delving into a decade-by-decade investigation of children's costume from 1860 to 1920, it is helpful to consider a number of social factors and generalizations regarding the everyday and special-occasion children's wear of the Victorian period. Much thought and care was given to the virtue of economy. The pages of women's periodicals were full of advice to mothers on how to dress the family well regardless of budget. Extending the life of children's clothing was one way to economize despite an initial outlay of funds. Knee protectors for boys' stockings, for example, could be made at home for an outlay of between eighteen and twenty five cents c.1900. Advice columnist Elizabeth Robinson Scovil reported in *Ladies' Home Journal*, April 1898, "they are said to make one pair of stockings last as long as five." All of this in spite of the fact that most children's hosiery could be purchased with "double knees." Socks for infants were regularly made at home, silk socks requiring two balls of knitting silk in 1898.

Nightwear

Warmth was a major consideration in cold climate homes without central heating. Flannel nightgowns were favored for sleepwear throughout the Victorian era and usually worn over a fresh but light undershirt. Cold-feet gowns (long nightdresses

Illustration of a simple negligée for a young child. *Godey's Lady's Book and Magazine*, June to December 1861.

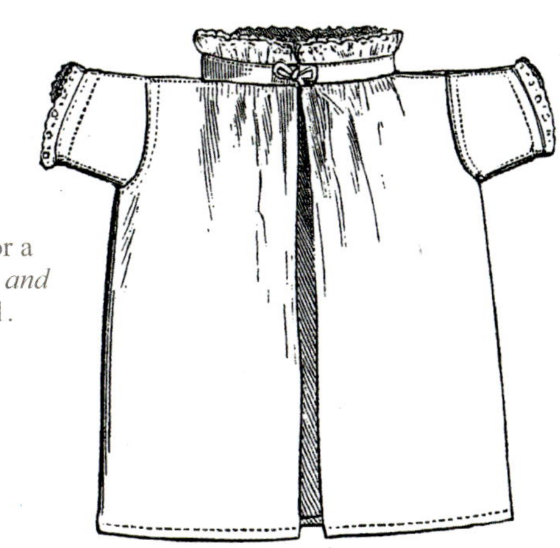

Fig. 10.—French *negligée* for a young child. To be made in cambric.

with button up flaps or drawstring casings at the hem) were recommended for restless sleepers who might throw off the covers during the night and become cold. Footed night drawers of flannel served a similar purpose and were furnished with a trap-door closure in the back. To save on washing, gray flannel was at times substituted for white.

Wrappers were worn over night dresses to provide warmth and were made of plain cloth throughout most of the Victorian era, but toward the end of the nineteenth century, chinchilla and crépon eiderdown became available. Four yards of fabric were estimated to make such a garment for a ten-year-old child.

Two-piece pajama sets in summer or winter fabrics did not become popular until the early twentieth century.

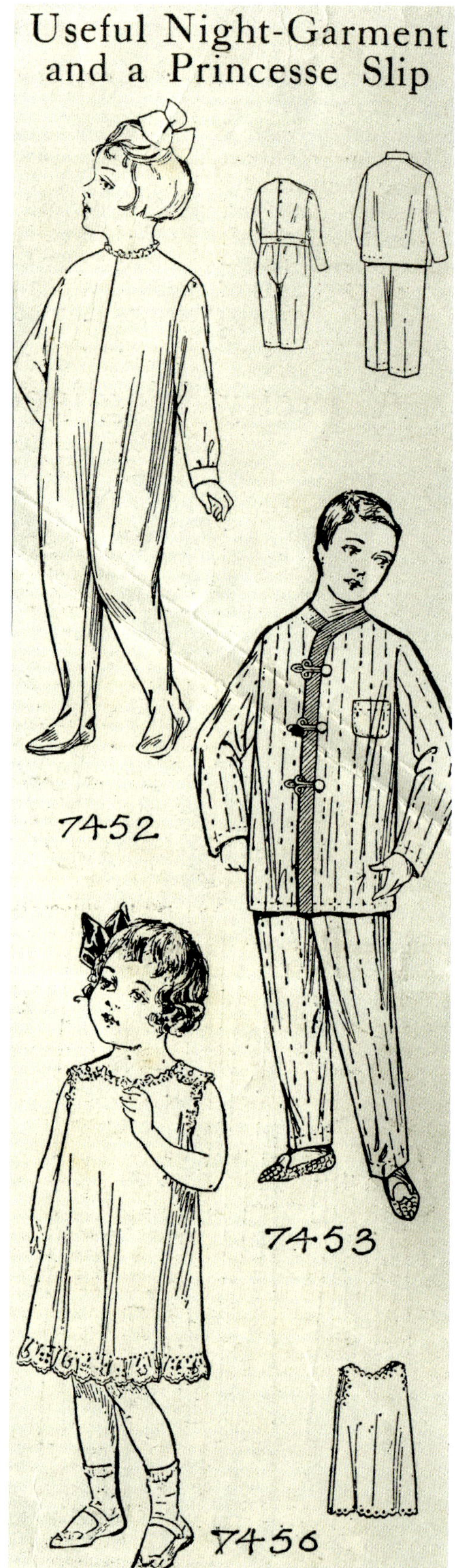

Patterns for these children's night-drawers, petticoat, and pajama sets could be obtained by sending ten cents to the publication. *Needlecraft Magazine*, December 1915.

Long and Short Clothes

Throughout the Victorian era, for the first five months or so, babies were dressed in what was known as long clothes, gowns that opened up the back and reached a foot or more beyond the baby's feet. Once the baby was able to crawl, long clothes became impractical and infants of both genders moved about in short clothes, dresses that reached the feet.

Expectant mothers could purchase layette sets containing ready-to-cut fabric for gowns, dresses, booties, bonnets, and carriage covers, pre-stamped with embroidery patterns, or start from scratch by purchasing separate patterns, fabric, and embroidery flosses to suit their individual taste.

Despite the apparent simplicity of infants' clothing, a number of style variations emerged, including a popular trend for finishing the bottom of a baby's skirt with a deep hem set below a cluster of pin tucks.

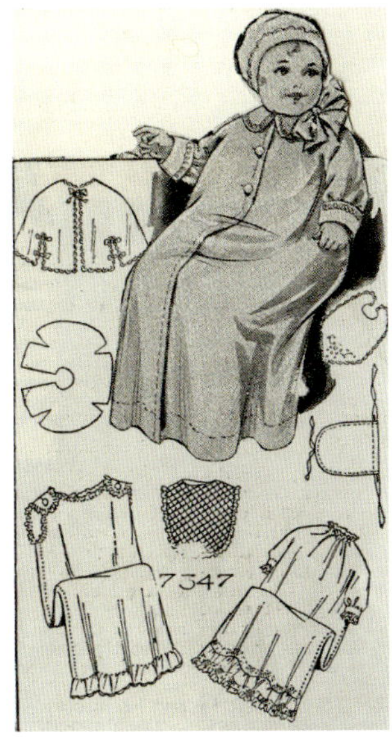

A sewing pattern package of infants' one-piece garments. *Needlecraft Magazine*, January 1916.

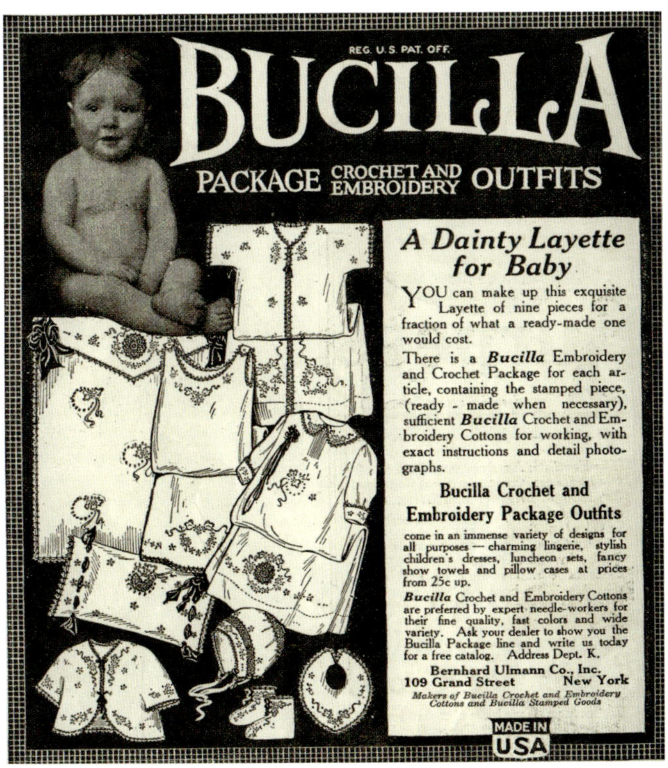

Ads for these step-saving Bucilla crochet packages appeared regularly in the pages of women's periodicals. *Needlecraft Magazine*, January 1916.

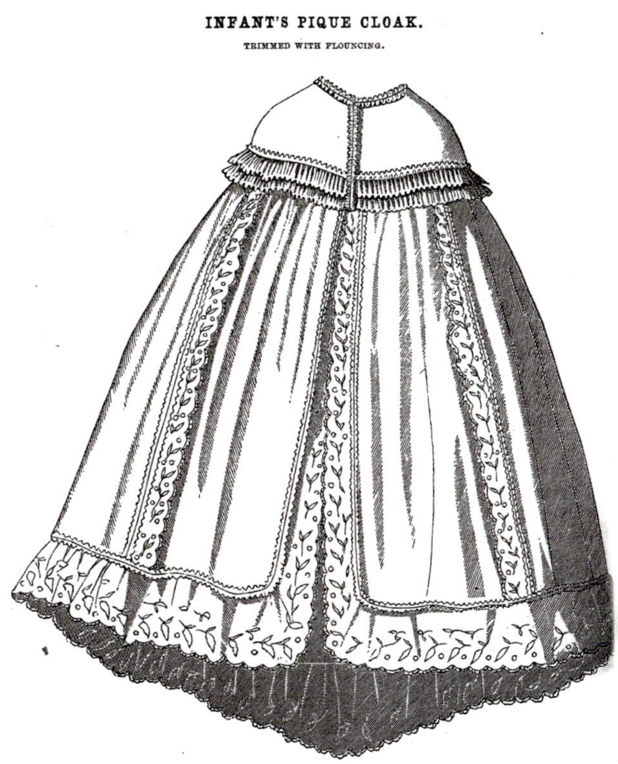

Infant's cape-like cloak trimmed with flounces. *Godey's Lady's Book and Magazine*, January to June 1861.

DRESS FOR A LITTLE BOY.

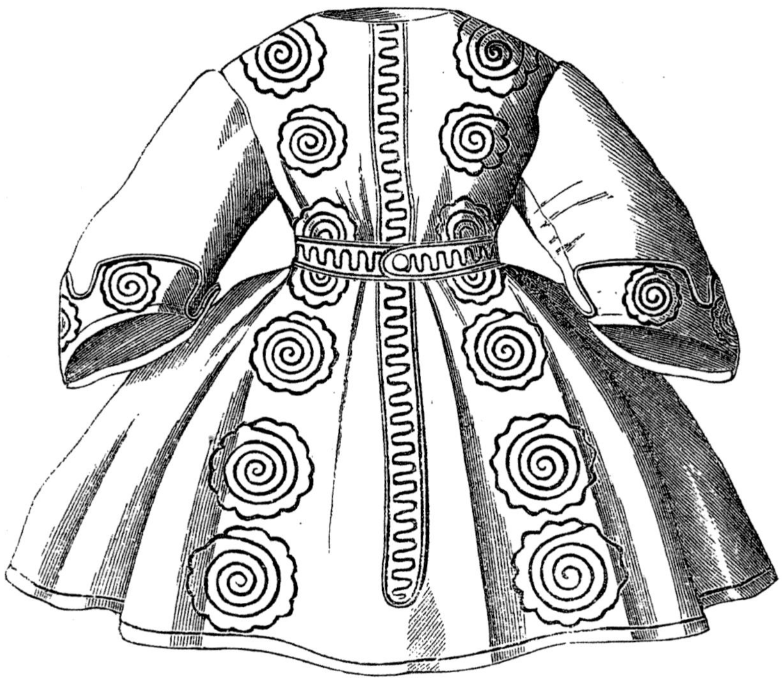

Dress for a little boy, full skirted with medallions of magenta braid on pearl colored poplin. *Godey's Lady's Book and Magazine*, January to June 1861.

INFANT'S SHORT DRESS.

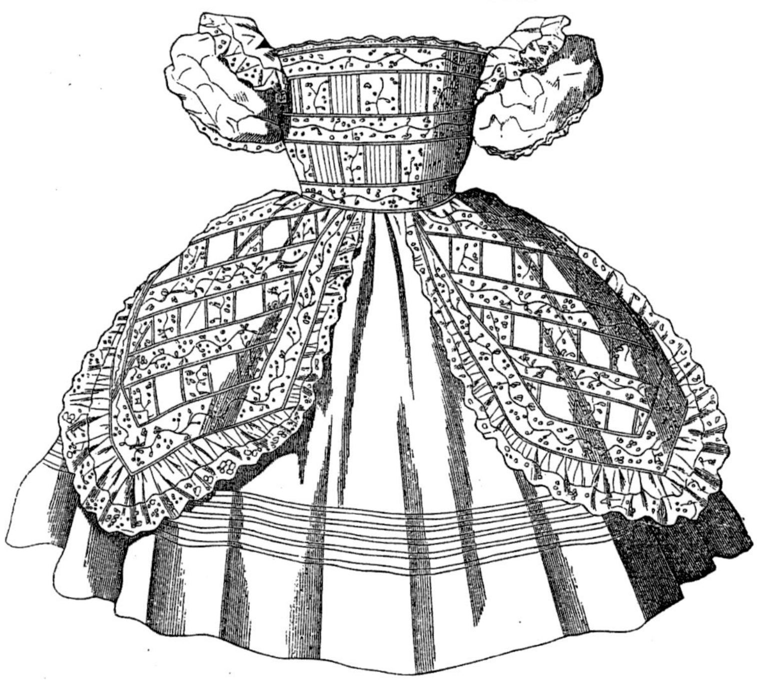

An infant's short dress of linen cambric, made special with lace insertion and trimmed with flouncing. *Godey's Lady's Book and Magazine*, January to June 1861.

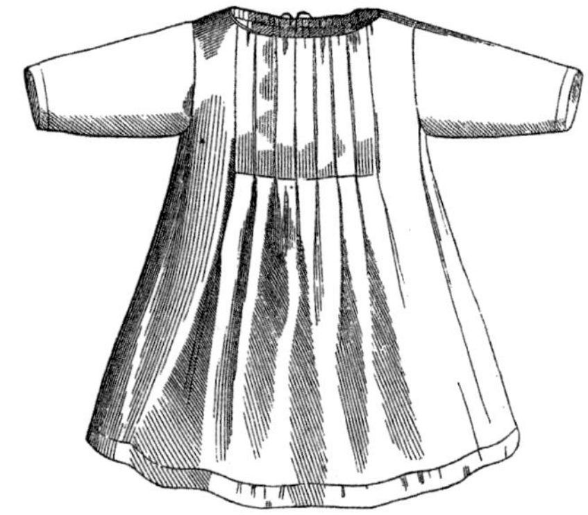

Pattern for an infant's plain morning slip. *Godey's Lady's Book and Magazine*, January to June 1861.

Fig. 3.

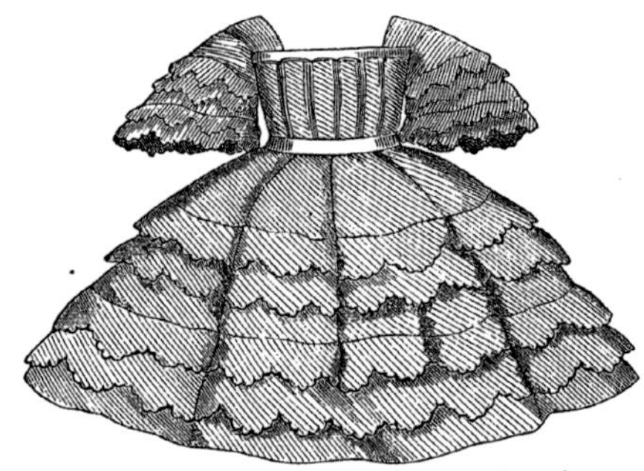

Extraordinarily fancy short dress for an infant, the skirt and sleeves described as having needle-worked scallops. *Godey's Lady's Book and Magazine*, January to June 1861.

Fig. 3.

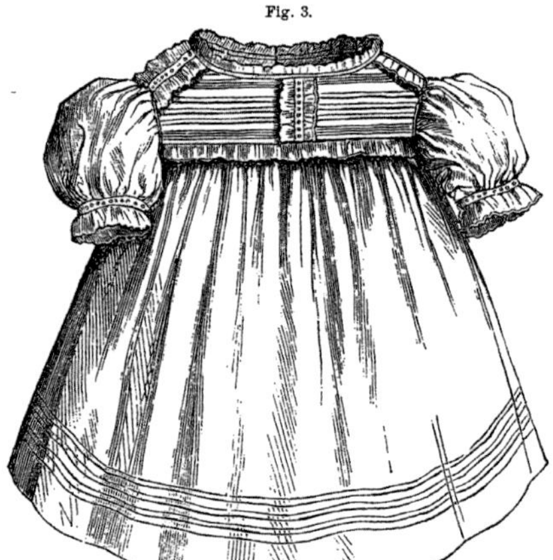

Trimmed with ruffling and narrow linen braid, this puffy sleeved dimity dress is described as a "morning slip for a child just walking." *Godey's Lady's Book and Magazine*, January to June 1861.

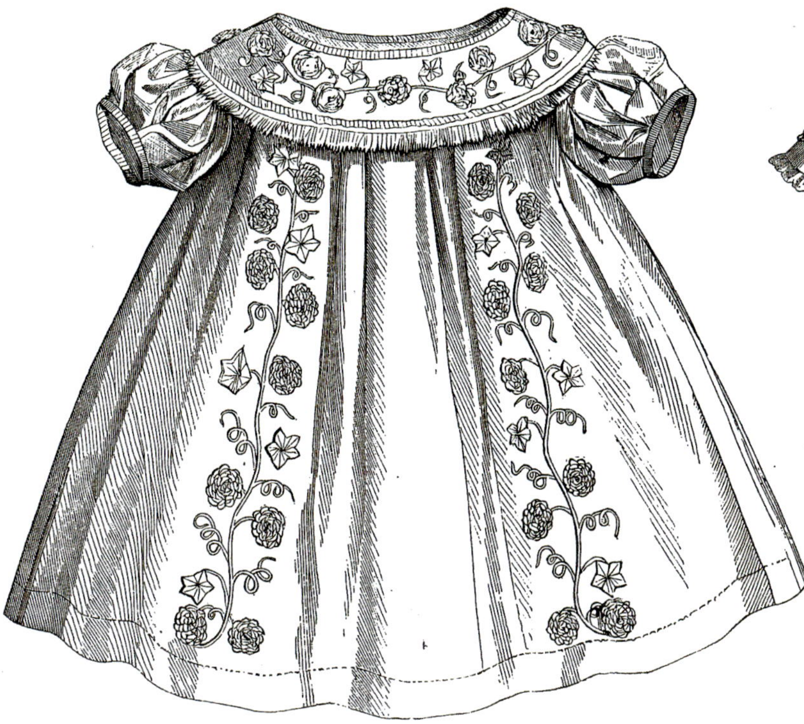

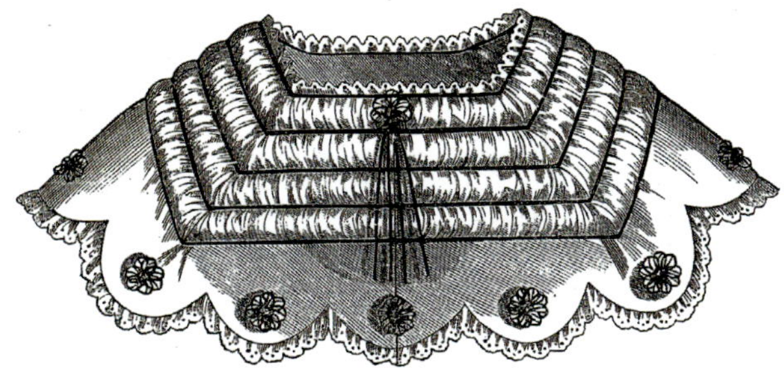

Illustration of a young child's striking bertha to be made of muslin with narrow black velvet ribbon trim. A lace-trimmed scalloped hem shows off a number of black velvet rosettes. *Godey's Lady's Book and Magazine*, June to December 1861.

Gender-neutral cambric dress for a child transitioning to short clothes. "The round yoke is covered by an embroidered bertha." *Godey's Lady's Book and Magazine*, June to December 1861.

NAME FOR MARKING.

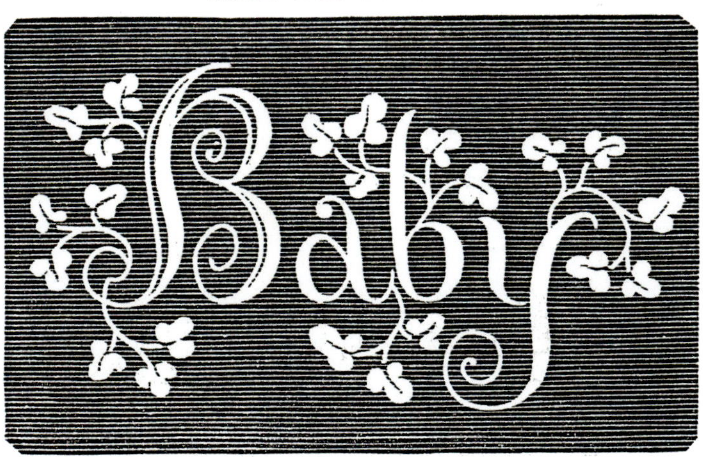

1860s embroidery illustration for the marking of baby's clothes. *Godey's Lady's Book and Magazine*, July to December 1861.

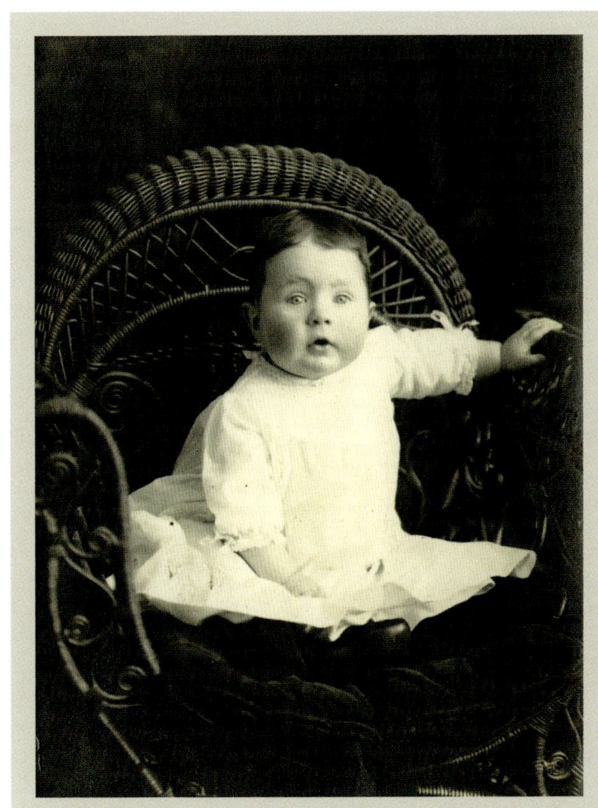

Infant Lorne O'Brian in short clothes c.1914.

Shoes

Imagine our pioneer foremothers preparing their little ones to venture outside and teaching them to count at the same time: "One, two, buckle my shoe," the rhyme goes as mother draws first one, then the other latchet or strap of her child's leather shoe through a buckle shaped to conform to the foot. "Three, four, shut the door." Mother instructs her child to close the door behind him as he leaves the house. "Five, six, pick up sticks." The lesson and the outing become fun for the child, and so it goes.

One of the first developmental stages for children is mastering the ability to walk. While few of us remember this accomplishment, many of us retain our early fascination with shoes. Bare feet are fine for languishing in earthy soil, sandy shores, or fields of clover, but when stepping out of our homes, propelling ourselves into the world around us, we require shoes.

Throughout the late Victorian era, manufacturers kept the public advised of their ability to produce the latest in fashionable footwear for boys, youth, misses, and children. Styles changed with the seasons utilizing such materials as authentic and imitation kangaroo, patent leather, calf, and chrome kid.

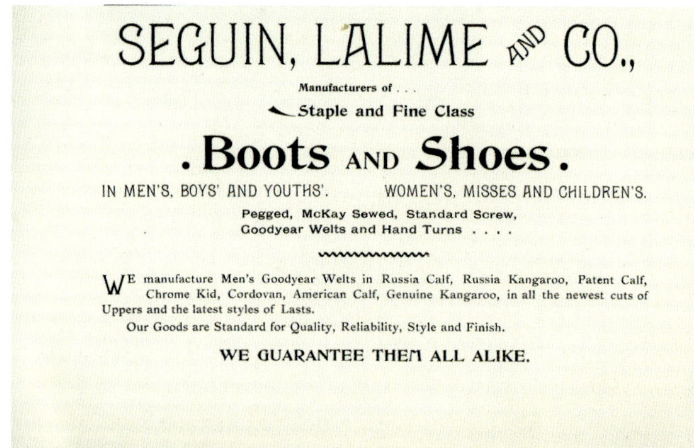

Canadian footwear manufacturer's advertisement for "staple and fine class" boots and shoes. *Canada and Her Commerce*, 1894.

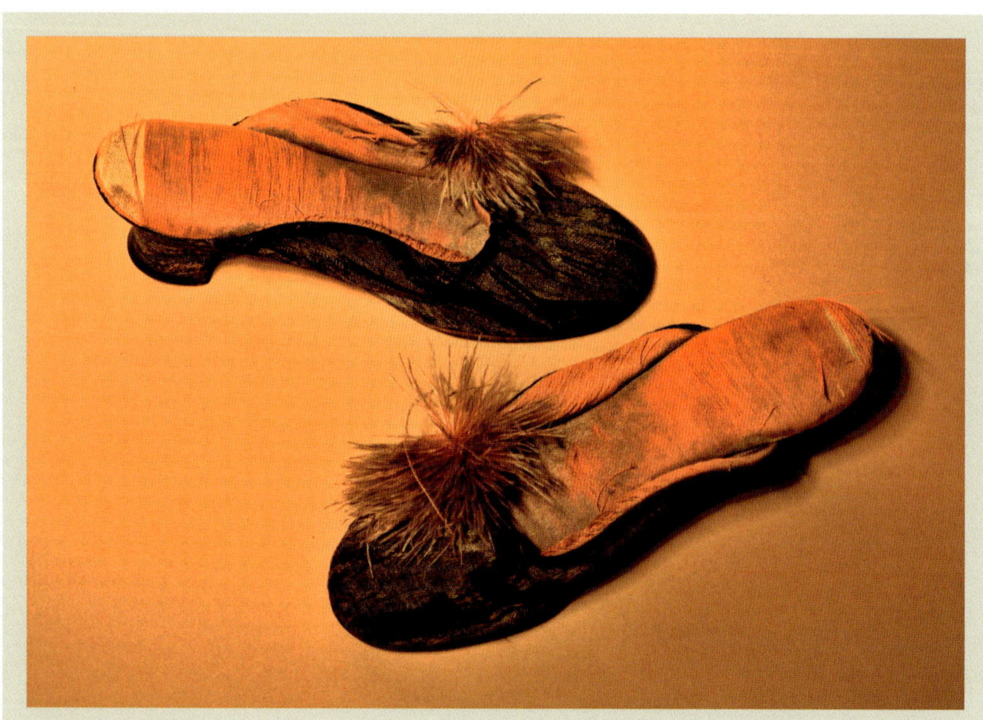

These girls' Victorian silk Louis heel slippers measure six inches from heel to toe.

Little Lids

Hats and bonnets of various styles graced the heads of little ones throughout the Victorian era and well into the twentieth century. No fashionable outfit was complete without a complementary head covering. Mothers kept up to date with the latest in lids, most of which could be made at home by following the descriptions outlined in fashion magazines. Instructions for the Napoleon hat, for example, which was described as being "pretty for a little boy three years old," was outlined in the February 1900, issue of *The Ladies' Home Journal*. Also known as a bicorne, this simple little cloth topper in red, navy blue, black, or dark green was trimmed with a bow of narrow ribbon placed in front and at each side where the brims meet.

The Millinery Herald and *The Monitor of Fashion for the Millinery Trade*— magazine-style publications supplied free of charge to hat makers in the late Victorian and early Edwardian era—informed the American trade on the latest fads, trends, and hat fancies to come out of Paris, while promoting a group of wholesalers ready to supply the necessary forms, trims, and importations.

In the history of children's hats, several classic styles such as the beret, the hood, and the skimmer are repeated. Yet, one style stands out: the beanie. This brimless, segmented style was easily made from remnants of felt, making it an inexpensive choice for boys who wanted to emulate their late Victorian working class dads while keeping their bean—slang for head—warm. Eventually, the beanie enjoyed collegiate status when it was used to represent school colors from the 1920s through the 1940s, and was even fitted with a novelty propeller for a time. Over time the beanie sprouted a brim and morphed into the baseball cap.

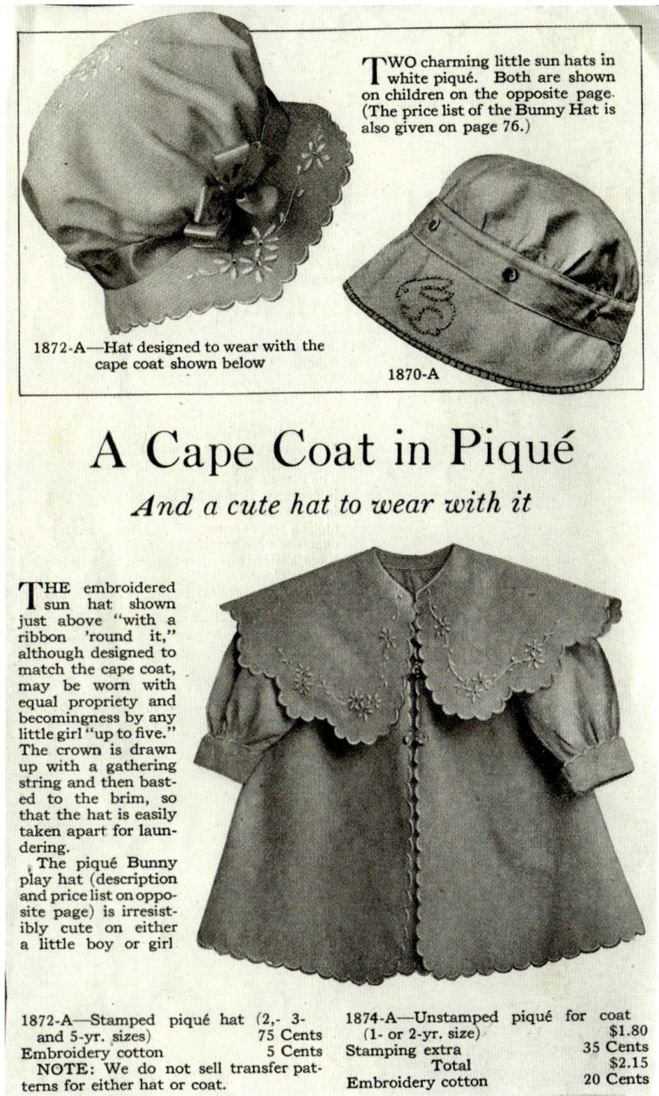

TWO charming little sun hats in white piqué. Both are shown on children on the opposite page. (The price list of the Bunny Hat is also given on page 76.)

1872-A—Hat designed to wear with the cape coat shown below

1870-A

A Cape Coat in Piqué

And a cute hat to wear with it

THE embroidered sun hat shown just above "with a ribbon 'round it," although designed to match the cape coat, may be worn with equal propriety and becomingness by any little girl "up to five." The crown is drawn up with a gathering string and then basted to the brim, so that the hat is easily taken apart for laundering.

The piqué Bunny play hat (description and price list on opposite page) is irresistibly cute on either a little boy or girl

1872-A—Stamped piqué hat (2,- 3- and 5-yr. sizes) 75 Cents
Embroidery cotton 5 Cents
NOTE: We do not sell transfer patterns for either hat or coat.

1874-A—Unstamped piqué for coat (1- or 2-yr. size) $1.80
Stamping extra 35 Cents
Total $2.15
Embroidery cotton 20 Cents

A cape coat and hats for youngsters up to five years. *Woman's Home Companion*, June 1919.

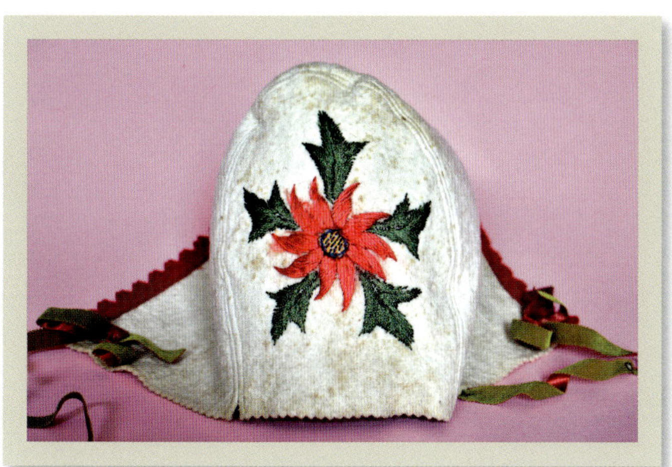

Victorian Christmas bonnet with embroidered poinsettia, red and green velvet ribbon ties.

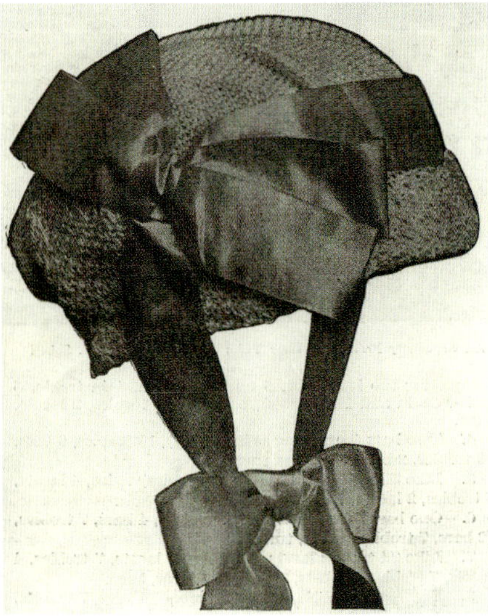

A ribbon-trimmed Gretchen cap to be crocheted with coarse silk-finished cotton. *Needlecraft Magazine*, July 1916.

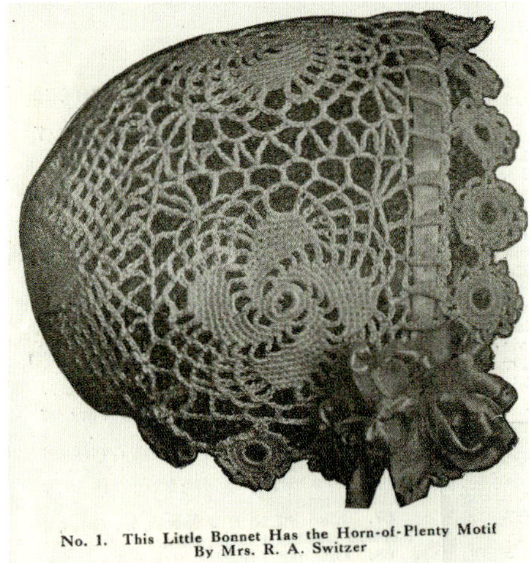

Illustration for crocheted baby bonnet in a horn of plenty motif. *Needlecraft Magazine*, July 1916.

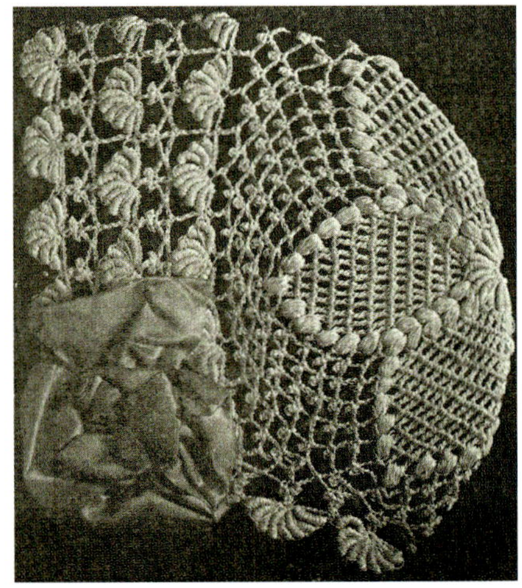

Illustration for a star crown crocheted baby bonnet. *Needlecraft Magazine*, March 1916.

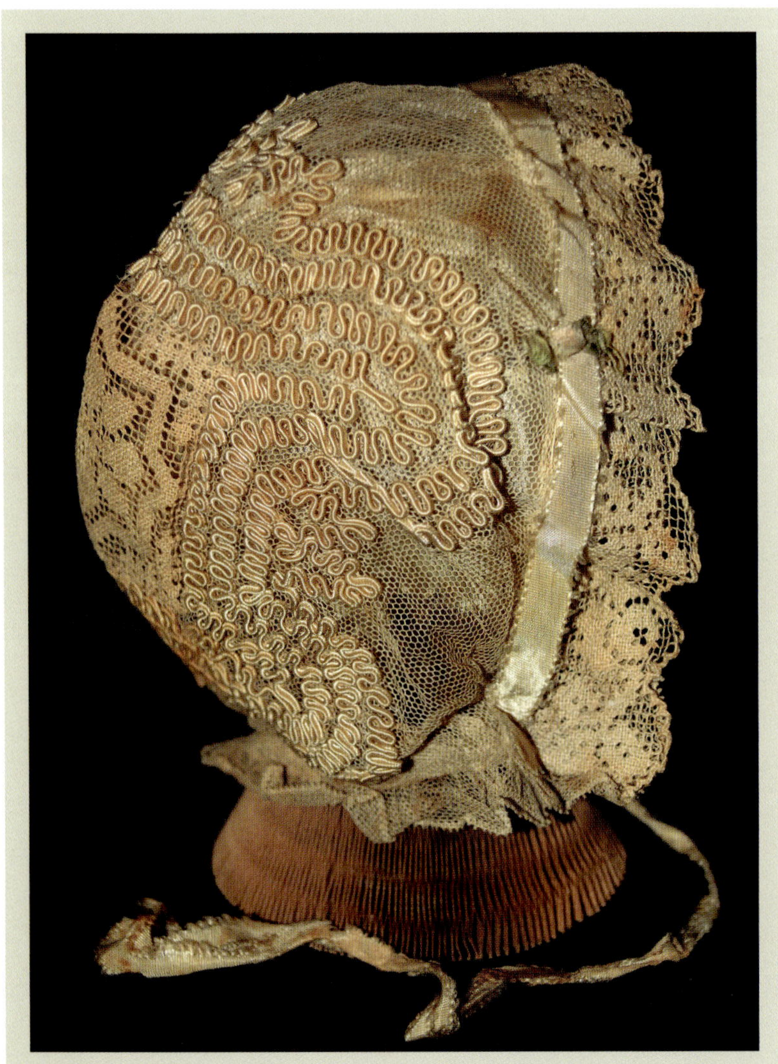

Star-patterned baby bonnet in fine crochet.

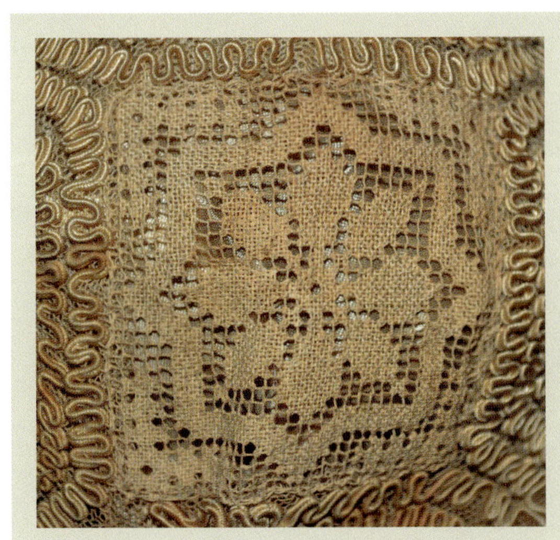

Back detail of star-patterend baby bonnet.

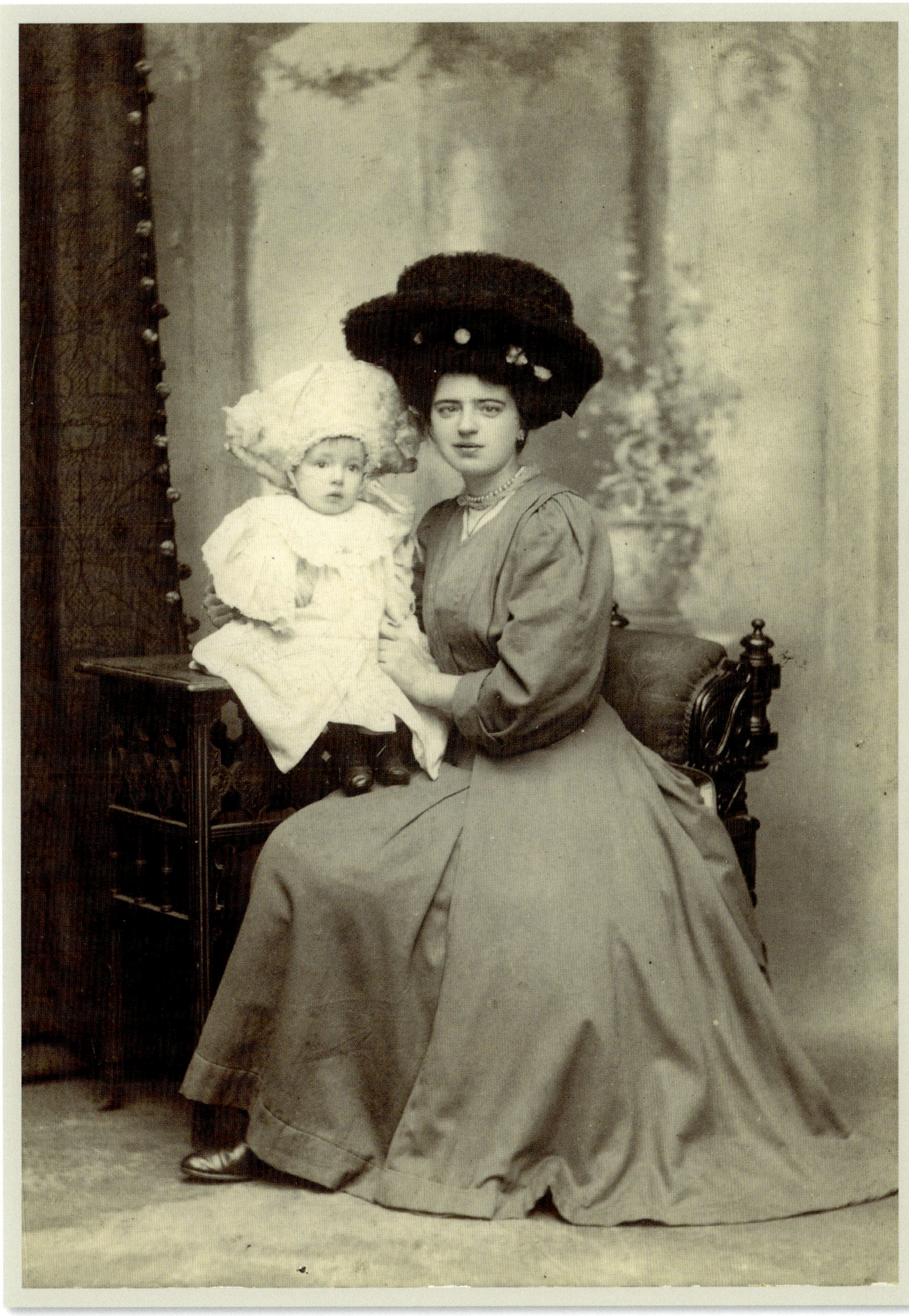

A fashionable Adeline Strachan, age eighteen years, poses with her infant brother James Jones, who sports an enormous, white frilly lingerie hat.

GLENGARRY CAP IN CROCHET.

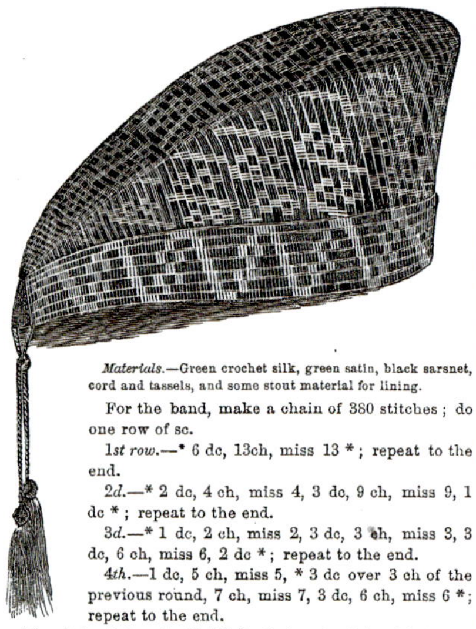

Materials.—Green crochet silk, green satin, black sarsnet, cord and tassels, and some stout material for lining.

For the band, make a chain of 380 stitches; do one row of sc.

1st row.—* 6 dc, 13ch, miss 13 *; repeat to the end.

2d.—* 2 dc, 4 ch, miss 4, 3 dc, 9 ch, miss 9, 1 dc *; repeat to the end.

3d.—* 1 dc, 2 ch, miss 2, 3 dc, 3 ch, miss 3, 3 dc, 6 ch, miss 6, 2 dc *; repeat to the end.

4th.—1 dc, 5 ch, miss 5, * 3 dc over 3 ch of the previous round, 7 ch, miss 7, 3 dc, 6 ch, miss 6 *; repeat to the end.

5th.—1 dc, 2 ch, miss 2, * 3 dc, 3 ch, miss 3 dc of last row, 3 dc, 3 ch, miss 3, 3 dc, 4 ch, miss 4 *; repeat to the end.

6th.—1 dc, 5 ch, miss 5, * 3 dc, 5 ch, miss 5, 3 dc, 8 ch, miss 8 *; repeat to the end.

7th.—7 dc coming on the 5 ch and a dc at each side, and 11 ch before the next dc. This is the last row of the band.

For the crown, make a chain of 140 stitches, and repeat the pattern on it as often as it will permit. These stitches form the extreme width of the crown. A piece of fourteen inches long must be made, which should require about seven repetitions of the pattern.

There now remains to be worked the piece between the band and the crown, and this is done by making a chain of 120 stitches, and doing one pattern; and three rows of the next on this, increasing three stitches at each end of every row. Then work each edge separately, doing first three patterns, then two, then one only; not decreasing all at once, but leaving a few stitches at the *inner* edge of every row.

To make up the cap, cut out the shape first in paper; then in fine tick, or any similar material. Cover this with black on one side, and with green satin on the other. The satin should be rather darker in color than the crochet, which is to be tacked over it. The corners of the oblong piece done for the crown must then be cut off, and all sewed firmly and neatly together. A piece of enamelled leather usually lines the band, and a cord and tassels finish the cap at the back of the head.

Pattern for a crocheted Glengarry cap. *Godey's Lady's Book and Magazine,* July to December 1861.

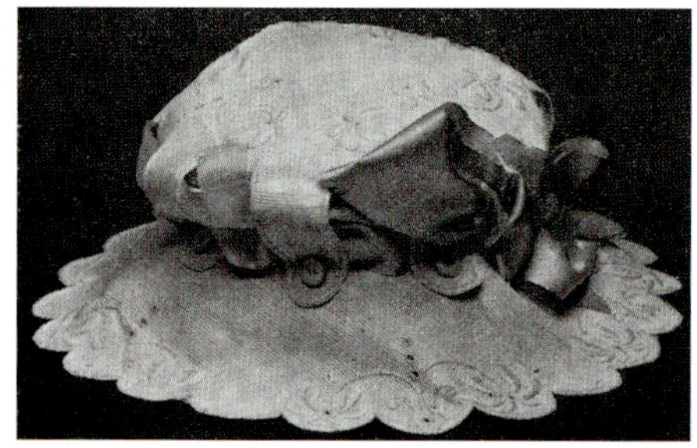

Child's ribbon-trimmed lingerie cap with button-on crown. *Needlecraft Magazine*, July 1915.

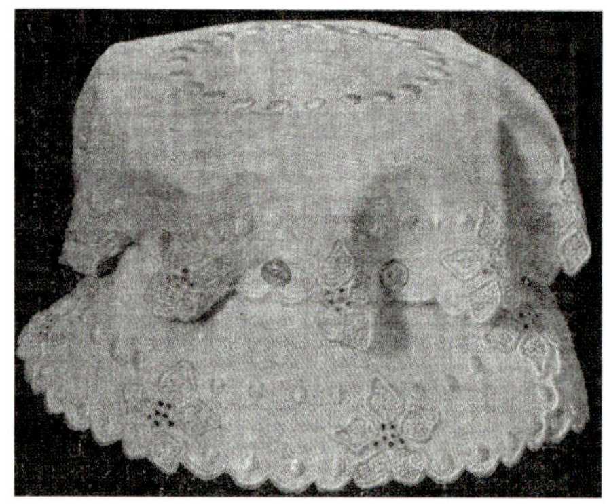

An alternate style of infant's lingerie cap. *Needlecraft Magazine*, June 1916.

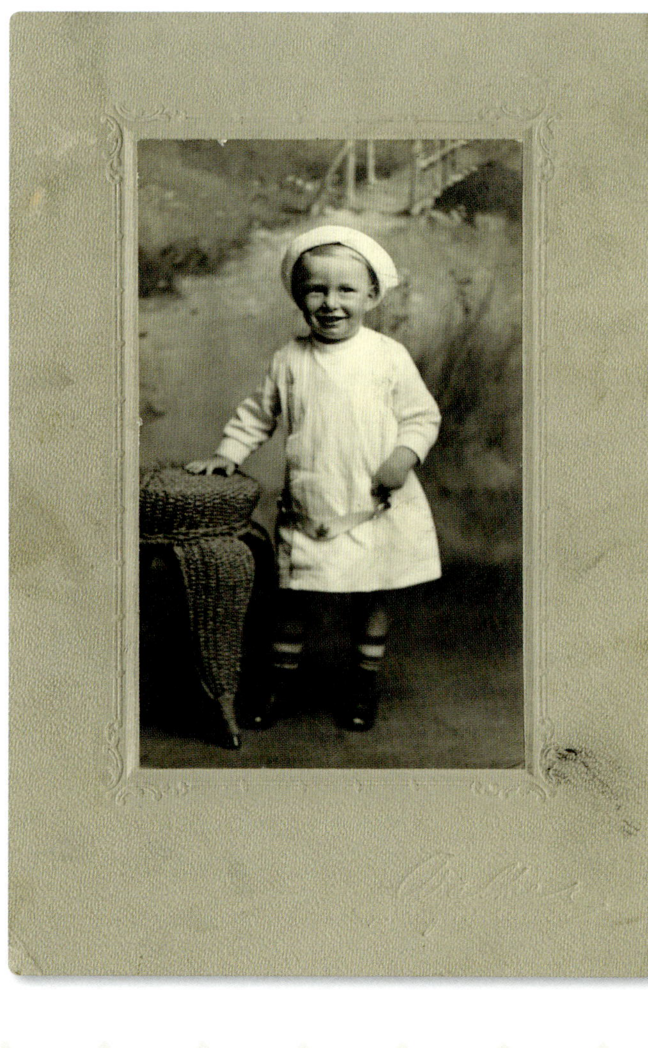

This tot is dressed simply in a crisp white dress and simply constructed fabric sailor hat.

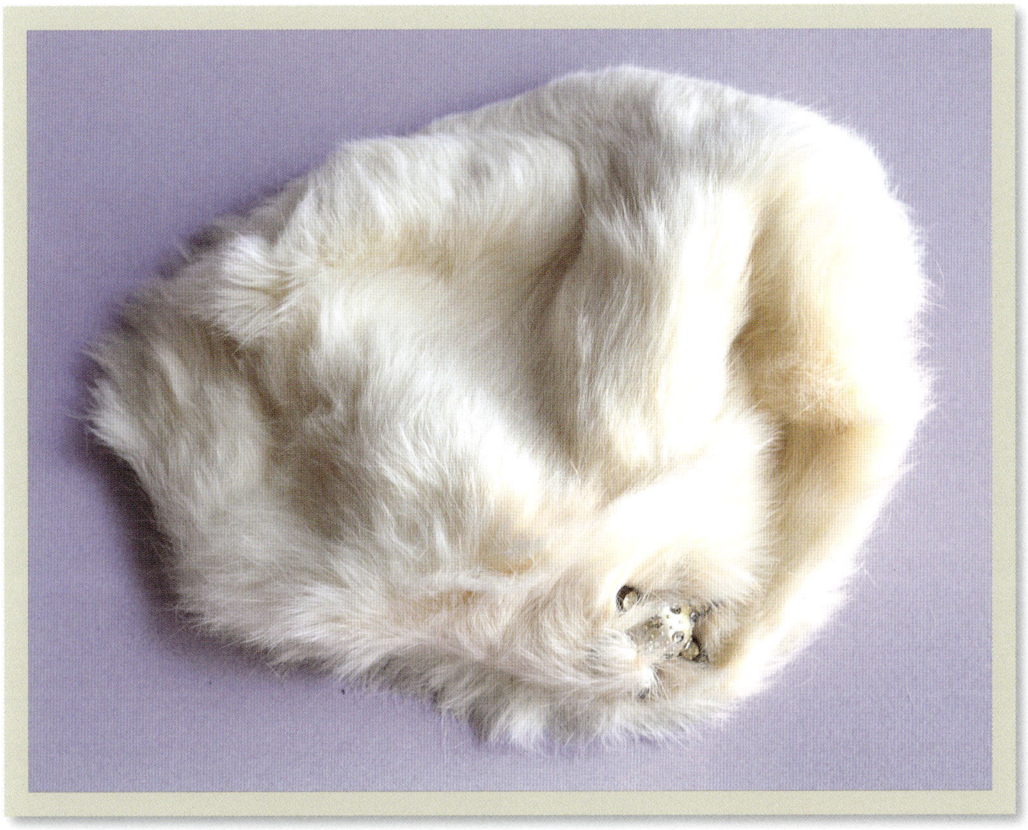

Child's white rabbit fur cap with star pin.

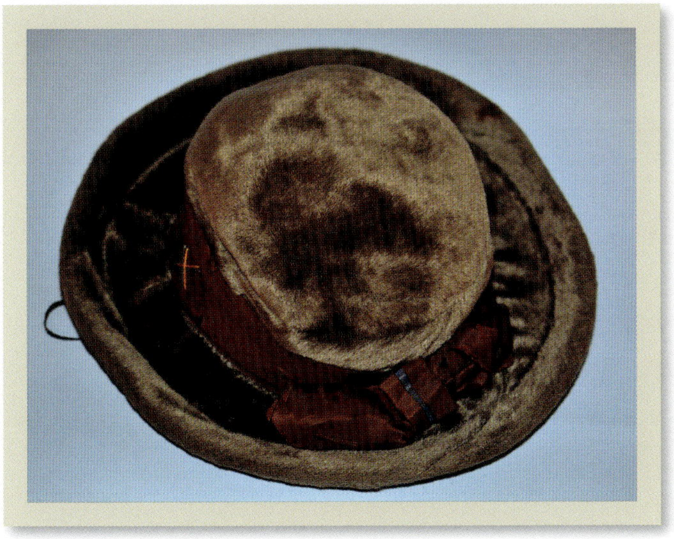

Child's beaverette rolled brim winter hat with silk ribbon band and elastic chin strap.

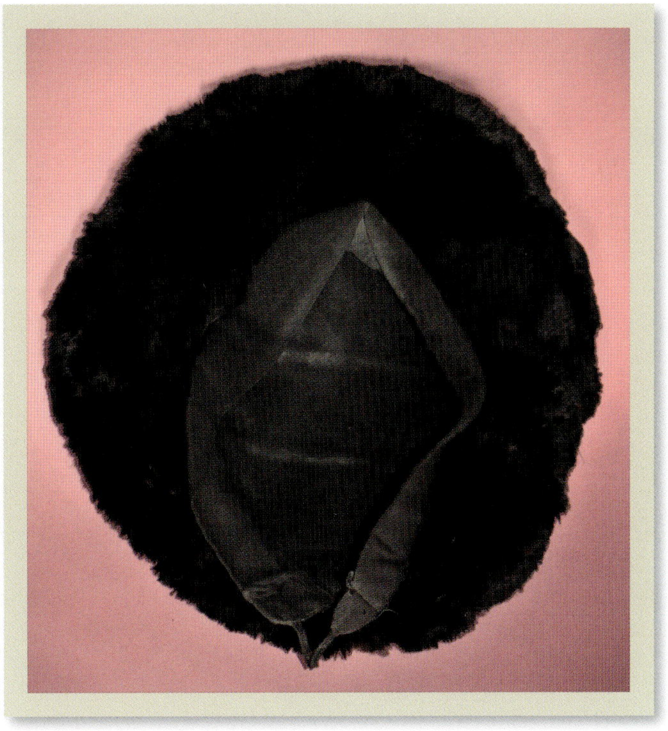

Child's black seal beret.

Child's formal bonnet c.1880.

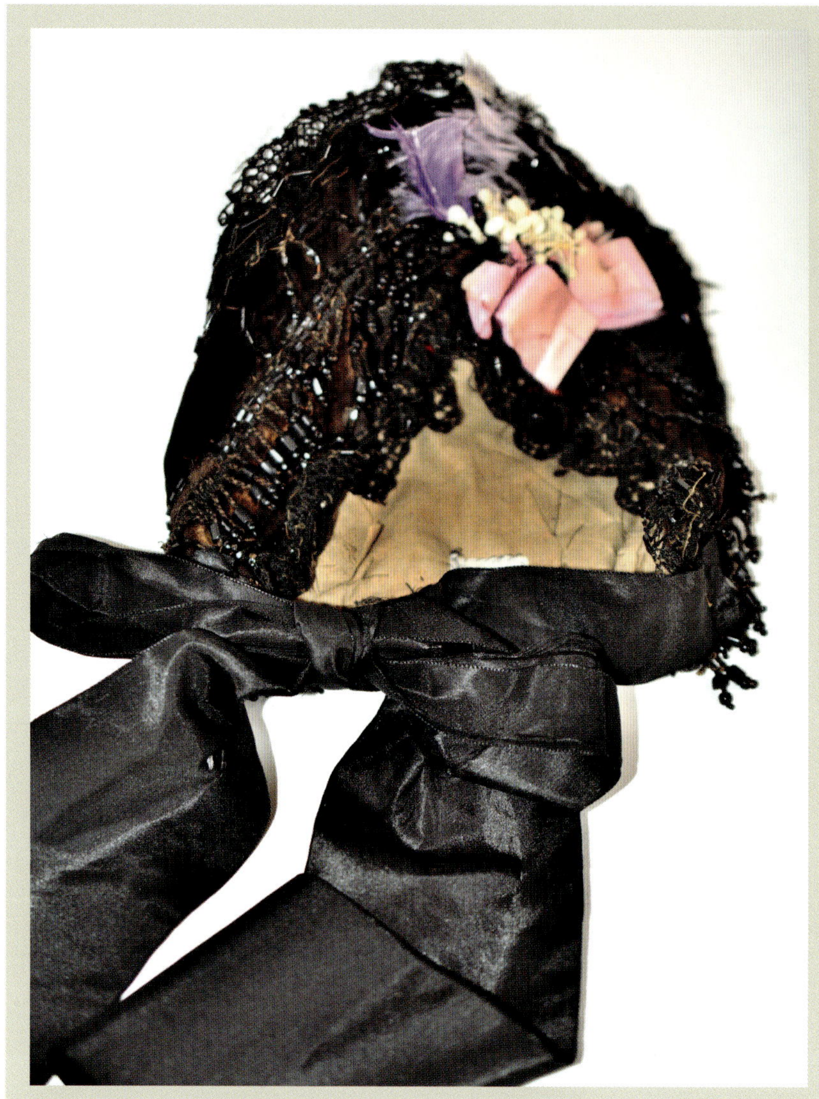

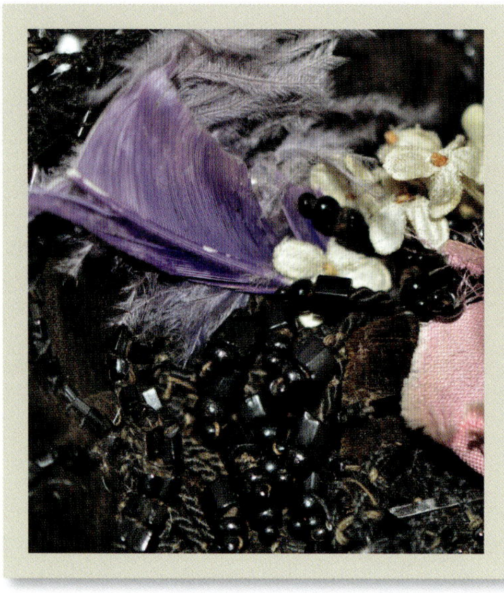

Detail: jet bead, feathers, fabric flowers, and ribbon trim.

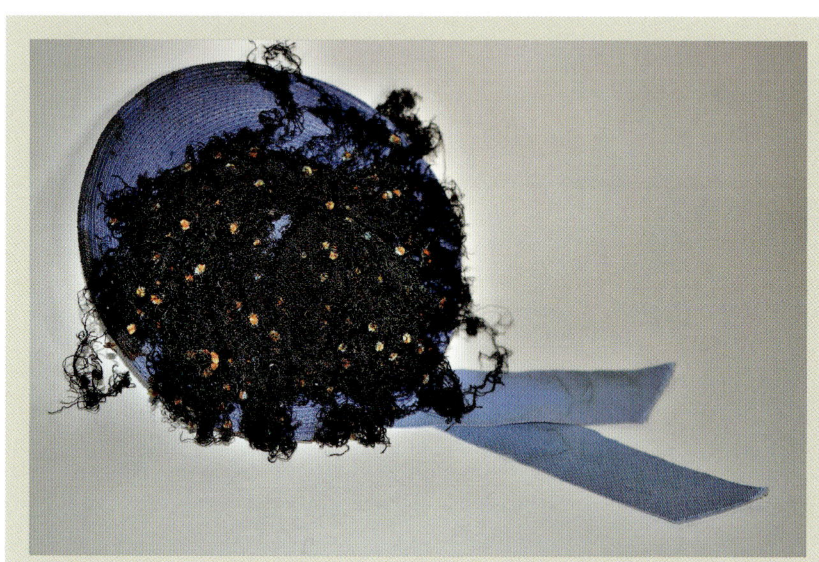

Young girl's blue straw bonnet with grosgrain flirtation ribbons, black net, and tiny straw flowers.

Gloves

Throughout the Victorian era, gloves were so ubiquitous that even dolls wore them, and glove boxes were incorporated into furniture design with hinged containers flanking the mirrors of dressers and dressing tables. Miniature versions of leather gloves styled for women were produced for children by famous glovers such as the Fownes Company.

Over the centuries, gloves have served as a practical covering for the hands, providing a barrier against excessive cold, heat, and wind as well as bacteria and viruses. Gloves lost part of their protective purpose as twentieth-century vaccines and antibiotics became available, but they maintained their sartorial intent for a time.

Children's leather gloves were popular during the Victorian age but were eventually replaced with less expensive hand-knit or machine-made woolen mittens, more suitable for outdoor winter activities. Hand-crocheted lace varieties also fell out of fashion, with cotton varieties standing in at graduations, religious observances, and weddings.

Gloves were originally the domain of gentlemen, but once the fairer sex adopted them as an adornment for the hands, they completely feminized them, going so far in Victorian times as to develop a method of communication with the fashionable accessory—a secret language similar to that of the fan.

In January 1887, *The New York Times* advised young maidens how to send love messages to a suitor in full view of their watchful chaperones. Observing that "certain old fogies go to balls and social gatherings merely to observe the conduct of young people," the newspaper advised that you could beckon a friend to follow you into the next room by striking both gloves against your left arm.

Twisting the fingers around the thumb of a glove communicated, "Be on your guard against my governor," while a careful smoothing of the gloves meant, "I love you still."

Someone even invented glove semaphore using a careful and elaborate knotting of the fringe that often trimmed a pair of young girl's gloves. Each knot stood for a single letter of the alphabet. Not surprisingly, this system did not catch on.

What did persist were the many social imperatives around the wearing of gloves. When the following verse—"If from 'glove' you take the letter 'G', then 'glove' is 'love' and that I send to thee"—accompanied a pair of gloves given as a Valentine's gift, the recipient was free to receive them as she would a marriage proposal.

When a popular young girl—most Victorian brides were married by the time they were eighteen—received such a gift from several suitors, she would wear the gloves from the gentleman of her choice at Easter to return the sentiment.

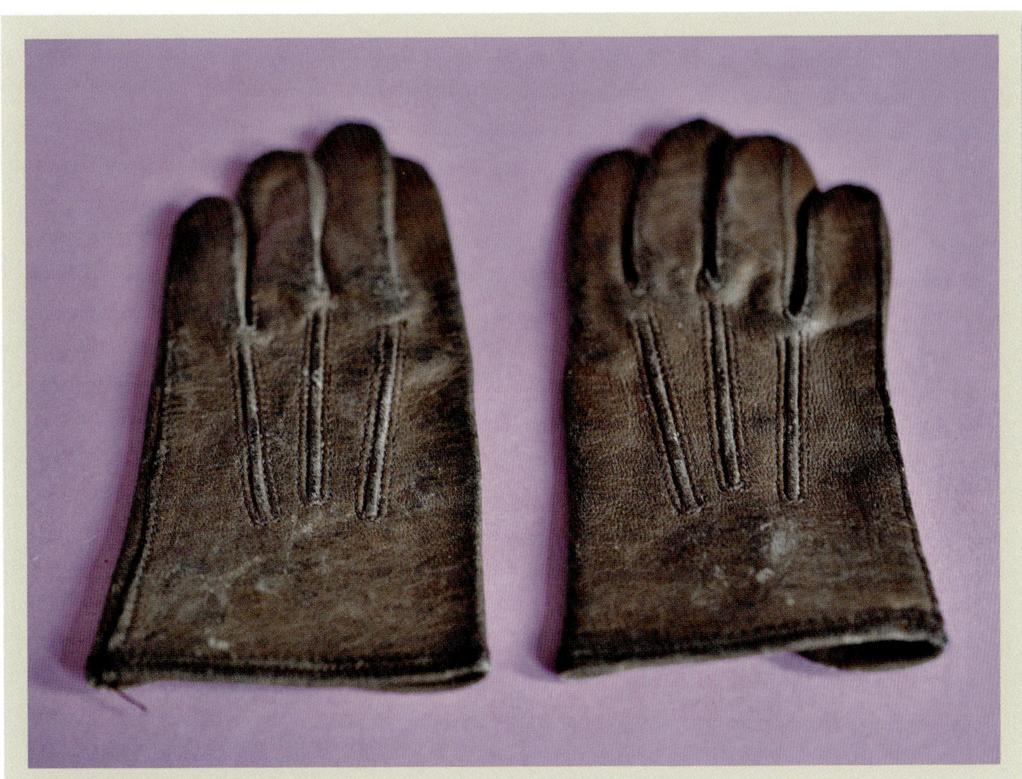

Child's leather gloves c.1910, originally owned by Ellen Daisy Grace Potter.

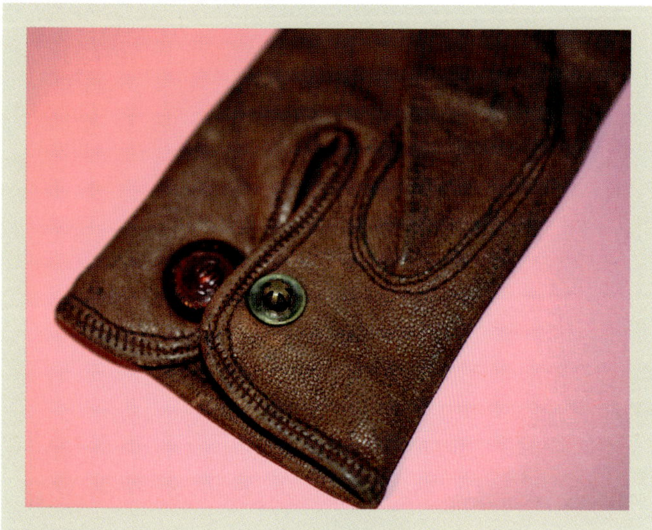

Snap detail.

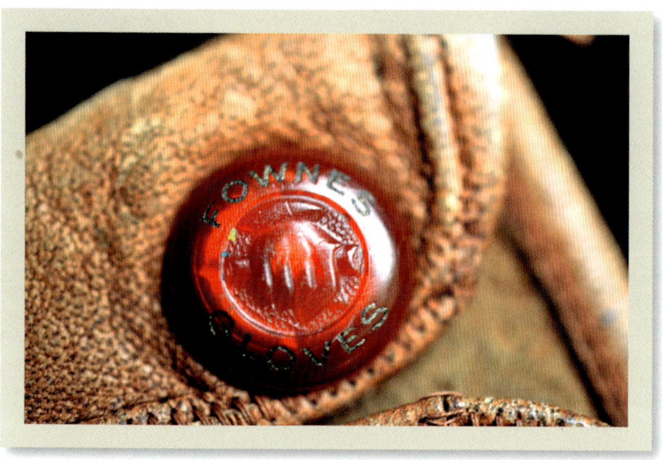

Glass button snap-cover with Fownes Co. logo. Fownes was named for its founder who established the London company in 1887.

Over time, this sentiment morphed into the giving of gloves at Valentine's Day as a love token. Later, when the giving and receiving of paper gloves replaced the real thing for February 14th observances, New Year's Day became the customary time of year to exchange gifts of gloves.

Perhaps the one surviving glove tradition in America is the debutante glove, an accessory *de rigeur* with maidens coming out to society at a debutante ball. This custom, derived from the English tradition of young ladies being presented to the British Court, came to America in 1748 when several aristocratic Philadelphia families held the first Dancing Assembly to formally introduce girls of marriageable age to suitors of a similar social standing.

Traditionally, debutantes wore over-the-elbow gloves made of white kid leather with a three-button wrist opening, known as a *mousquetaire* through which they might extract their hand without removing the glove.

> "No display of period costume, with the exception of undergarments, is complete without gloves."—Donna Young, costume collector

The popular nineteenth-century American novelist Louisa May Alcott found how much gloves can reveal about a person so intriguing that she built a story, "The Baron's Gloves," around this very notion. When a pair of monogrammed gloves, scented with violets and adorned with a coat-of-arms, drops from a balcony above, Amy, the protagonist, examines them in an effort to understand who might have lost or tossed them. Discovering a little hole fretted by a ring on the third finger, she exclaims, "handsome hands wore these; I would like to see the man."

Collectors and costumers are equally curious about the gloves they stumble across today at flea markets, antique stores, and grandmother's attic. Where were the gloves worn? What costumes did they accessorize? To whom did they belong?

Glove collecting is not new. According to Linda Baumgarten in her 2002 book, *What Clothes Reveal,* Horace Walpole, the fourth Earl of Oxford—an eighteenth-century author, antiquarian, and politician—collected old costume to help him understand the people of the past. His collection boasted embroidered gloves that once belonged to King James I.

While modern collectors will find some eighteenth- and nineteenth-century children's gloves still in circulation, twentieth-century examples are much more abundant. They can be an easy and inexpensive entrée into the world of antique costume collecting. Their small size allows for relatively easy storage and display, and iconic examples, emblematic of a particular historic period, can stand in for an entire costume that may be more difficult to obtain, conserve, or exhibit.

The Museum of Fine Arts in Boston houses numerous fine examples including a pair of children's black silk knitted gloves.

Some kinds of gloves are elusive. Those made of lace, net, satin, silk, taffeta, and velvet soiled quickly and could just as easily be damaged through laundering as through snags and tears, so relatively few have survived. Even sturdier leather and fur examples tend to dry and crack over time, and many were discarded and replaced rather than preserved.

Gloves fell out of fashion two generations ago, marking them as a novelty artifact with many vintage costume collectors who are only beginning to appreciate this personal item of apparel for its variety of workmanship and design. The

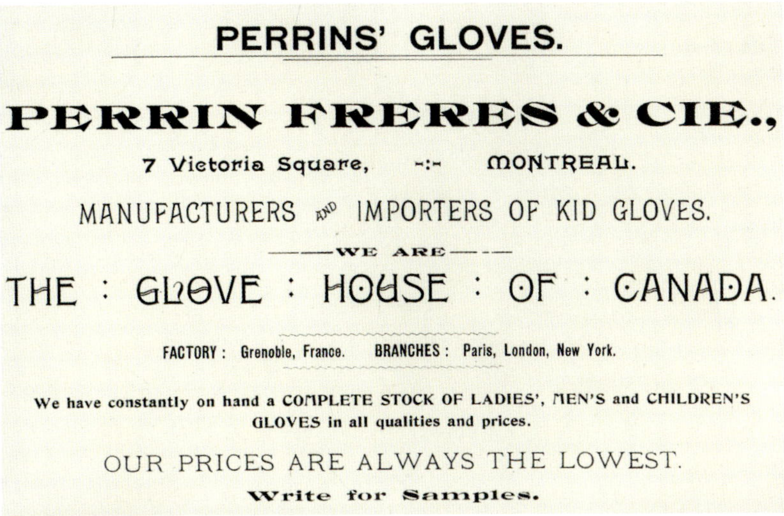

1894 advertisement for Perrin Brothers and Company glove manufacturers and importers. *Canada and Her Commerce*, 1894.

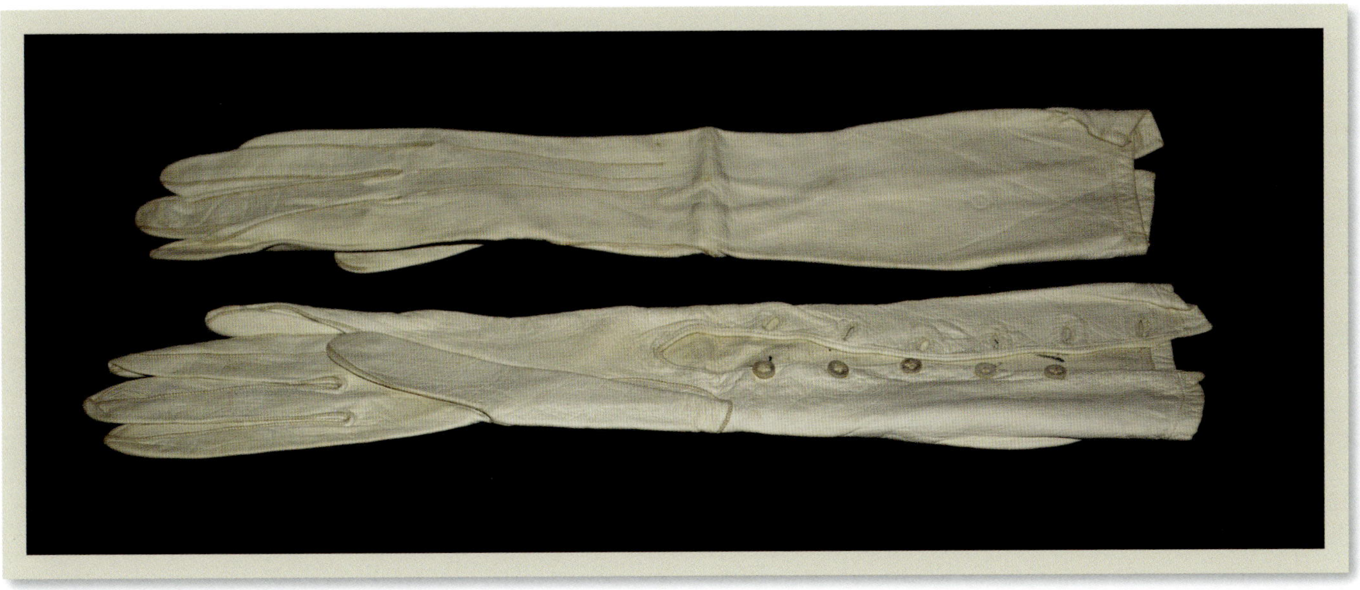

Teen girl's white kid leather gloves with button closure.

monetary value of more recent vintage gloves varies. Nice examples can be found for between $5 and $100.

Throughout the twentieth century, gloves saw many style changes and innovations—most notably the use of synthetic materials. The finest examples can carry famous designer labels.

Many factors affect the deterioration of textiles over time including exposure to light, heat, humidity, soil, chemicals, animals, and pests, but gloves are especially susceptible to damage because they may be exposed to the oils secreted by human hands. Children's gloves in particular often sacrifice themselves during play or when protecting little hands from injury.

While it is possible to remove dirt and stains from period silks, linens, cottons, and other fabrics, and to restore cracked and dried leathers to a softer condition, it is best to consult a professional conservator before attempting to launder or repair an antique glove. The same rule applies to any vintage textile, as unskilled cleaning may further damage costume artifacts.

Pack gloves and other aged textiles flat between sheets of acid-free tissue paper following museum standards for storage and display. Easy to follow guidelines can be found on the Textile Museum's website: www.museum.gwu.edu.

Collars and Cuffs

Numerous collar styles, either detachable or integral to the garment, characterized children's costume, particularly in the Victorian and Edwardian eras. Collar styles varied in size, shape, and fabrication, many with their own additional adornments.

Collars helped to define a desired silhouette and served a number of practical purposes. White collars drew the eye to the face and created a pleasing contrast to the primary textile of the garment. Detachable collar and cuff sets, which could be removed for laundering, protected the portions of a garment that soiled easily. Fur kept necks warm in winter and reflected one's social status in summer.

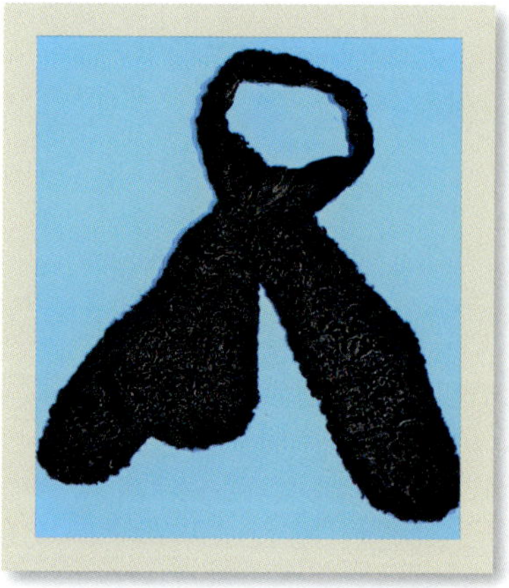

Child's black astrakhan neck piece, late Victorian.

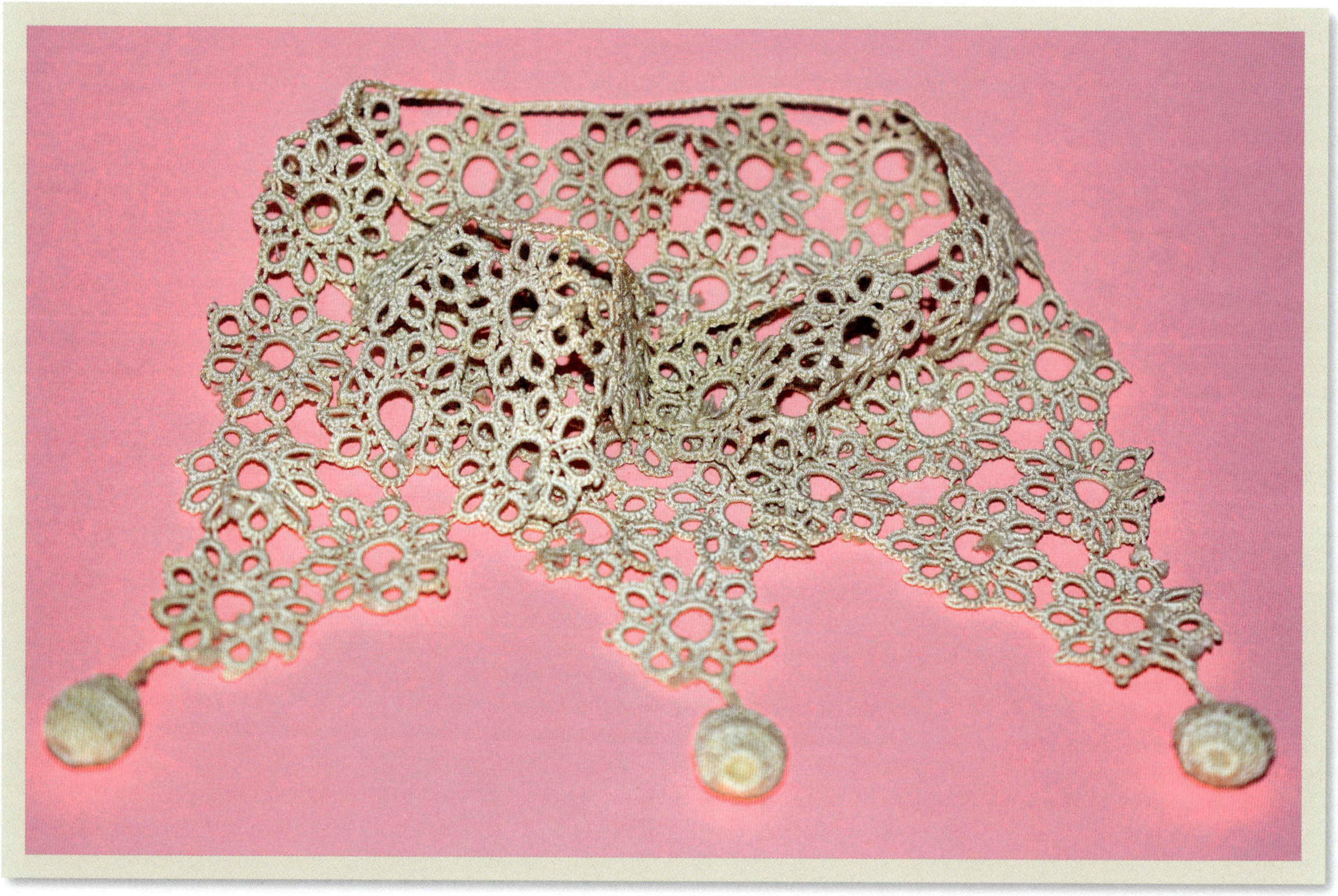

Child's hand-worked detachable lace collar.

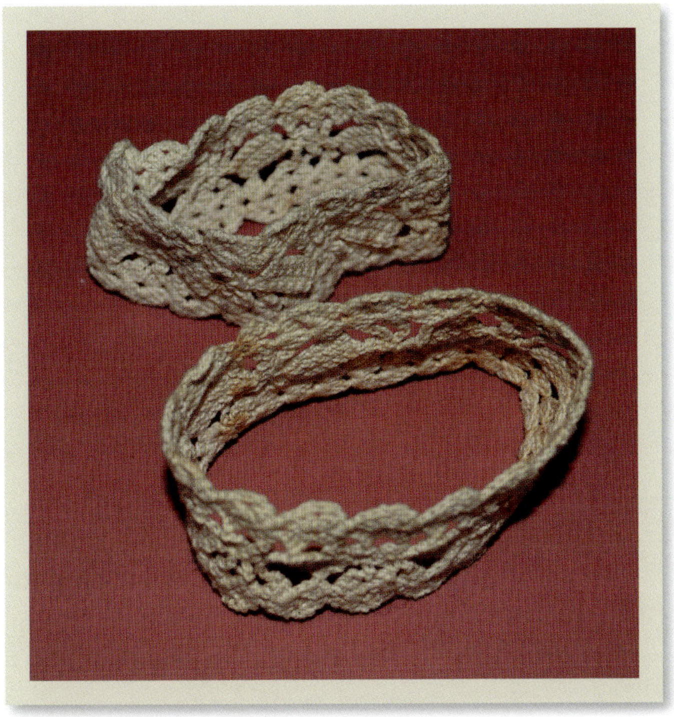

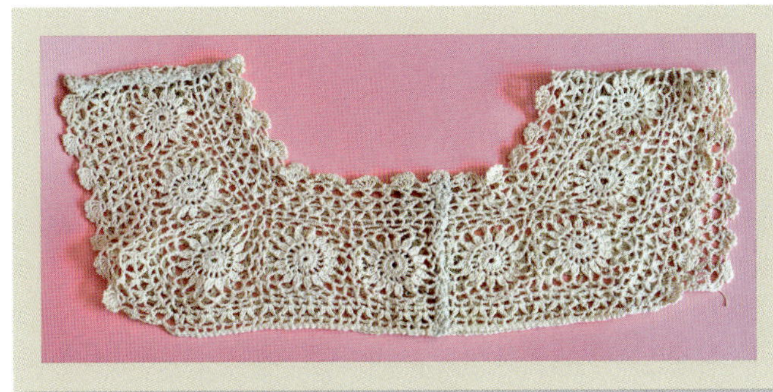

Boy's detachable lace-edged square collar.

Child's hand-crocheted lace cuffs, late Victorian.

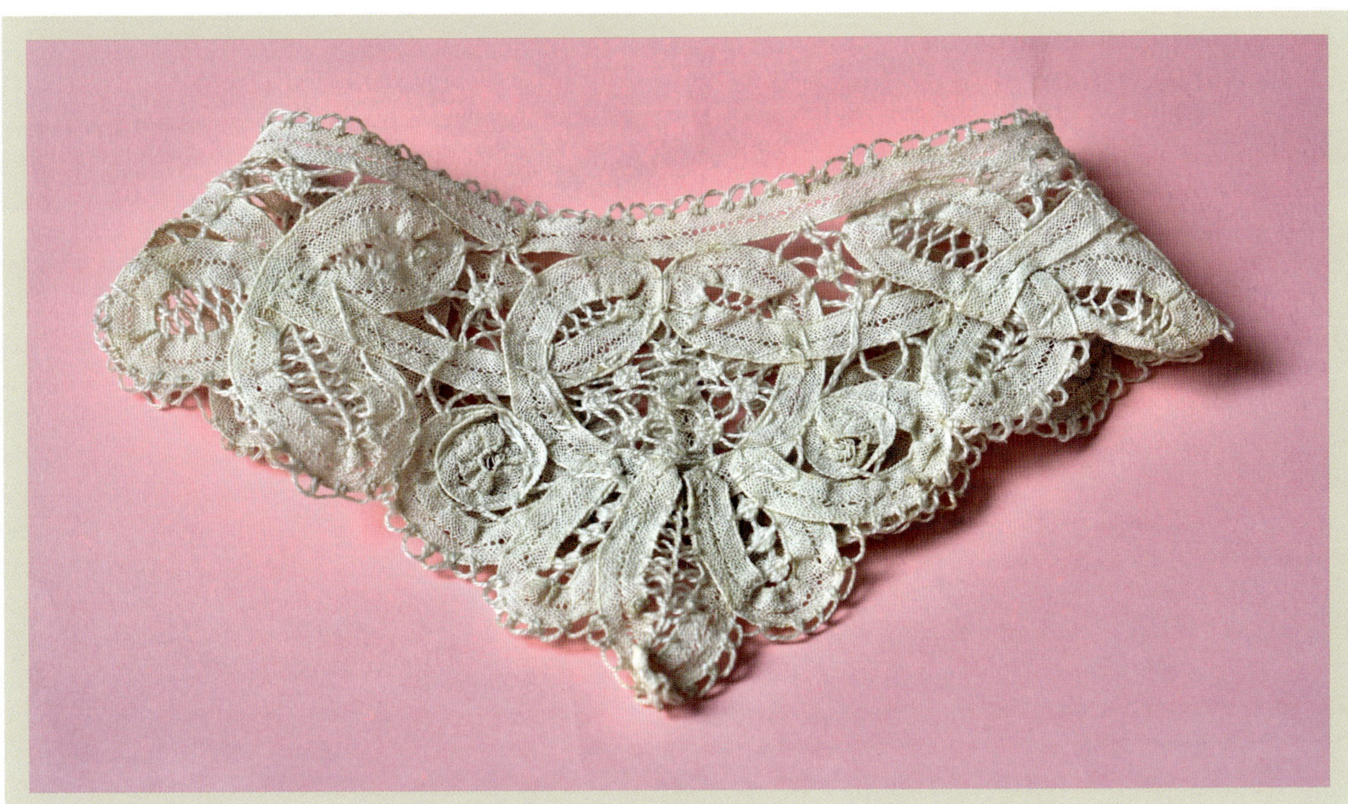

Delicate tape lace collar.

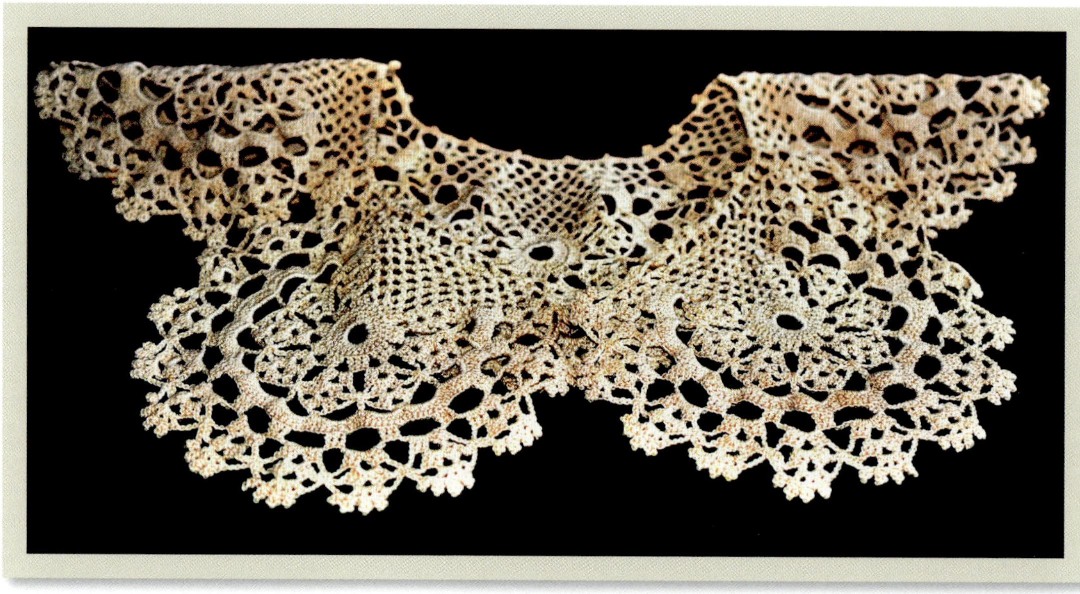

Boy's hand-crocheted collar.

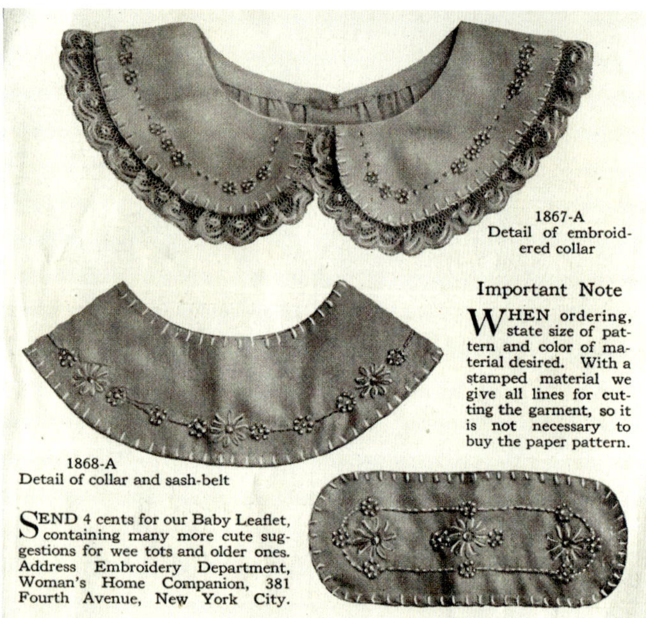

1867-A
Detail of embroidered collar

Important Note

WHEN ordering, state size of pattern and color of material desired. With a stamped material we give all lines for cutting the garment, so it is not necessary to buy the paper pattern.

1868-A
Detail of collar and sash-belt

SEND 4 cents for our Baby Leaflet, containing many more cute suggestions for wee tots and older ones. Address Embroidery Department, Woman's Home Companion, 381 Fourth Avenue, New York City.

Pattern for a young child's embroidered collar, cuffs, and sash belt featured in the June 1919 issue of *Woman's Home Companion*.

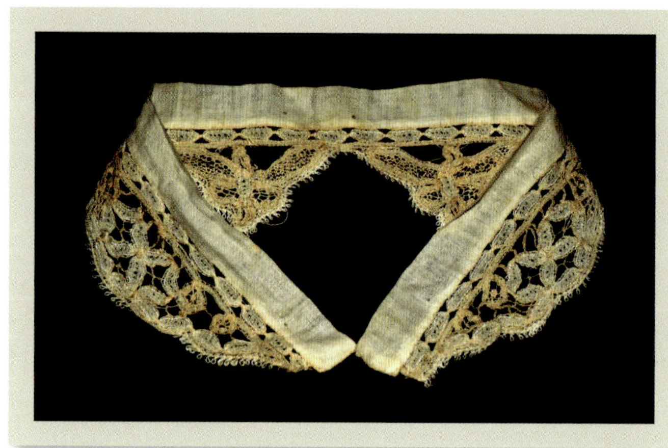

Infant's ecru-colored, handmade tape lace collar.

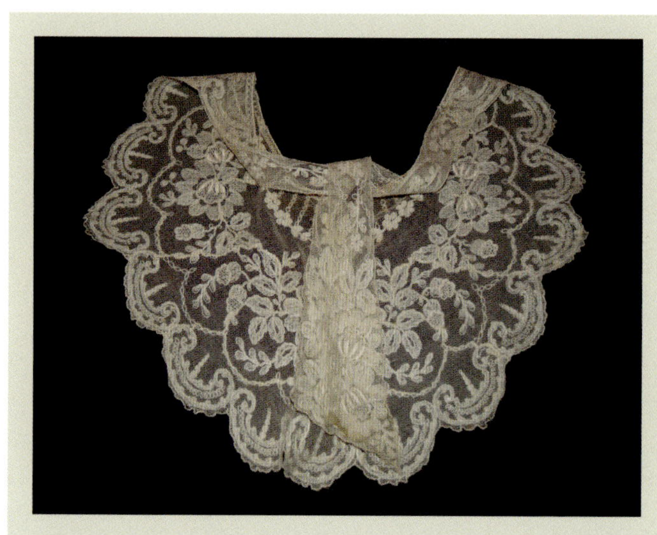

Floral patterned Victorian collar of net lace.

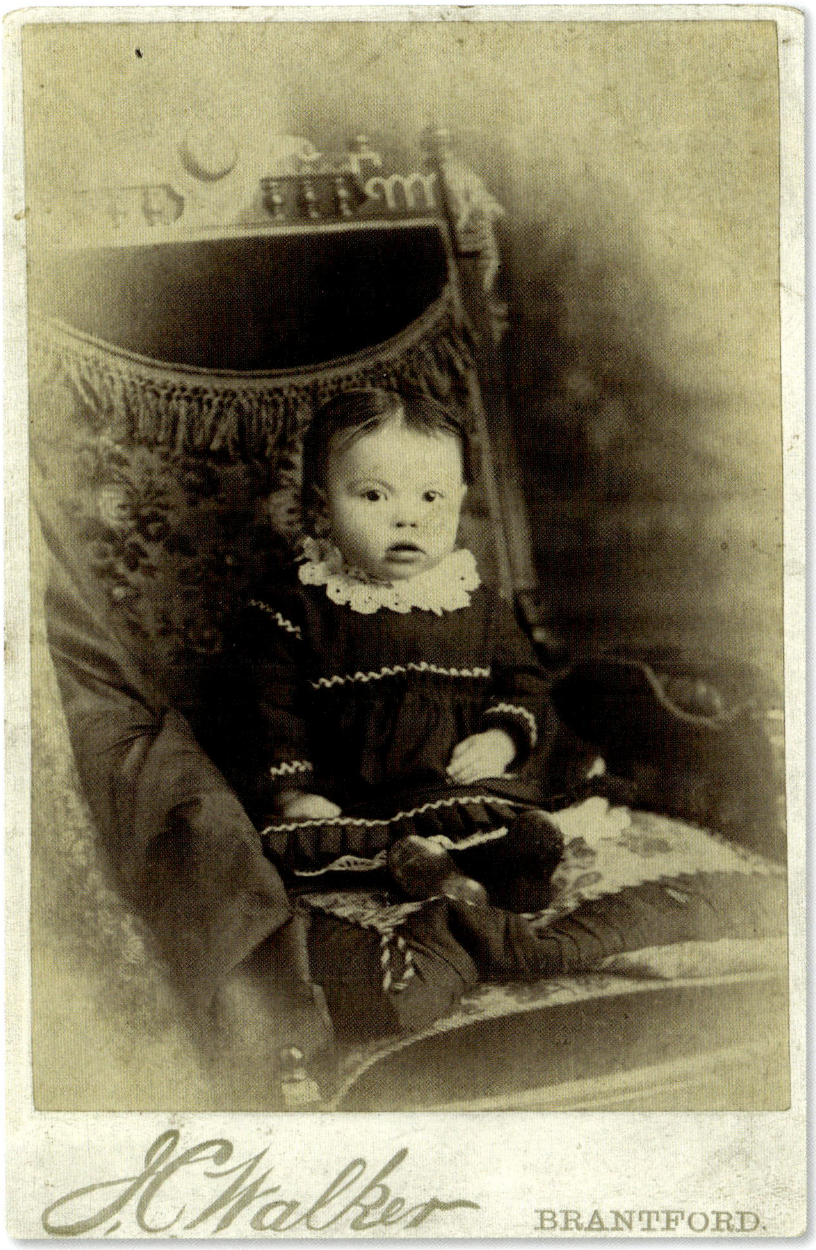

This dress's pleated hem and rickrack trim are in keeping with late nineteenth-century styling. The contrast collar appears to be a hand-crocheted adornment.

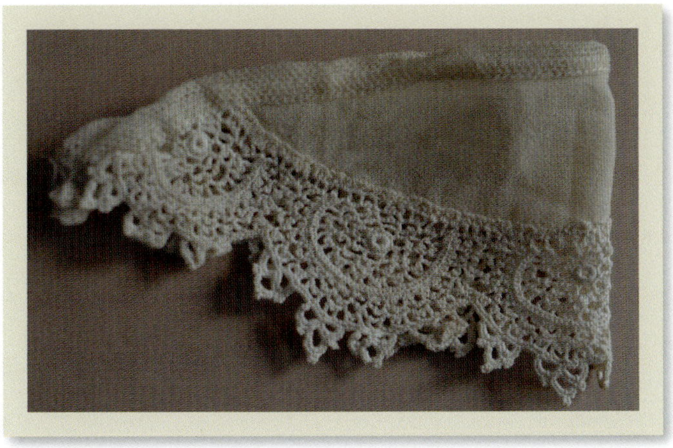

Young child's lace embellishment for dress and blouse shoulders.

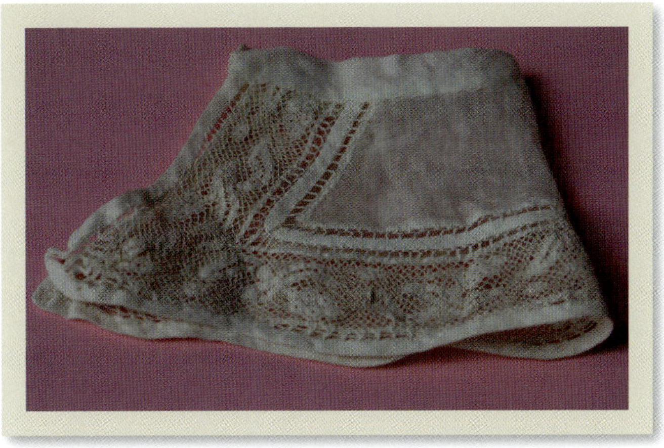

Boy's detachable cotton wrist cuff with crocheted lace insertion.

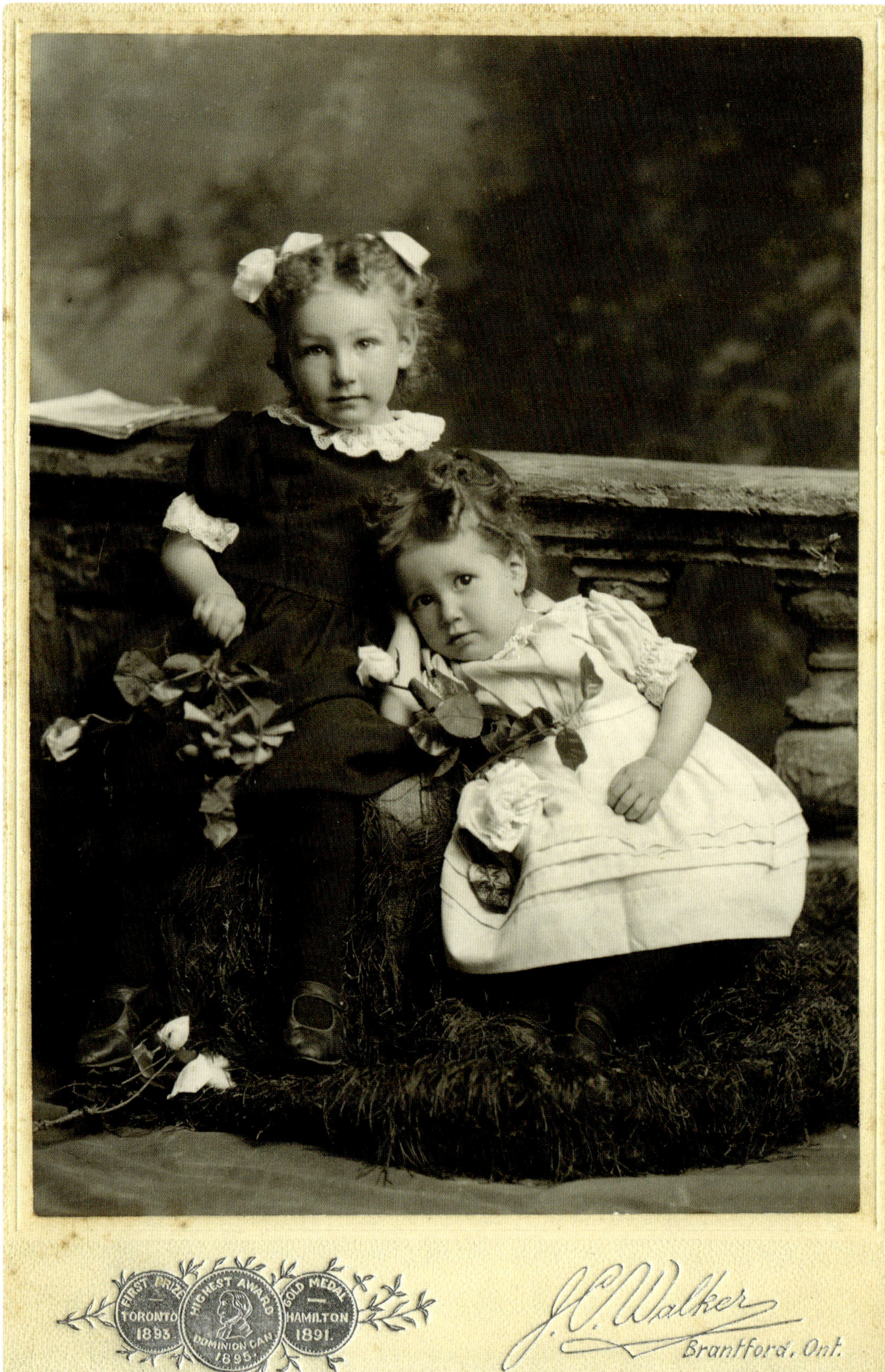

This beautifully posed early twentieth-century portrait demonstrates the fashion for short-sleeved dresses with clearly defined waists below close-fitting bodices. The contrast collar and cuff set provides a striking contrast to the dark-colored dress on the left.

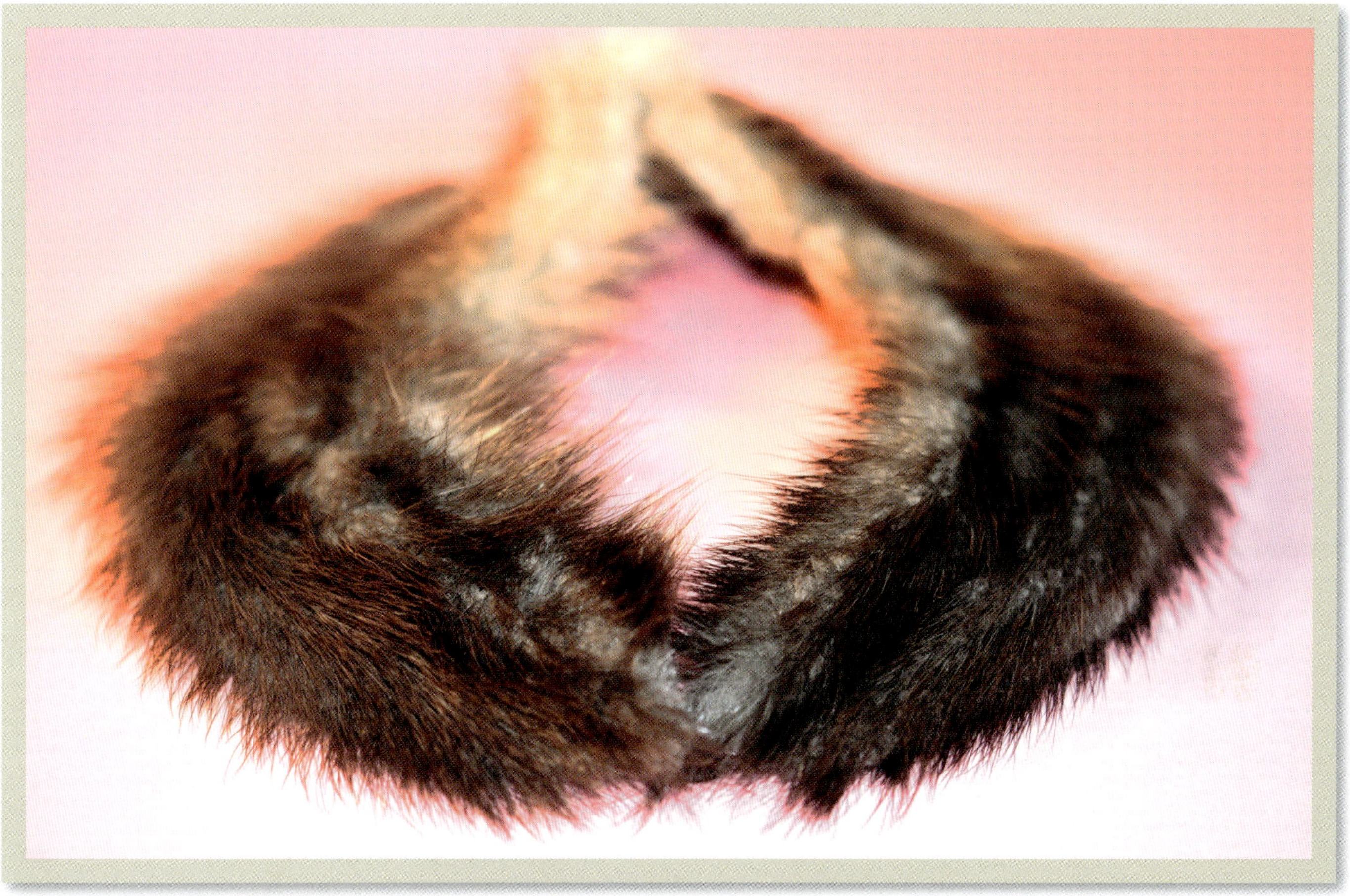

Child's neckpiece of blue mink, originally owned by Ellen Daisy Grace Potter.

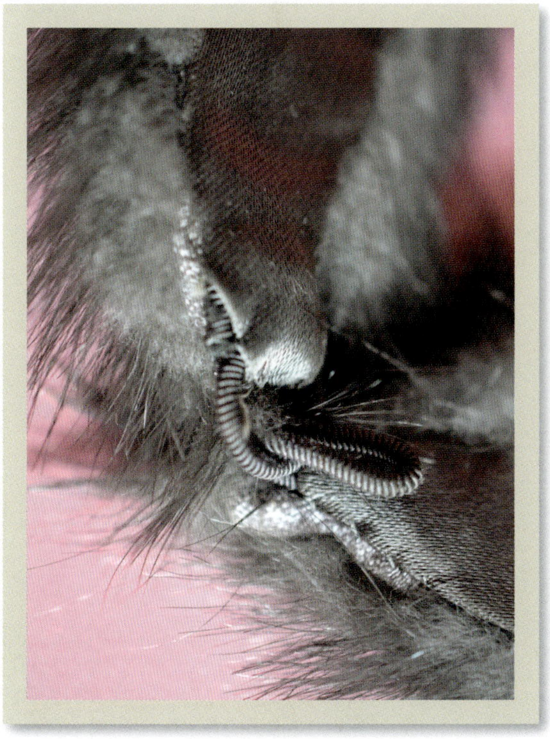

Detail: hook and eye closure.

Reticules, Handbags, and Purses

Named for the fashionable sixth child of Queen Victoria, one of the many popular handbags or workbags that could be made at home was the Princess Louise drawstring crochet bag. The simple pattern was usually made up of fine crochet cotton and lined with remnants of silk. While the versatile purse sometimes served as an opera bag for adult women, it was also a young girl's carryall for bits of frippery and handwork. Patterns published in 1916 and 1917 are still being made up today and sold online.

Young children's purses often hung from shoulder straps while those for misses resembled the beaded and ornamental handbags adult women carried. These generally dangled from the wrist or finger.

Victorian child's commercially made purse, sequined on a metal frame with a swirl of fur.

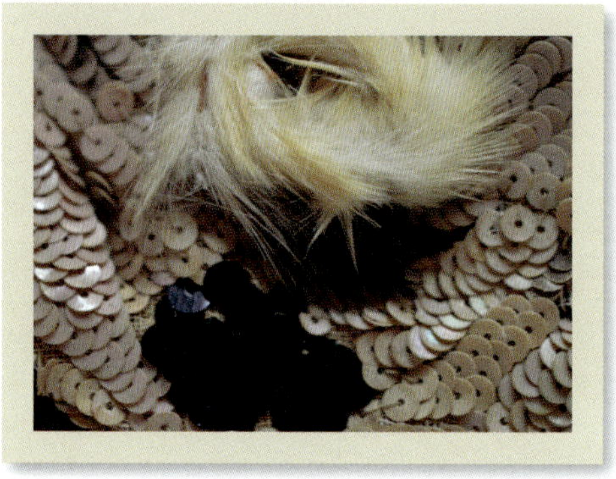

Detail.

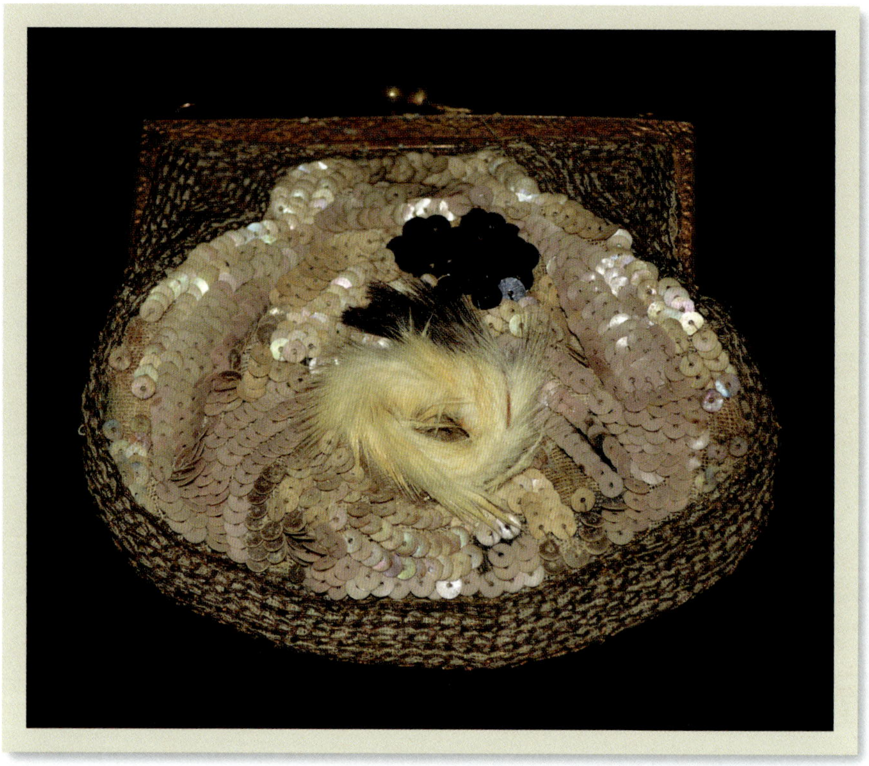

Ornamental beaded handbag with finger loop.

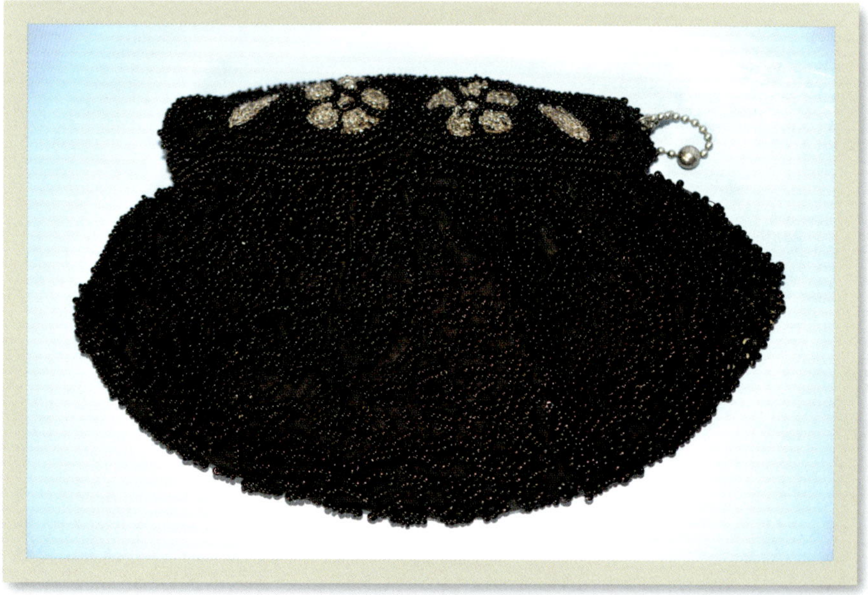

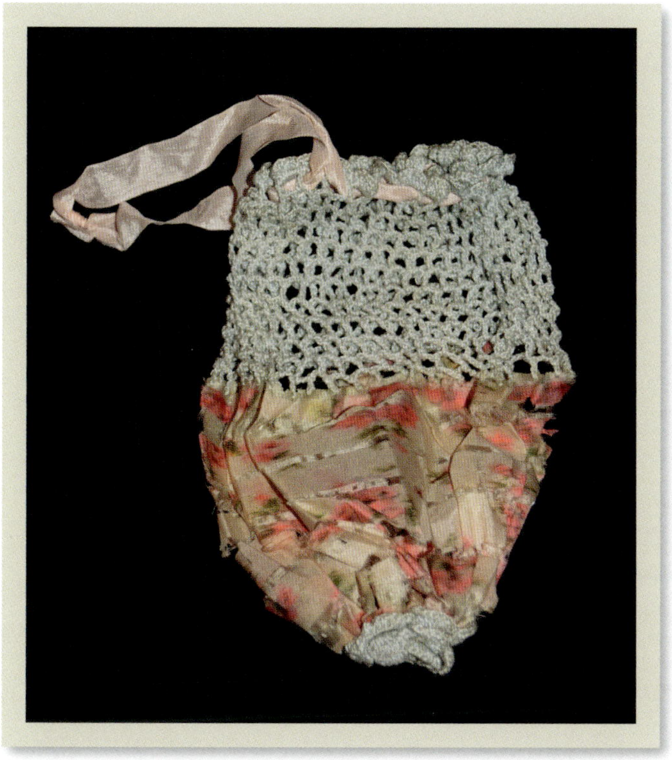

Reticule, homemade with silk ribbon base and crocheted top.

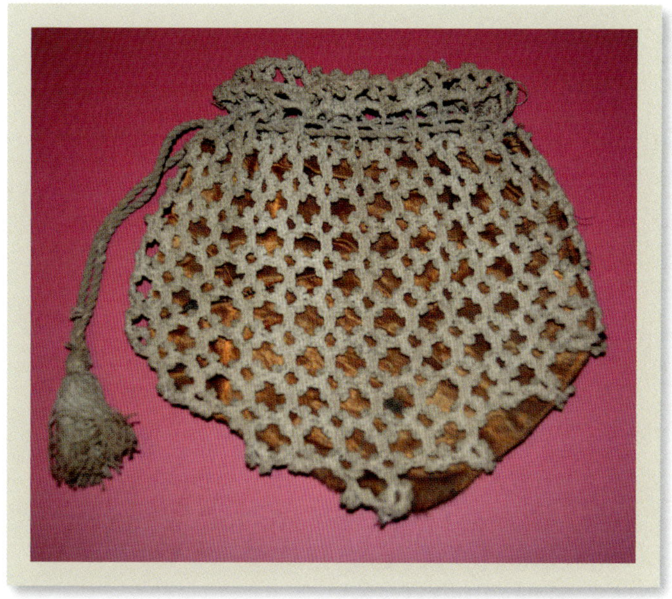

Hand-crocheted Princess Louise drawstring bag with copper colored silk lining.

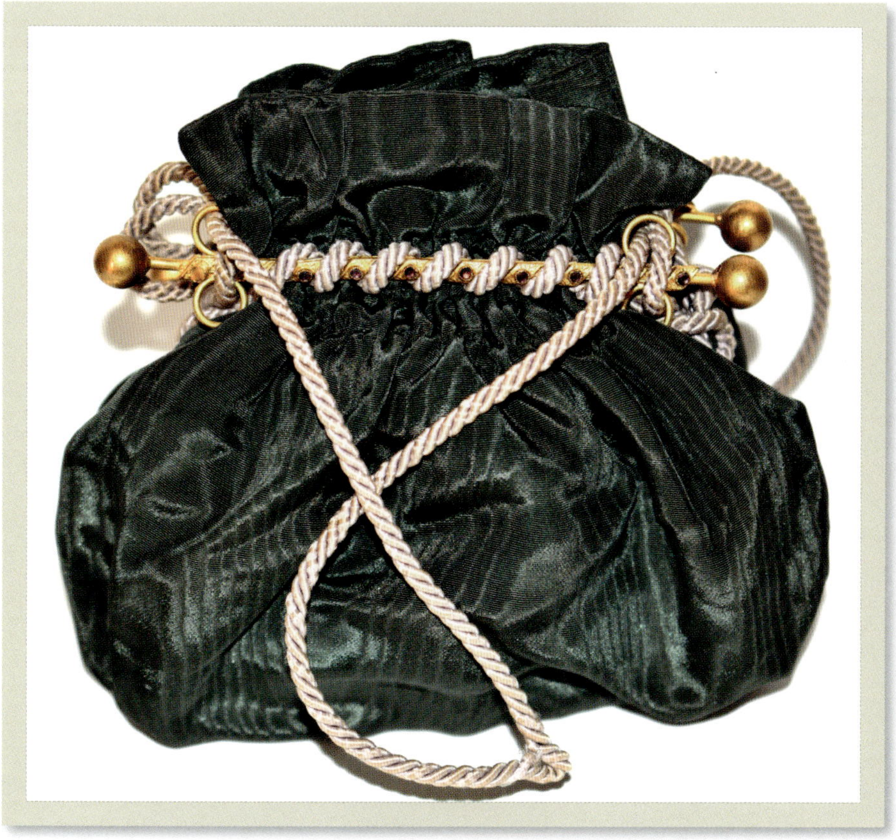

Jewel-handled moire silk wrist bag.

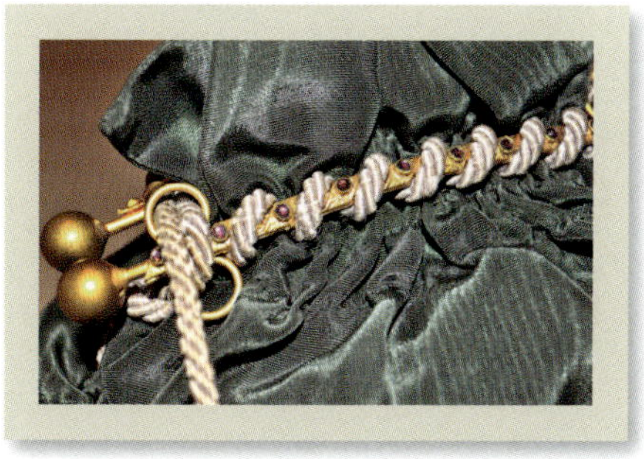

Detail.

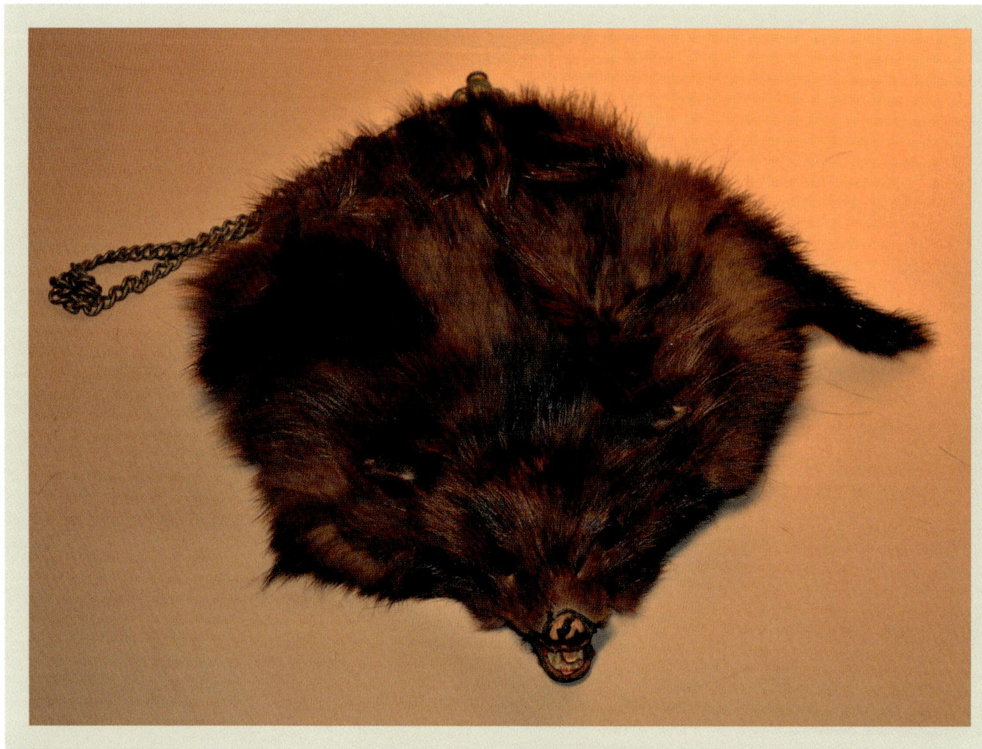

This child's purse is an example of the Victorian obsession with taxidermy.

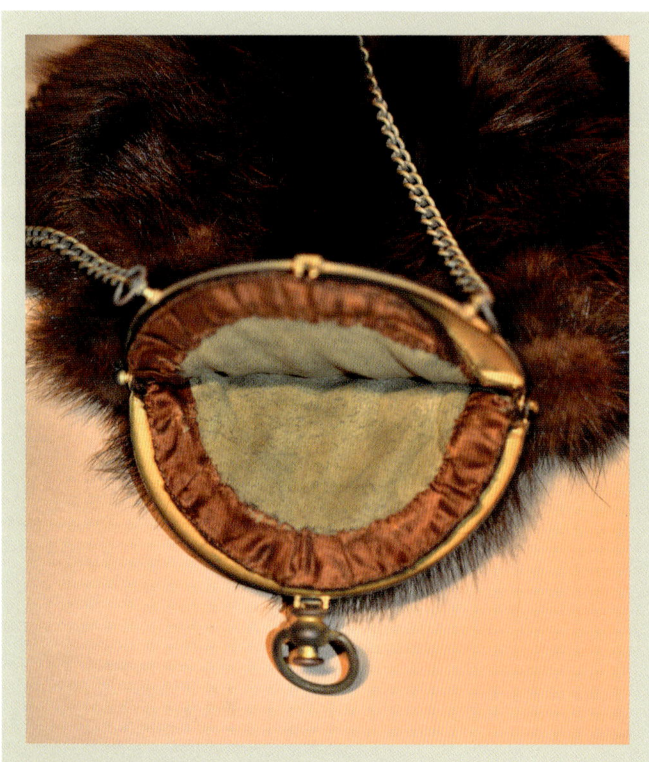

Detail: interior.

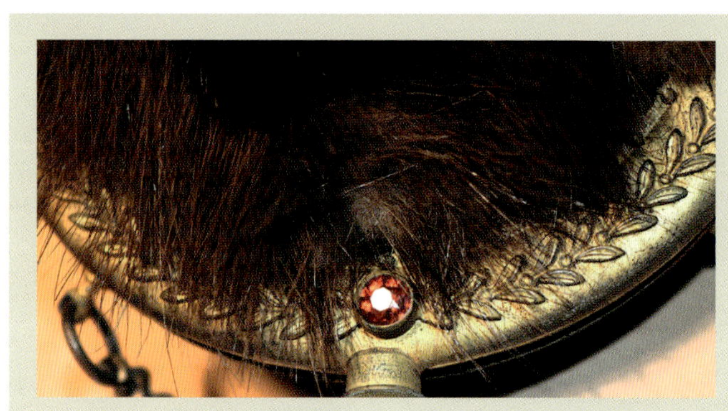

Detail: metal clasp, faux-jewel adornment.

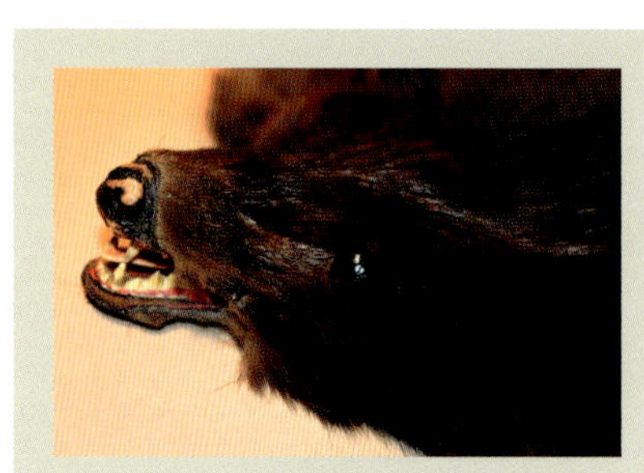

Detail: face with snout, complete with teeth.

Parasols and Umbrellas

One of the most compelling accoutrements of Victorian costume is the parasol. Fashioned of cotton, eyelet, taffeta, silk, or lace on a frame of wood or steel, they bring to mind romantic images of Victorian and Edwardian children strolling parks and sidewalks in elaborate walking costumes. Try to imagine an 1870s Easter parade, mothers and daughters in their finery with the sauciness of colorful parasols floating atop handles of wood, bamboo, tortoiseshell, ivory, bakelite, or glass.

During the mid-Victorian period, parasols and umbrellas formed such an integral part of the female costume that it became commonplace for gentlemen to complain of their hats being knocked off while strolling in public. Yet parasols and umbrellas performed a practical purpose. Upper class female fashion, comprised of expensive and somewhat delicate textiles, required protection from the elements. Aesthetically, an open parasol balanced the wide and/or bustled skirts of the 1860s and 1870s, and, it can be argued, the open umbrella or parasol performed a social function as well, marking an individual's territory or separation from others (particularly gentlemen).

A parasol was a serviceable accessory, prone to damage through exposure to sunlight as well as repeated manipulation when opening and closing the portable handheld device. In relation to the number of Victorian parasols produced, few have survived in good condition.

Parasols can be distinguished from umbrellas primarily through the shape of their handles—stick-straight for parasols, bent for umbrellas. This is a general rule with a number of exceptions. Determining the length of the shaft and the dimension of the canopy can help in dating parasols, but children's parasols are easily recognizable by their size. Fashion plates are an ideal reference for dating early pieces.

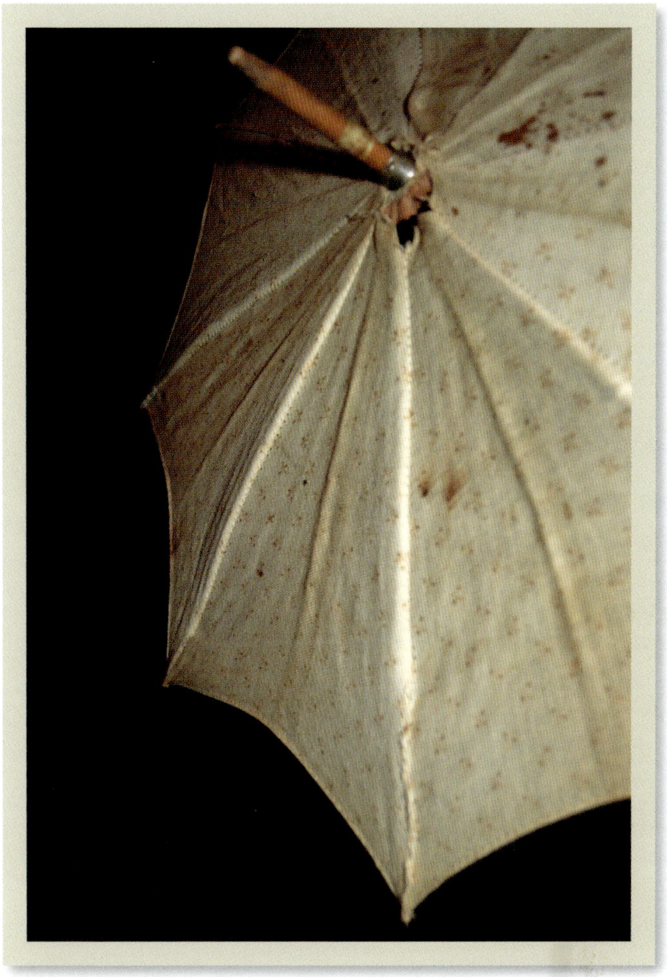

C.1885: A young girl's calico parasol; wooden handle, metal frame.

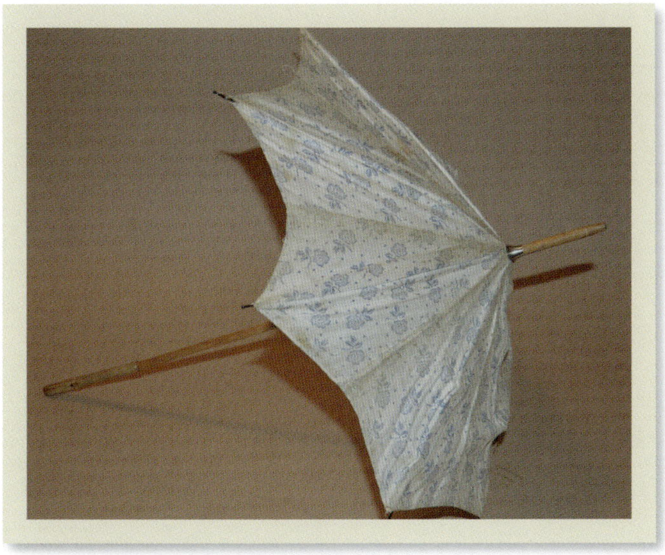

Similar, floral-patterned cotton parasol.

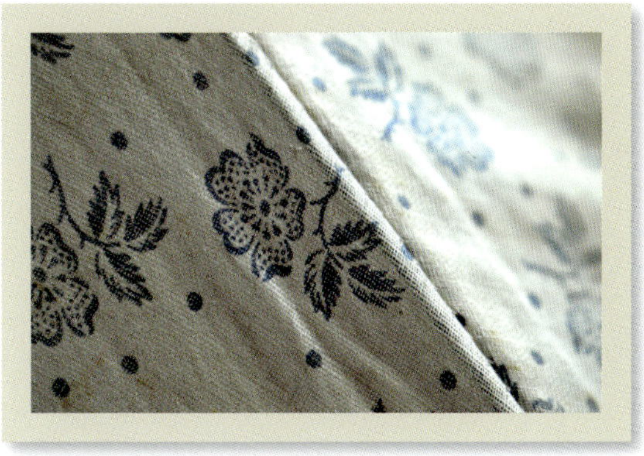

Textile detail.

Teen girl's ruffle edged fine cotton Victorian parasol.

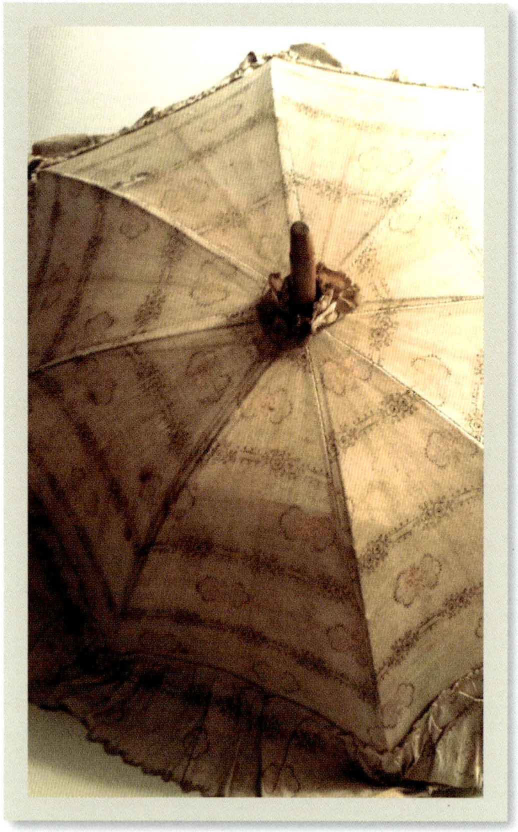

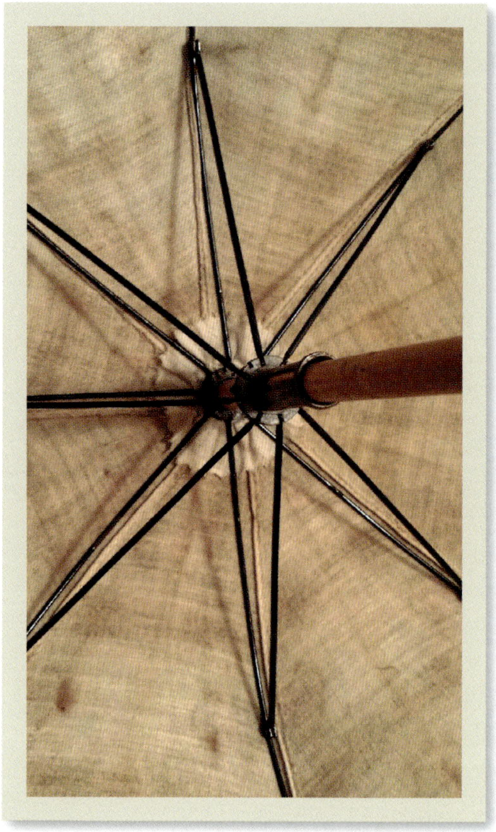

Interior.

Older girl's art deco parasol.

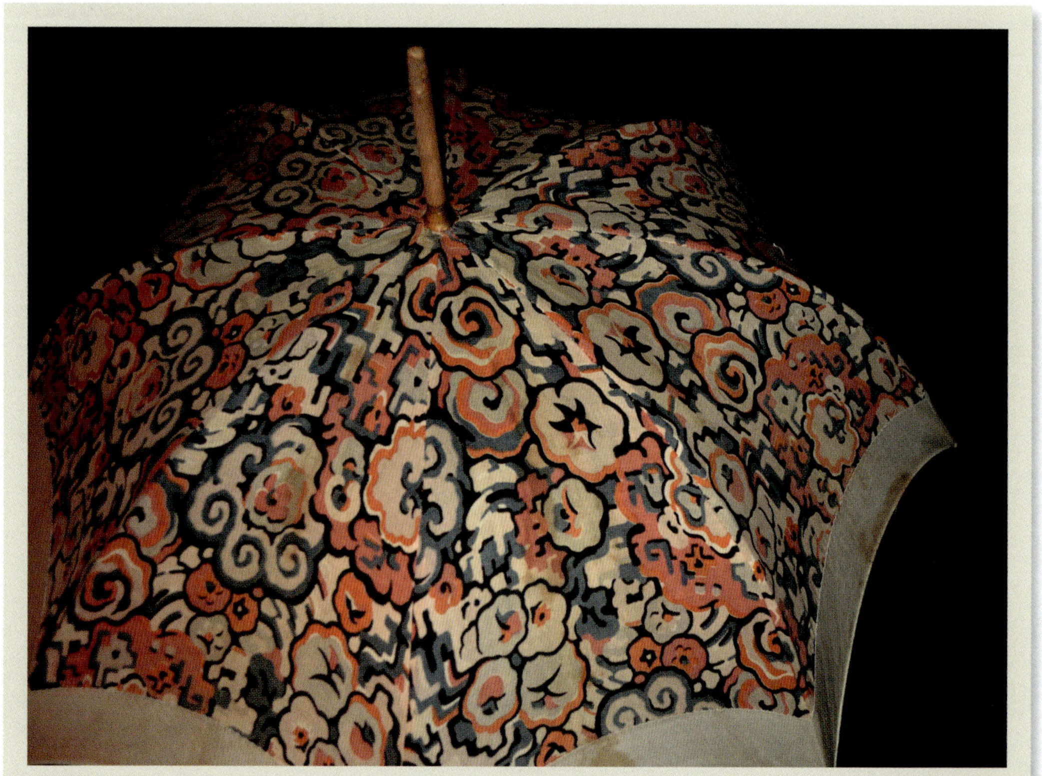

Bibs and Bib Pins

> "Very small people object quite decidedly to wearing an ordinary eating bib at meals.... Let mothers provide bibs decorated with scenes from Mother Goose, or any sketches naturally attractive to children, and see how quickly objections to those useful bits of apparel will disappear."—Mildred E. Bateman, *Needlecraft Magazine*, April 1916

The arrival of a new member of the family has always been met with the giving of gifts, none more practical or easier to produce than the simple bib. Quilted varieties were preferred, as these were the most absorbent; but quilted or plain, all were made beautiful through the application of embroidery and at one time, even jewels. "A pin with the birthstone for the month in which the baby was born would be an appropriate gift," wrote *Ladies' Home Journal* advice columnist Elizabeth Robinson Scovil in May 1901. "At times two pins are given and are used to catch up the full sleeves at the shoulder."|

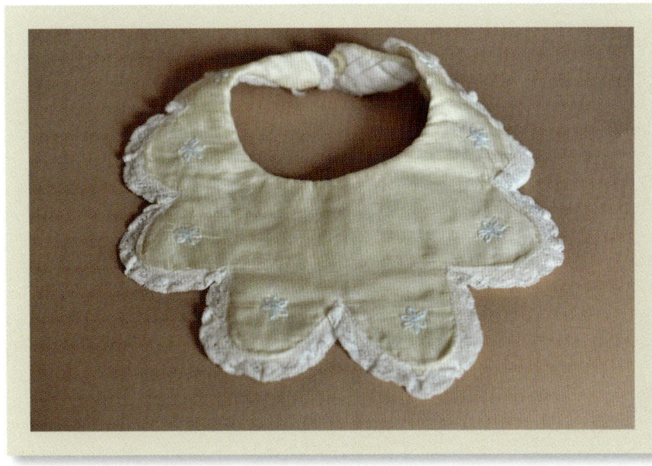

Yellow silk padded bib, lace-trimmed with hand embroidery, Victorian.

CHILD'S BIB IN CROCHET.

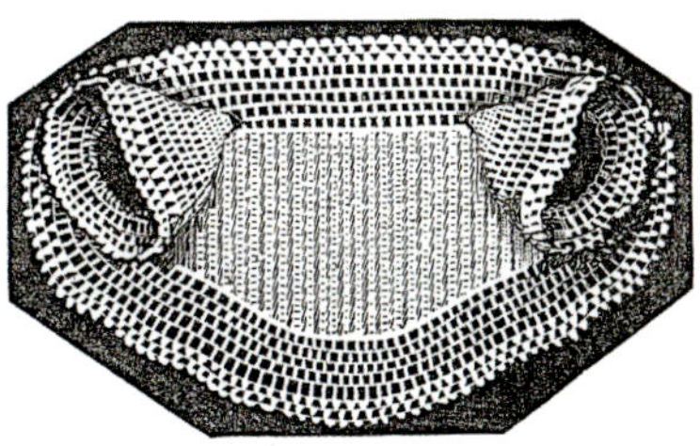

This illustration for a bib with sleeves appeared in an 1861 issue of *Godey's Lady's Book*.

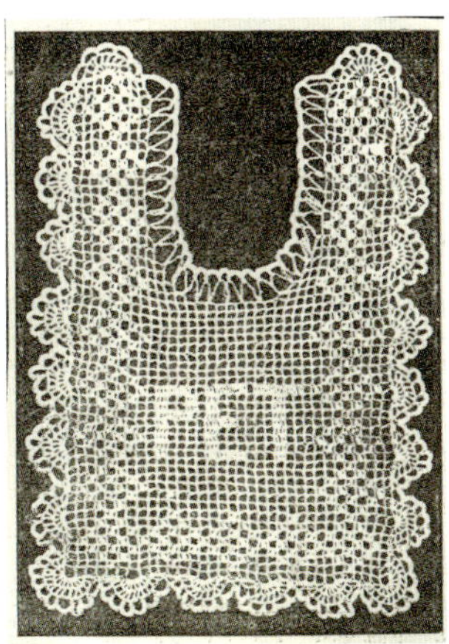

Crocheted bib pattern. *Godey's Lady's Book and Magazine*, Vol. LXIII, July to December 1861.

NEW STYLE OF INFANT'S CROCHET BIB.

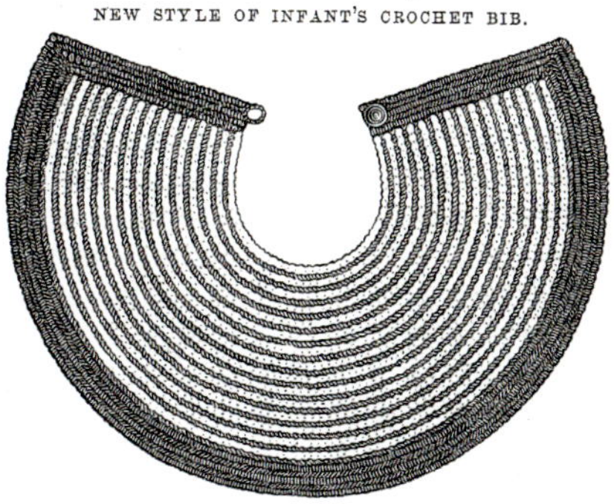

Crocheted bib pattern in the style of concentric half-circles. *Godey's Lady's Book and Magazine*, Vol. LXIII, July to December 1861.

CROCHET BIB.

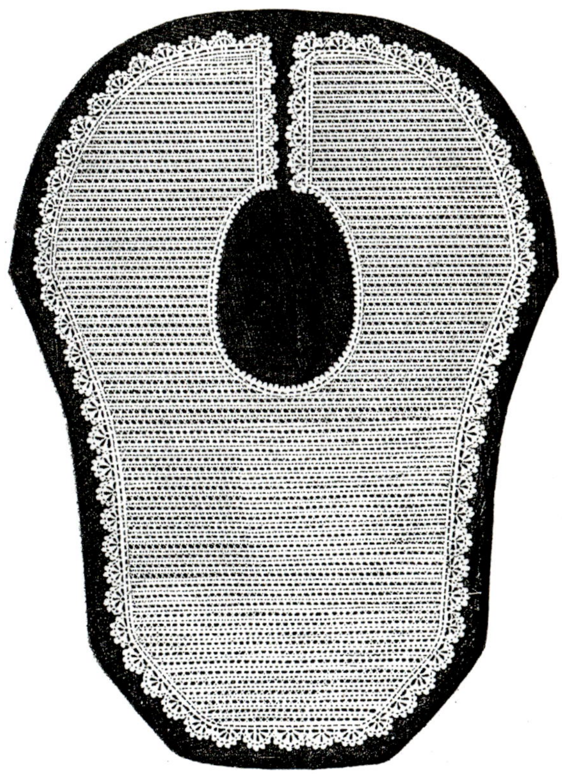

Fancy crocheted baby's bib. *Needlecraft Magazine*, February 1915.

Undergarments

"Graceful girls become graceful women."—Ferris company corset advertisement, *Needlecraft Magazine*, April 1915

Complicated undergarments were as essential for children as they were for adult women. In 1897 an ad placed by the Ferris Bros. Corset Manufacturers of New York offered "Good Sense Corset Waists" for babies, claiming the pearl button garments would support the body healthfully and comfortably. The device was also designed to hold baby's other garments secure.

A study of advertising copy for children's undergarments during Victorian times reveals a preoccupation with the supposed health benefits of the various elements of underclothing. In an age when coughs and colds often proved fatal to children, advertisers used terms like "life-preserving," "blessing," "ventilating," and "healthful" to sell girls' and boys' waists, undershirts, and suspenders to caring mothers.

As a nod to dress reform and the corset controversy, phrases such as "good sense" and "thinking women" targeted buyers of waists that still looked very much like corsets.

Some companies offered incentives such as a free child-sized undershirt with the purchase of an adult garment or a miniature sample for dolly.

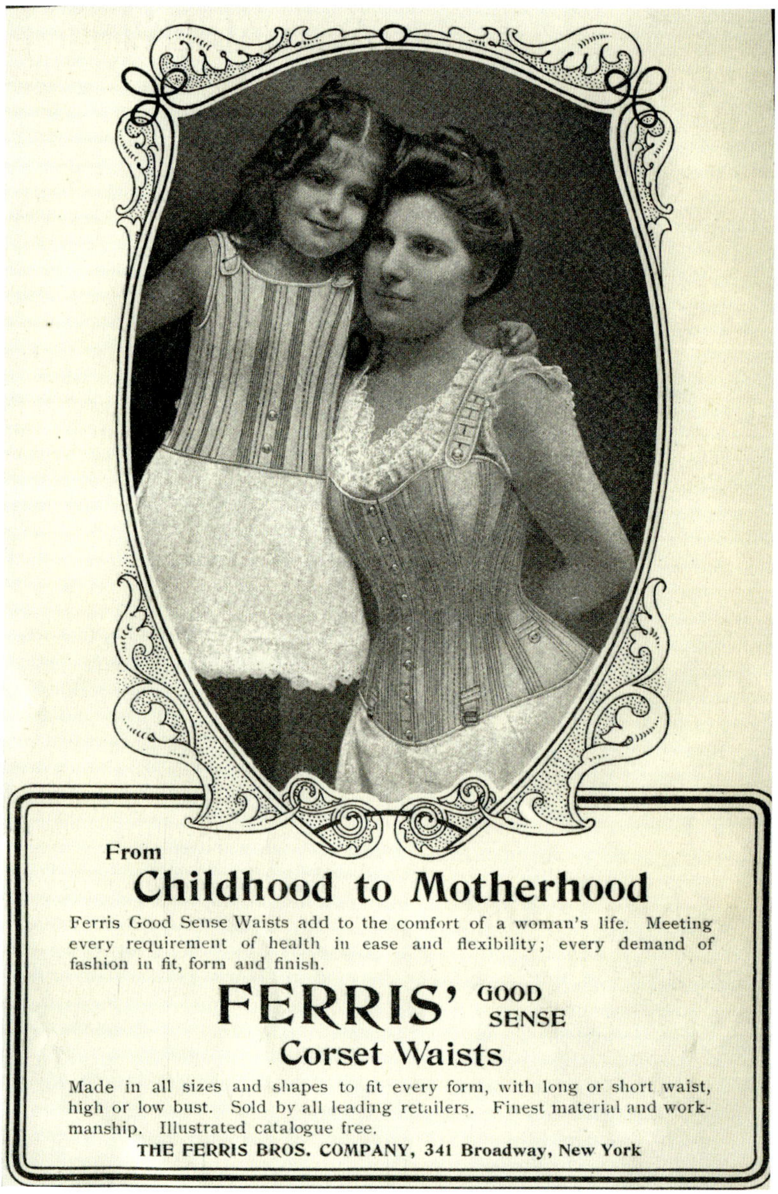

Ferris Company advertisement for corset waists. *Ladies' Home Journal*, May 1901.

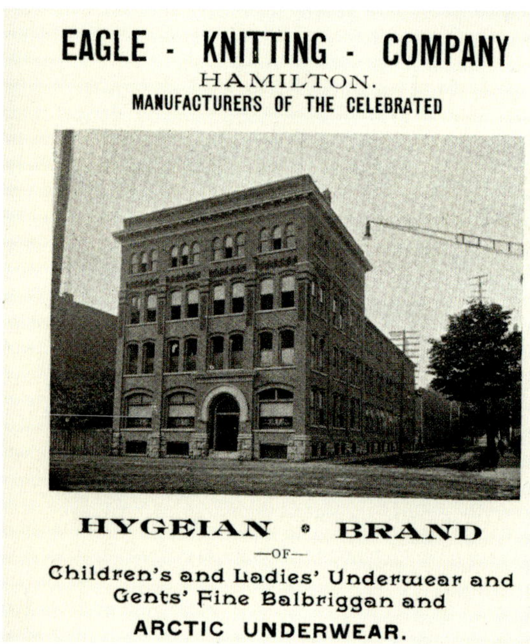

Nineteenth-century advertisement for a Hamilton Ontario Knitting company specializing in children's undergarments. *Canada and Her Commerce*, 1894.

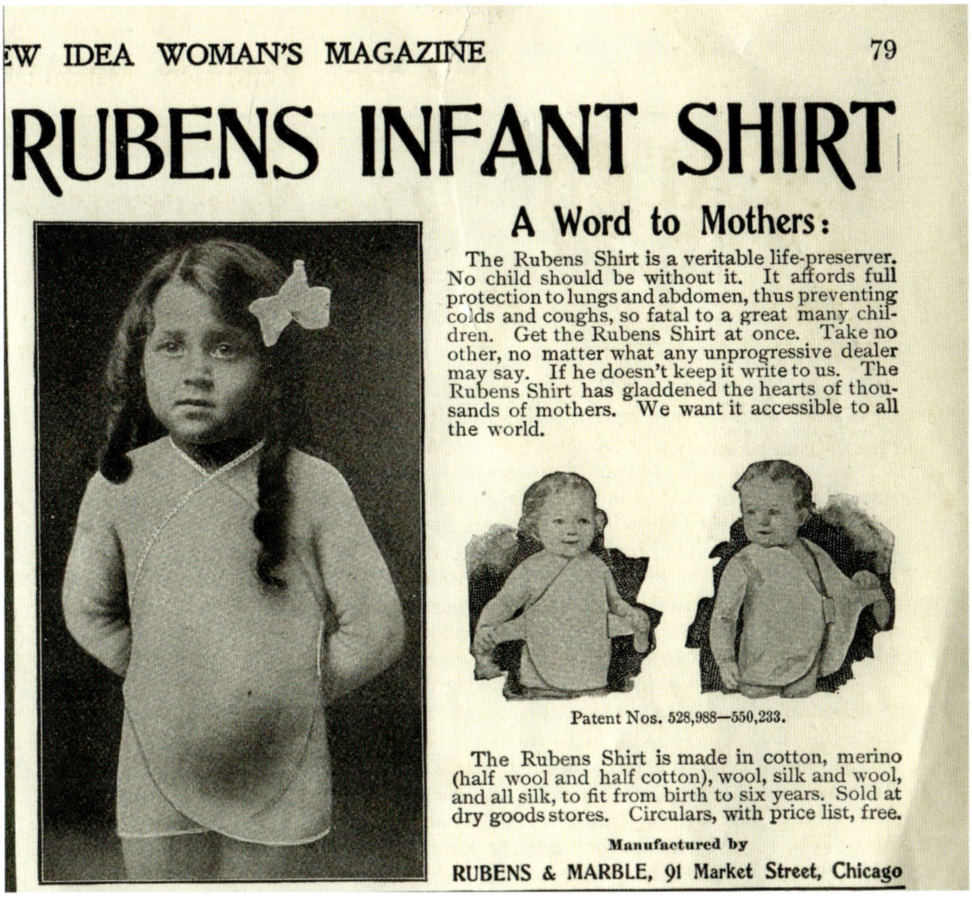

An advertisement c.1908 from *New Idea Woman's Magazine* makes the bold statement that this cotton/merino wool blend infant's shirt will protect a child's lungs and abdomen from fatal ailments.

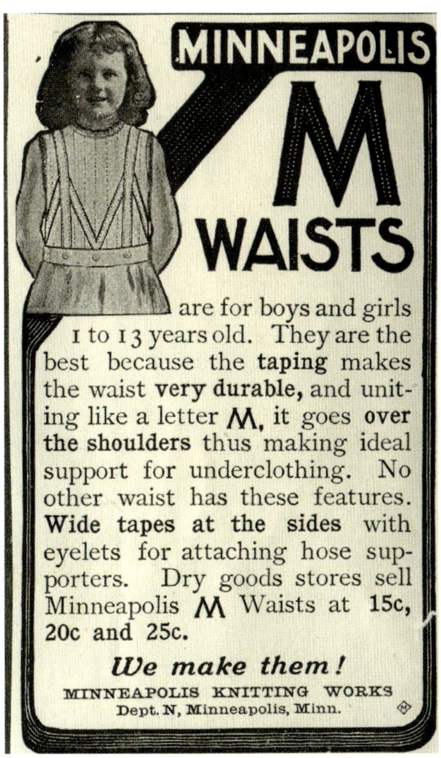

These early twentieth-century over-the-shoulder waists featured eyelets for attaching stockings and other undergarments.

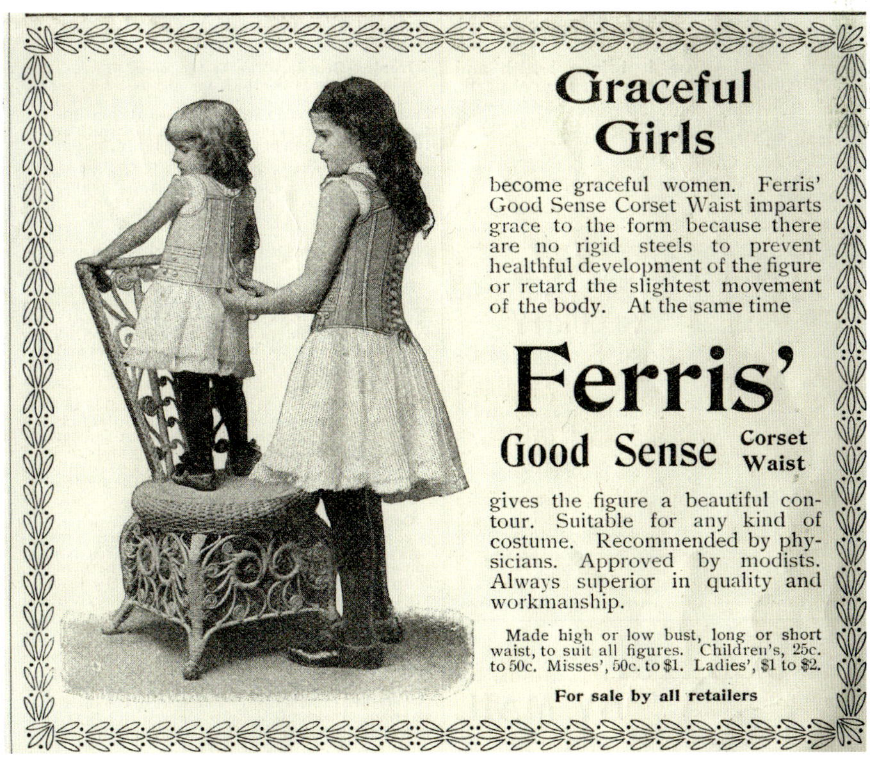

A Ferris Waist's advertisement in *Needlecraft Magazine*, October 1915.

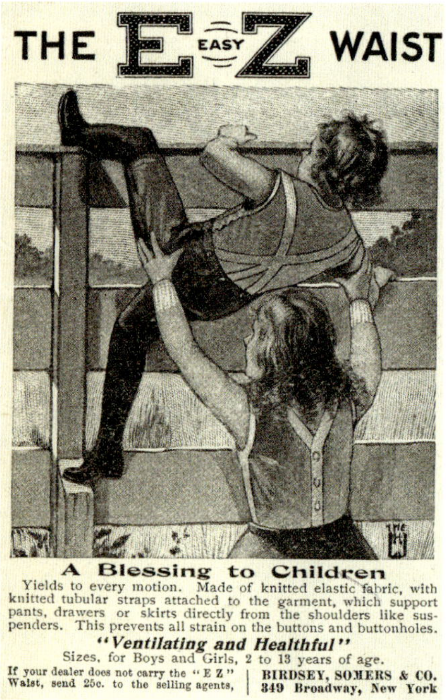

This E Z Waist advertisement attempts to show the product's suitability for active children.

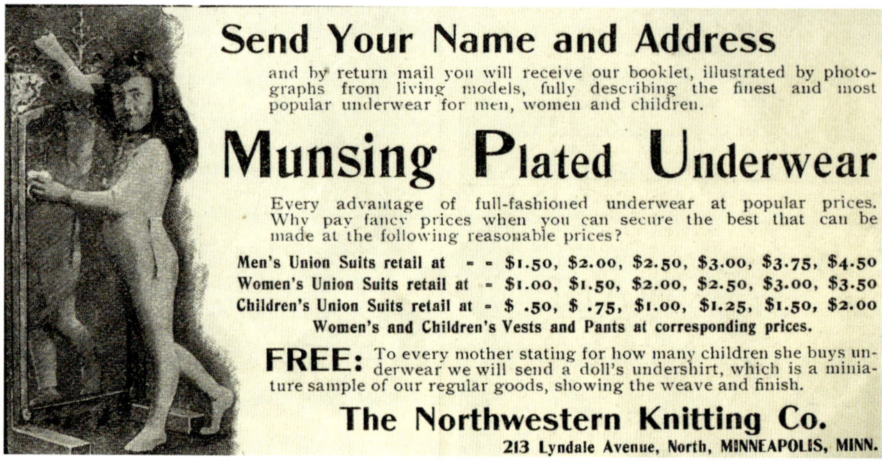

Northwestern Knitting Co. ad for children's underwear.

An endearing ad by the Root Manufacturing Co. showing a young girl telling her dolly, "You must wear this too."

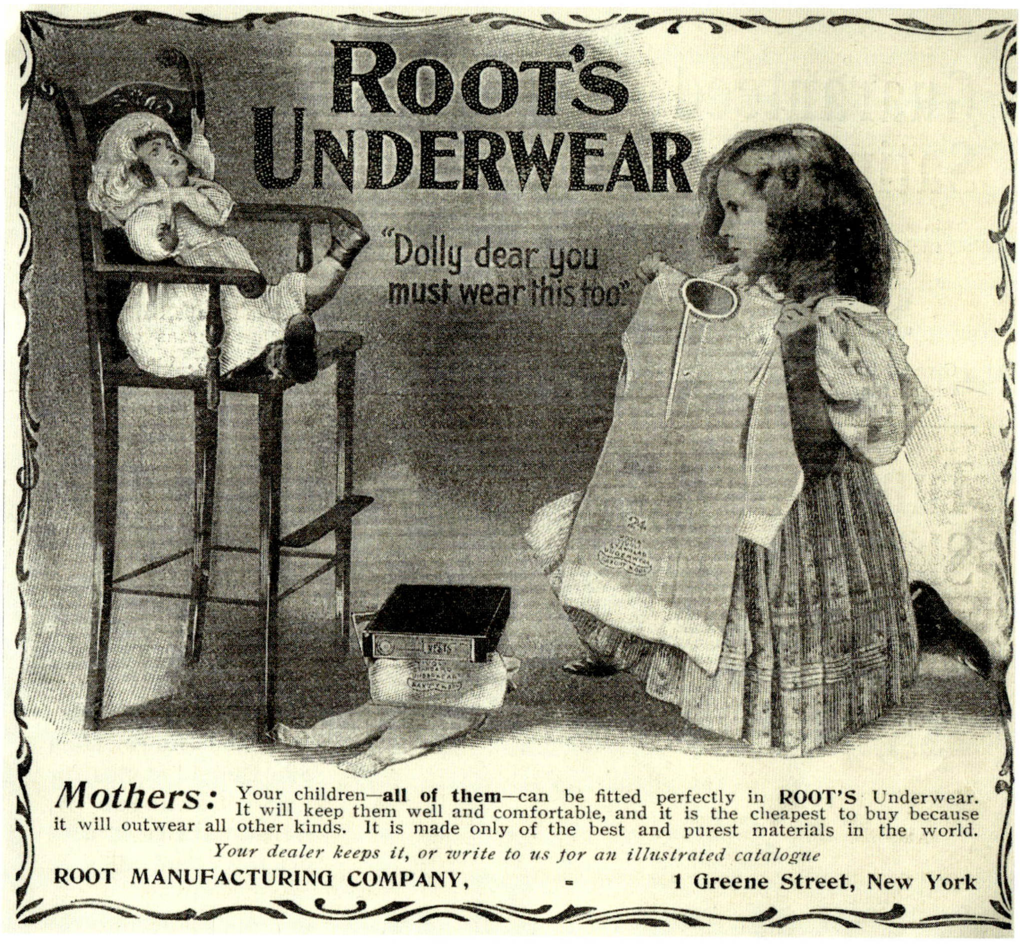

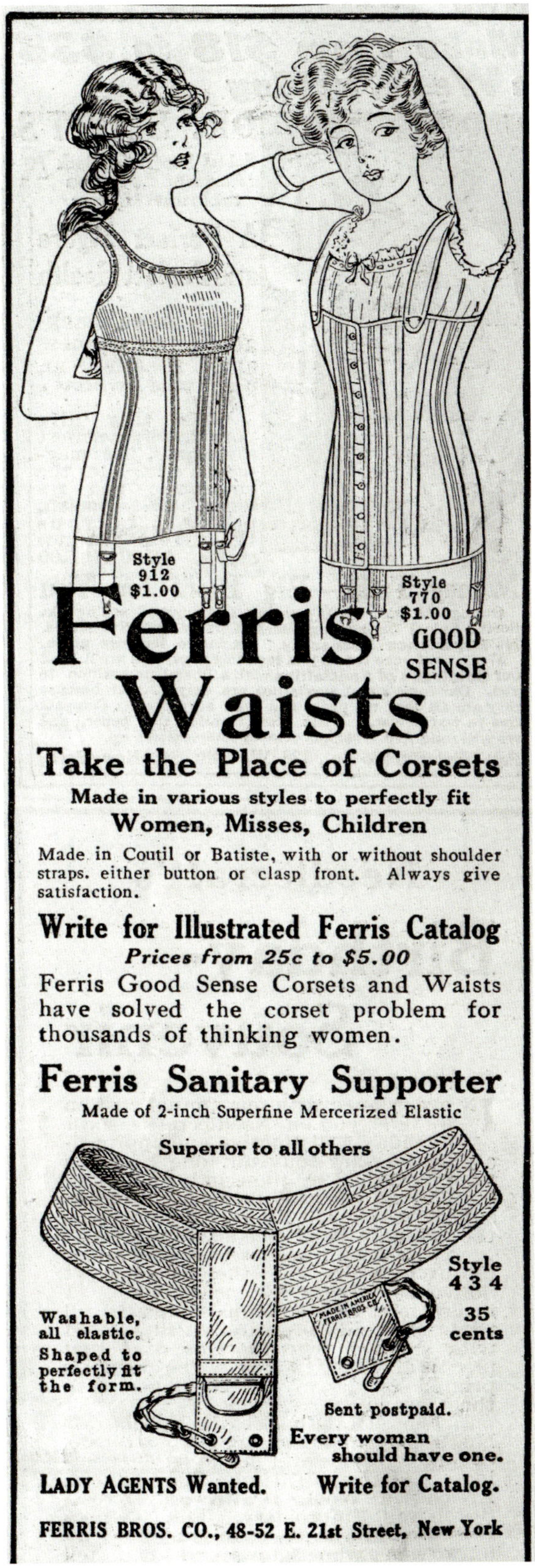

A Ferris Bros. Co. ad for women's and children's waists, which look very much like corsets. The ad also features a request for lady agents under an illustration of a sanitary supporter.

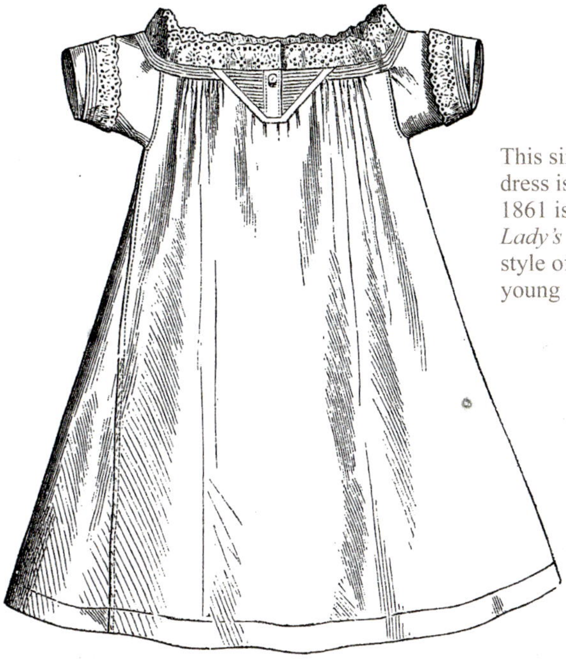

This simple, lace-trimmed dress is described in an 1861 issue of *Godey's Lady's Book* as a "new style of chemise for a young lady."

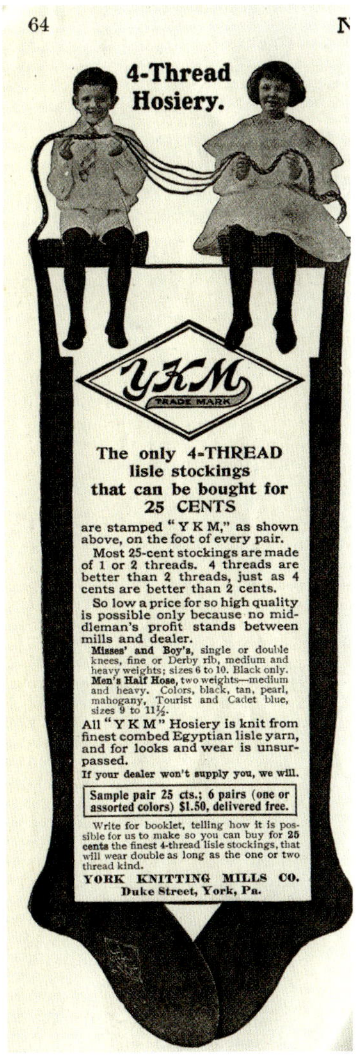

This York Knitting Mills ad for lisle stockings appeared in the October 1903 issue of *New Idea Magazine*.

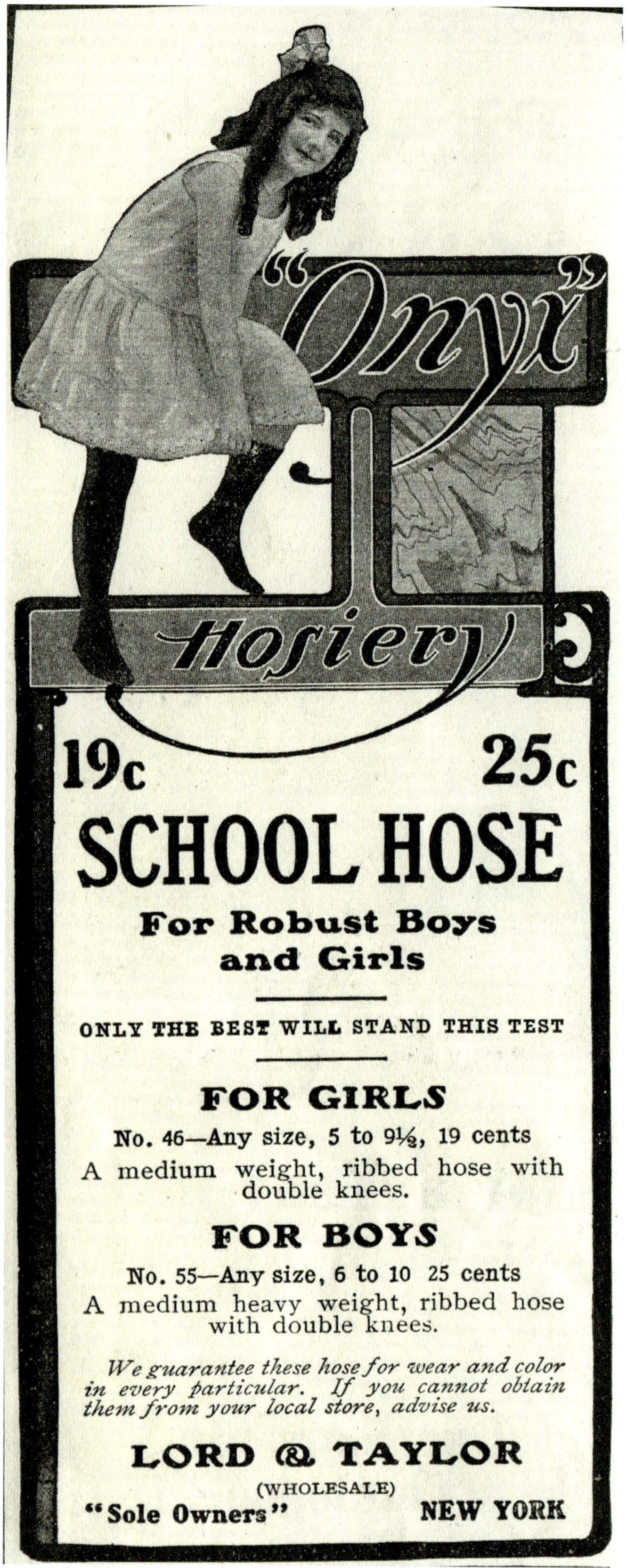
"Onyx"
Hosiery
19c
25c
SCHOOL HOSE
For Robust Boys and Girls
ONLY THE BEST WILL STAND THIS TEST
FOR GIRLS
No. 46—Any size, 5 to 9½, 19 cents
A medium weight, ribbed hose with double knees.
FOR BOYS
No. 55—Any size, 6 to 10 25 cents
A medium heavy weight, ribbed hose with double knees.
We guarantee these hose for wear and color in every particular. If you cannot obtain them from your local store, advise us.
LORD & TAYLOR
(WHOLESALE)
"Sole Owners"
NEW YORK

Advertisement for Onyx Hosiery. *New Idea Magazine*, October 1903.

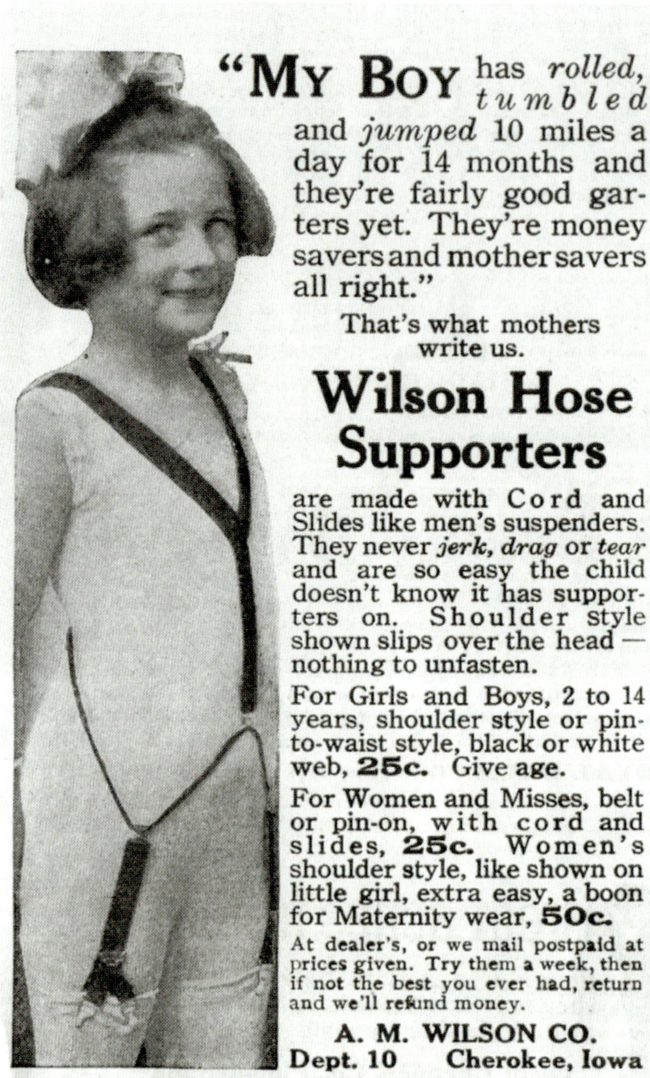
"MY BOY has rolled, tumbled and jumped 10 miles a day for 14 months and they're fairly good garters yet. They're money savers and mother savers all right."
That's what mothers write us.
Wilson Hose Supporters
are made with Cord and Slides like men's suspenders. They never jerk, drag or tear and are so easy the child doesn't know it has supporters on. Shoulder style shown slips over the head — nothing to unfasten.
For Girls and Boys, 2 to 14 years, shoulder style or pin-to-waist style, black or white web, 25c. Give age.
For Women and Misses, belt or pin-on, with cord and slides, 25c. Women's shoulder style, like shown on little girl, extra easy, a boon for Maternity wear, 50c.
At dealer's, or we mail postpaid at prices given. Try them a week, then if not the best you ever had, return and we'll refund money.
A. M. WILSON CO.
Dept. 10 Cherokee, Iowa

Advertisement for Wilson Hose Supporters. *The Modern Priscilla Magazine*, April 1913.

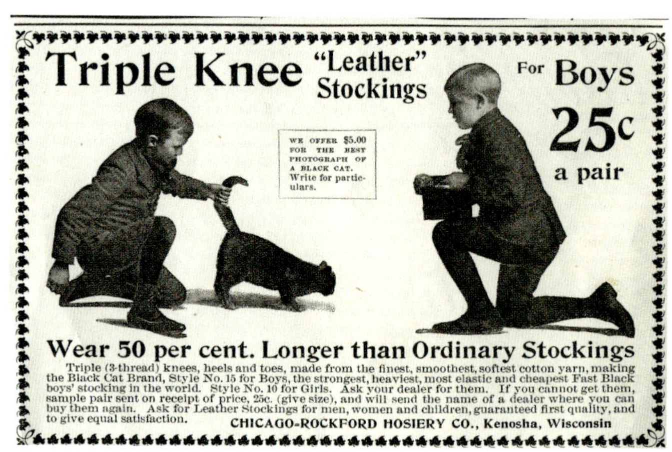

Early twentieth-century advertisement for triple knee stockings at twenty five cents a pair. *New Idea Magazine*, 1903.

Sourcing Historic Children's Costume

In the absence of early extant examples of any given item, historians look to the illustration of artifacts in art, advertising, and photography as well as citations in early letters and official documents for an accurate understanding of the material culture of earlier times. *Darlings of Dress* undertakes a comprehensive investigation of children's clothing 1860—1920 through the examination of period studio portraits and amateur photographs, magazine and catalog illustrations, advertisements, and sewing patterns, in addition to examples of museum-quality garments and accessories.

Nineteenth-century examples of children's clothing are fairly abundant, as are those of the last century. Two of the best ways to source them are through vintage clothing dealers and by contacting local museums regarding deaccessioning sales and procedures.

Clothing lots of estate auctions are another good prospect, as the monetary value of individual pieces is insignificant and articles of clothing are unlikely to be sold separately.

Photographic Portraiture

> "Portraiture wants what cannot be had: life to stop without being dead. It's an art with a built in condition of failure. And that's why it is so interesting."—Debra Brehmer, Portrait Society Gallery director

In her essay entitled "Every Portrait Tells a Lie," gallery director Debra Brehmer purports that all portrait photography involves an attempt to create an idealized image, with the result that the finished product contains the imprint not of "who we are, but who we hope to be. *(Portrait Society Essays*, October 2010, portraitsocietygallery.com)."

Anyone who has ever taken pains with their appearance before sitting to be photographed, or discarded an image of themselves after it was printed, would likely agree. Note the popularity of today's selfie sticks.

Photography is a process in which practitioner and subject conspire to create a stable representation of a transitory moment in one's life that is neither constant nor dispassionate.

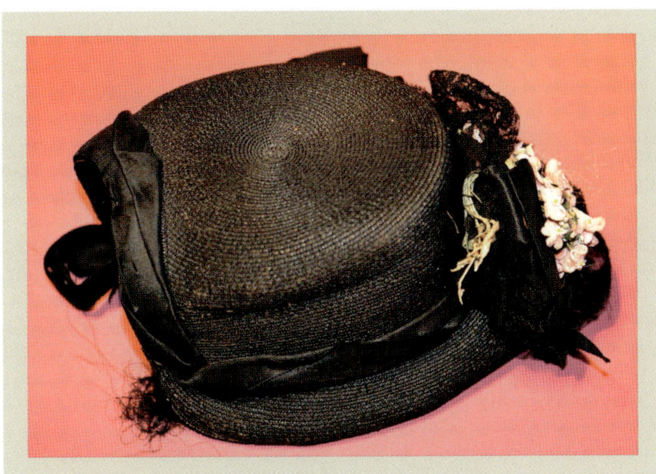

Girl's black straw bonnet with floral trim.

Detail.

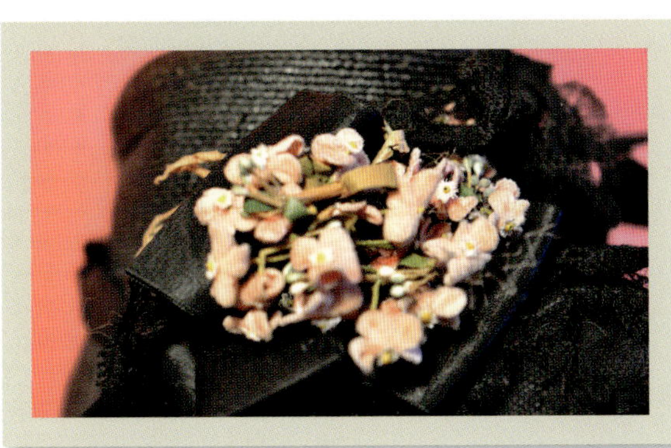

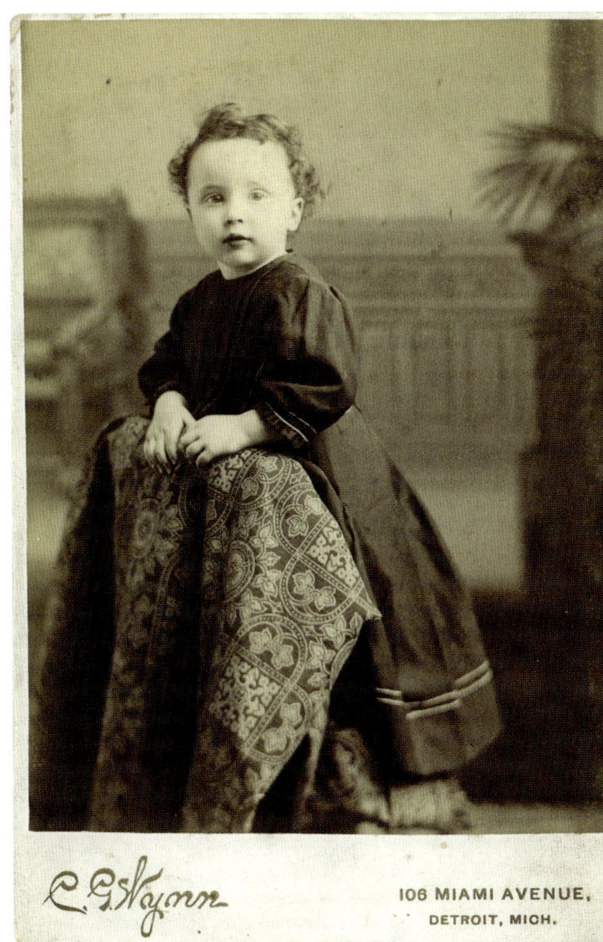

A bright-eyed Victorian toddler poses in her best dress for a Detroit photographer.

The pair work in concert to reflect, disclose, or enhance a desirable truth while concealing, ignoring, or diminishing an undesirable one.

What the onlooker sees when the process is complete depends largely upon what the subject and the photographer have chosen to reveal through the manipulation of dress, posture, and expression on the one hand, and lighting, backdrop, and timing on the other. Not all variables can be controlled, however, and some veracity of personality or genuine emotion may shine through. The subjects' attitudes toward the experience and their feelings toward the photographer will factor into the resulting image in a variety of ways to a greater or lesser degree.

Anxiety, vanity, excitement, or impatience, for example, will produce physical manifestations—facial flushing, muscle tension, excessive blinking—which the photographer may or may not coax the subject to correct. It can be argued that costume as well plays an important and often overlooked role in the attitude of the sitter, and hence the resultant image.

The question becomes, how do we assess the photographs of children in the context of our subject: historic children's costume 1860 to 1920? Photographic advancements over this sixty-year period make for some diversity in the look of the subject matter. Despite advances in photography from the early daguerreotypes, by 1900, color photography remained undeveloped. Studio portraits, however, were sometimes hand-colored to add vibrancy and authenticity.

Victorian and Edwardian Portrait Photos

Wander the stalls of any flea market or spend enough time in an antiques mall and you'll find them—sepia-tinted photographs, encased in frames or decorative mounts, depicting children in beautiful period costume with intricate embellishments and lavish detail. Less expensive, more durable, and easier to store than many of the delicate vintage costumes they depict, period portrait photos provide an accurate record of Victorian and Edwardian children's fashion and can form an exciting collection unto themselves.

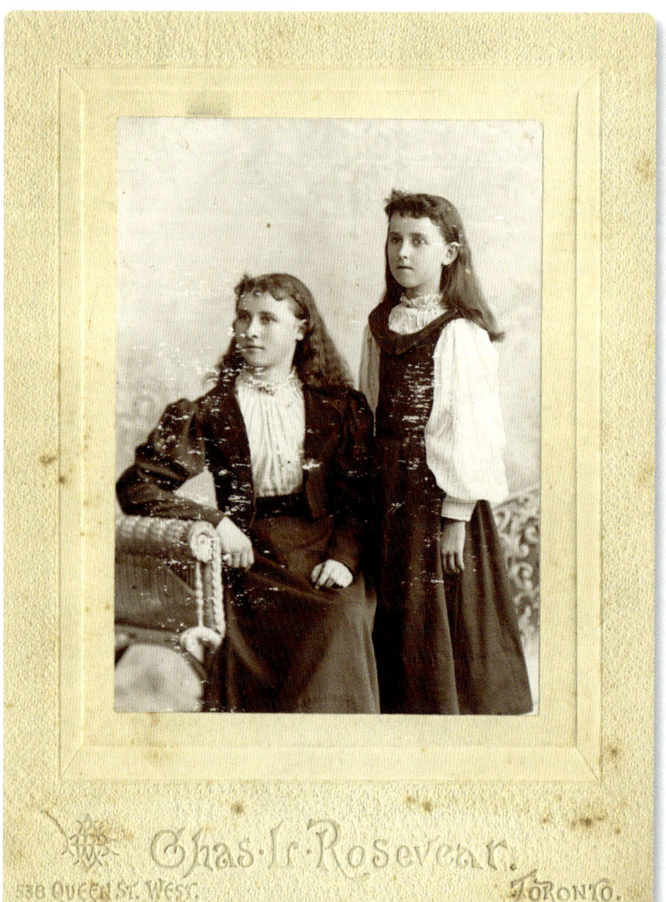

This late Victorian portrait of sisters was styled by a Toronto photographer at a time when the city was known as "Toronto the Good."

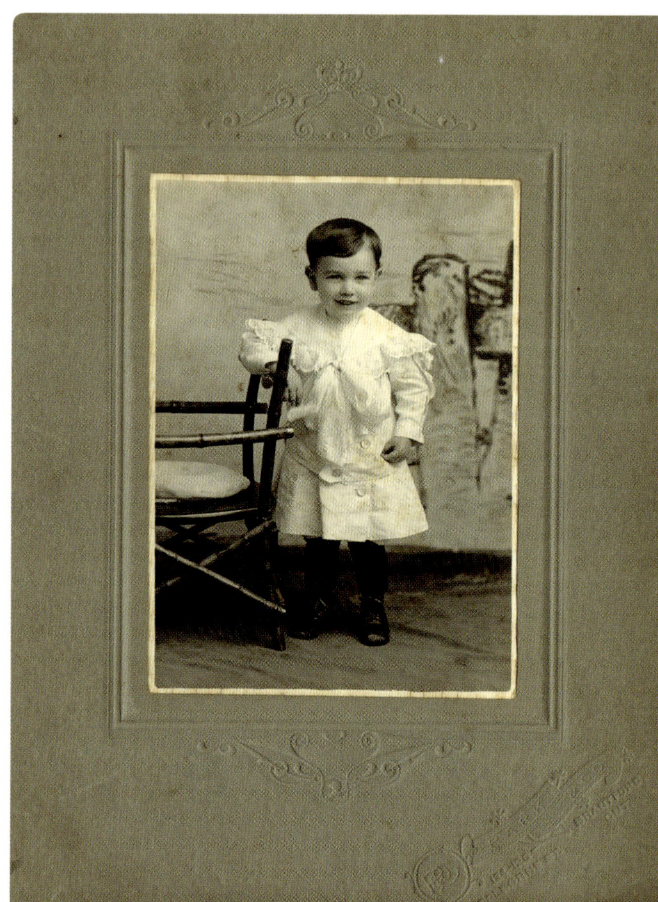

However it was achieved, this portrait has captured a sense of timeless boyishness.

Recognizable by their size, rigidity, and subject matter, Victorian and Edwardian portrait photos are always posed, never candid. Their images represent real people, fashionably attired in the exquisite fashions of a bygone era in a way that fashion plates and periodicals of the time do not.

During the Victorian and Edwardian eras, portrait photos of children, particularly the small *Cartes-de-Visite*, were taken and then exchanged between family members and friends as tokens of affection. They record special occasions like christenings and coming of age—even death.

Hidden Mother Photographs

A game of "dead or alive" is being played on a number of Internet photography sites that feature Victorian "hidden mother" tintype and cabinet card photographs. Viewers speculate as to whether the mothers—who are disguised as chairs or covered with a large textile—are holding live children or having a photograph taken as a last farewell to an infant or child who has perished. The fascination with these decidedly creepy photographs is growing, and while many depict children in "best dress" I have chosen not to include such photographs.

Not all hidden mother images fall into the category of post mortem portraiture, nor are all of the women shrouded in the photographs necessarily mothers of the subjects. Often, in the early days of photography, the duty of holding a young child still while maintaining a pose through lengthy exposure times fell to a nanny or even the photographer's assistant.

The resulting image, when cropped or matted for enclosure in a frame or locket, would appear as if the child was photographed against a textile backdrop; the complete images were likely never intended to be viewed in their original format.

Identifying Historic Portrait Photos

• Cabinet cards: Card-mounted, usually 4.25" x 6.5" in size, sometimes imprinted with a photographer's name and address.

• *Cartes-de-visite*: Card-mounted, usually 2.5" x 4" in size. Often found with decorative, and/or hand-colored mounts.

• Paper prints: Thin paper prints pasted to cardboard backings.

• Postcards: Personal snapshot images printed on postcard stock.

• Hand-colored prints: Many early black-and-white photos were hand-tinted with watercolors.

Care and Preservation of Antique Photos

Pollutants as well as light, moisture, or excessive dryness can damage photographic images and the material they are mounted on. Ideally, prints should be preserved individually in acid-free envelopes, then grouped together upright in cardboard or metal boxes made for archival storage.

Self-sealing food storage bags made of polyurethane can also be used to protect old photos. The American National Standards Institute (ANSI) recommends storage at temperatures of fifteen to twenty-five degrees Celcius with a relative humidity of thirty to fifty percent. If framing your original prints, use an acid-free window mat as a spacer to prevent direct contact with the cover glass.

While the photos will require careful handling and preservation, the images they represent can and should be copied and used in a variety of ways.

Style Progression, Embracing Change Through Dress

Patterning Fashion

One of the many ways couture fashion trickles from the runways of Paris, New York, and Milan, to the closets of everywoman is through the manufacture of sewing patterns. These charming artifacts of period design constitute one of the most accurate, accessible, and inexpensive resources for those interested in historic children's fashion.

Home sewers have Ebenezer Butterick to thank for the first graded and paper printed patterns in 1863. While rare antique patterns from this period create interest, retro and vintage sewing patterns are more widely sought after today, with good condition iconic specimens fetching relatively high prices.

The Delineator Magazine, published monthly from 1873–1937 by the Butterick Pattern Company, offered the most *au courant* clothing designs of their day, along with patterns and instructions, making the most up-to-date European fashions accessible to American home sewers.

Butterick Pattern Company sketch artists attended the seasonal Paris showings enabling the magazine to report on

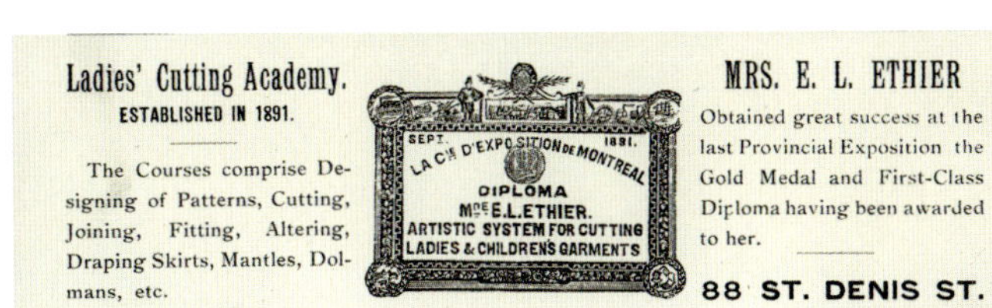

Advertisement for a pattern cutting academy, offering diploma courses in the "Artistic system for cutting Ladies' and Children's Garments." *Canada and Her Commerce*, 1894.

the latest creations by such notable designers as Paul Poiret, Lucien Lelong, Lucile, Louise, Boulanger, and Molyneux, offering American readers advice on what fabrics the garments were constructed of, how they were embellished, and where they could be worn.

The monthly periodical supported home and family values to the extent that for a time, it established a child rescue program, offering profiles of orphaned and neglected children whom readers could apply to adopt or otherwise support.

Cut Out for Fashion

With two-dimensional cardboard figures as easy to dress as three dimensional dolls, it is no surprise that cut-outs or paper dolls have been a favorite with children for over a century. Cut-outs were sold as books, with cardstock dolls incorporated into the covers. Their outlines were perforated enabling little hands to remove them. Idealized paper outfits, usually with fold-over tabs, filled the pages.

Paper dolls were made available in a number of styles representing fashions for brides, celebrities, teens, and children. Like trade cards, many of these were offered as advertising incentives as early as the 1880s.

Formal Attire

Fashionable dress for children was a Victorian and Edwardian social imperative, as important as manners, deportment, and cleanliness. As with adults, the appropriateness of a child's dress depended upon one's social standing and functions as well as time of day and prevailing sartorial trends. For upper and middle-class families, morning clothes carried one throughout the day, while evening dress was required for dinner and during the "candlelight" hours. Servants, on the other hand, which included girls as young as eight years old, often resided with their employers and were required to wear uniforms.

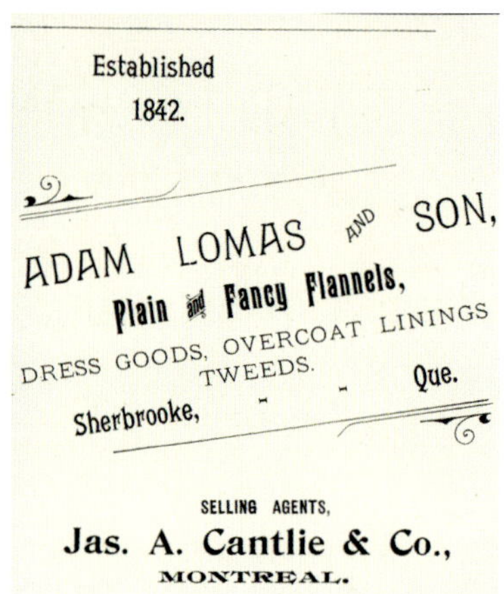

Sherbrooke, Quebec, textile company advertisement. *Canada and Her Commerce*, 1894.

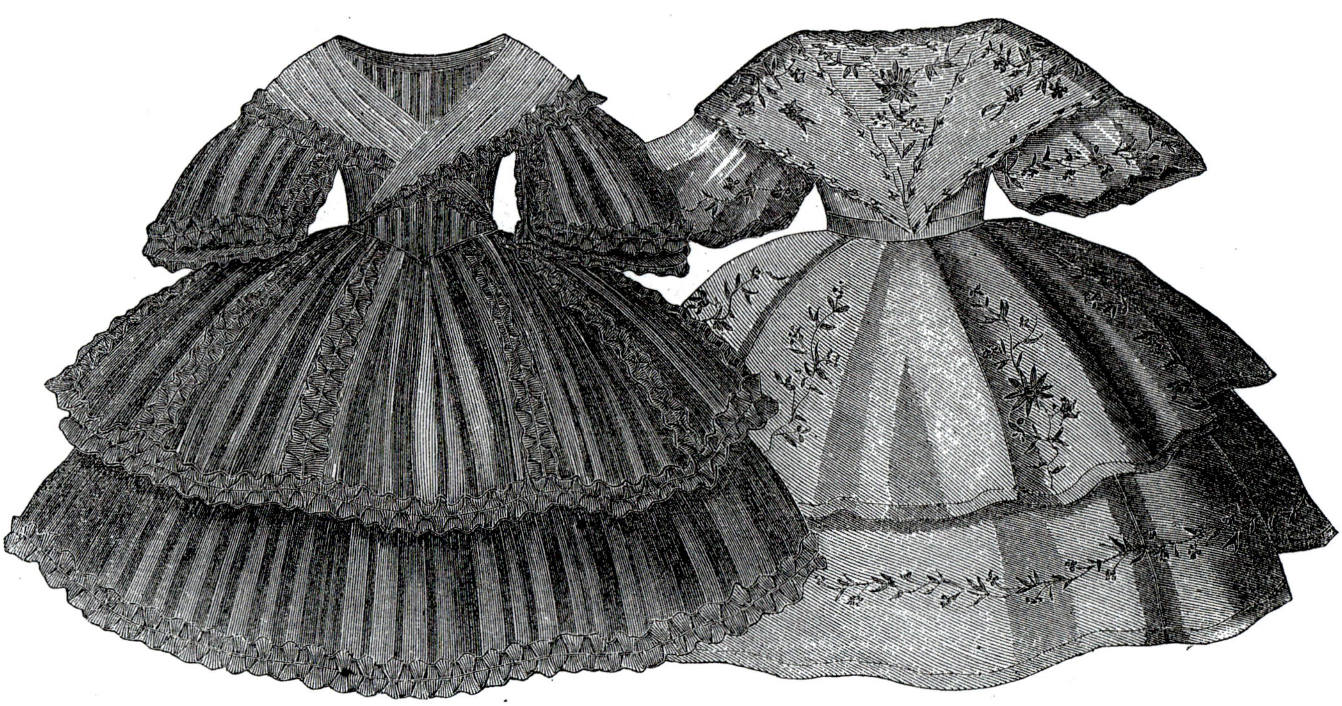

Pattern illustrations for fancy, full-skirted dresses for formal occasions, the first of striped poplin, the second of French Merino embroidered with silk. *Godey's Lady's Book and Magazine*, January to June 1861.

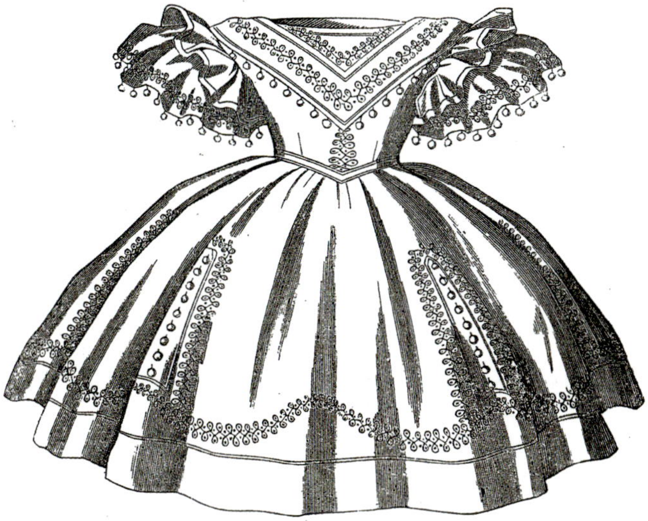

Drop buttons and gold embroidery embellish this 1860s party dress for a little girl. *Godey's Lady's Book and Magazine*, January to June 1861.

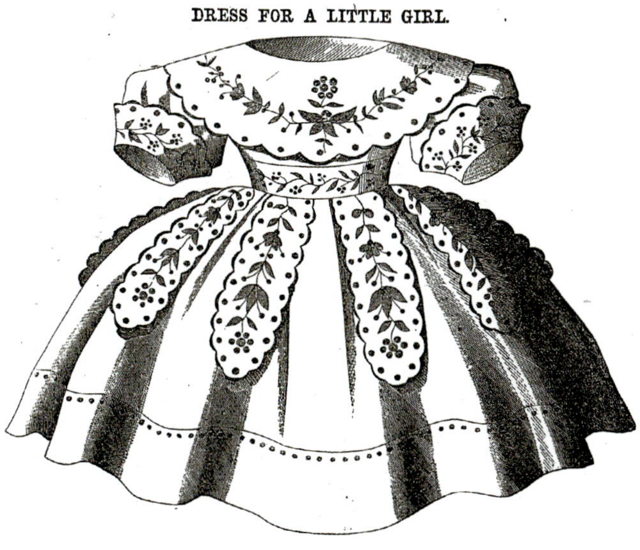

Dress illustration described as being made of French Merino in rose or blue with silk embroidered collar, cuffs, lappets, and waistband. *Godey's Lady's Book and Magazine*. January to June 1861.

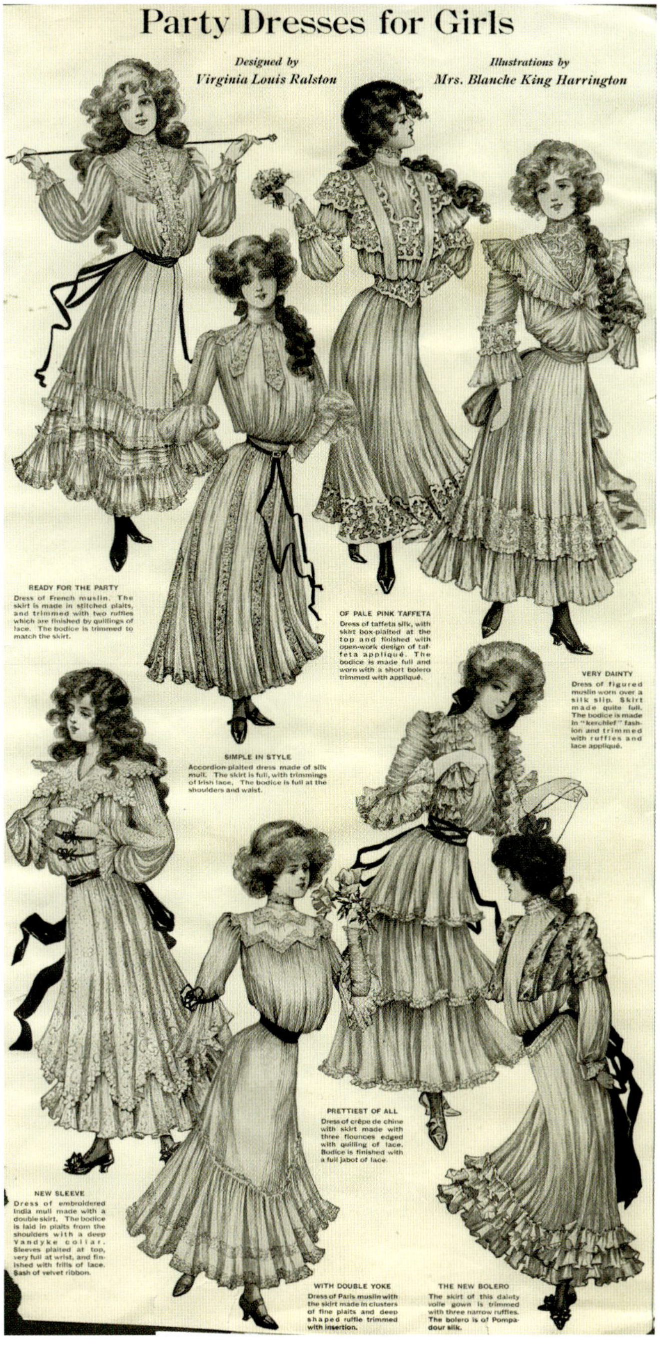

Party Dresses for Girls

Designed by Virginia Louis Ralston

Illustrations by Mrs. Blanche King Harrington

READY FOR THE PARTY

Dress of French muslin. The skirt is made in stitched plaits, and trimmed with two ruffles which are finished by quillings of lace. The bodice is trimmed to match the skirt.

OF PALE PINK TAFFETA

Dress of taffeta silk, with skirt box-plaited at the top and finished with open-work design of taffeta appliqué. The bodice is made full and worn with a short bolero trimmed with appliqué.

VERY DAINTY

Dress of figured muslin worn over a silk slip. Skirt made quite full. The bodice is made in "kerchief" fashion and trimmed with ruffles and lace appliqué.

SIMPLE IN STYLE

Accordion-plaited dress made of silk mull. The skirt is full, with trimmings of Irish lace. The bodice is full at the shoulders and waist.

NEW SLEEVE

Dress of embroidered India mull made with a double skirt. The bodice is laid in plaits from the shoulders with a deep Vandyke collar. Sleeves plaited at top, very full at wrist, and finished with frills of lace. Sash of velvet ribbon.

PRETTIEST OF ALL

Dress of crêpe de chine with skirt made with three flounces edged with quilling of lace. Bodice is finished with a full jabot of lace.

WITH DOUBLE YOKE

Dress of Paris muslin with the skirt made in clusters of fine plaits and deep shaped ruffle trimmed with insertion.

THE NEW BOLERO

The skirt of this dainty voile gown is trimmed with three narrow ruffles. The bolero is of Pompadour silk.

Eight frilly late-Victorian delights; party dressing for older girls. *Ladies' Home Journal*, October 1901.

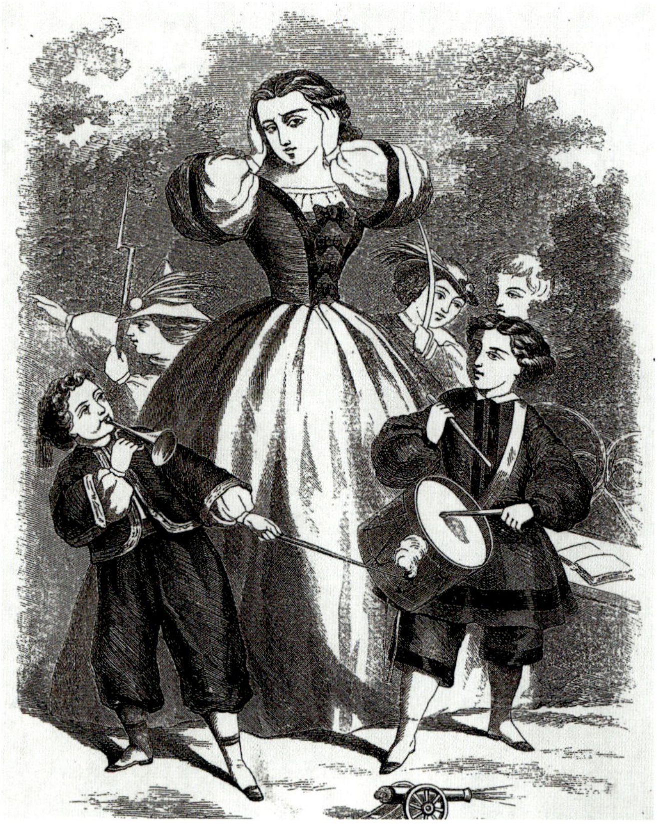

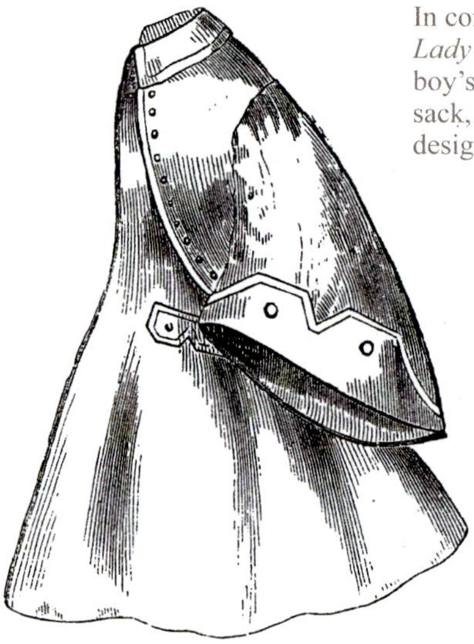

In contrast, the 1864 *Godey's Lady's Book* describes this boy's jacket, called the Elgin sack, as being "especially designed for home wear."

These tykes are dressed to be seen and heard at a Fourth of July celebration. *Godey's Lady's Book*, 1864.

The Fancy Dress Ball

Incredibly, fancy dress balls were attended not only by adults but also upper-class children, in part because many a masquerade began with a series of *tableaux vivants*, which depending upon the historical re-enactment might require the participation of the younger set.

Well-conceived elaborate costumes based on historical characters, current events, Greek mythology, or whimsical themes were elaborately constructed, complete with head pieces and accessories ranging from wildly wonderful hats, shoes, and stockings to fabricated props.

Some estates, such as Pointe-Claire, Quebec's former Mull Hall, were built with spaces that functioned at times as private ballrooms. Laurabelle MacLean, who spent some of her childhood at Mull Hall, remembered riding the dumbwaiter between the kitchen and upper level and peeking into the conservatory to gaze at the costumed guests when grand parties were held.

Like the estate of auto baron Robert Samuel McLaughlin in Oshawa, Ontario, many well-to-do families kept dressmakers employed on site. Their duties would extend to creating and re-creating seasonal garments for each member of the family, based upon their social calendar. Samantha George, curator of Parkwood Estate, explains that special occasion garments worn once by an older child would be refashioned for a younger sibling.

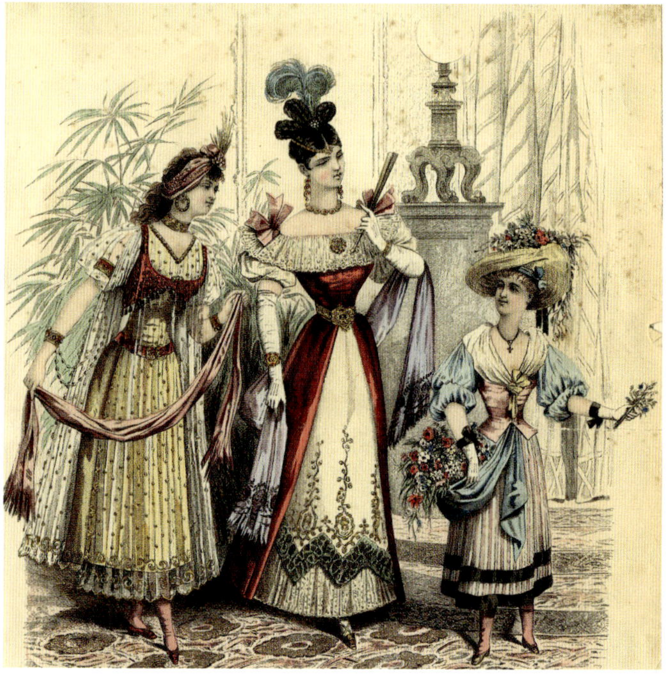

Fashion plate of two women attired in ball gowns and evening headdresses, and a girl in a colorful "flower seller" ensemble, appropriate for a child's fancy dress costume.

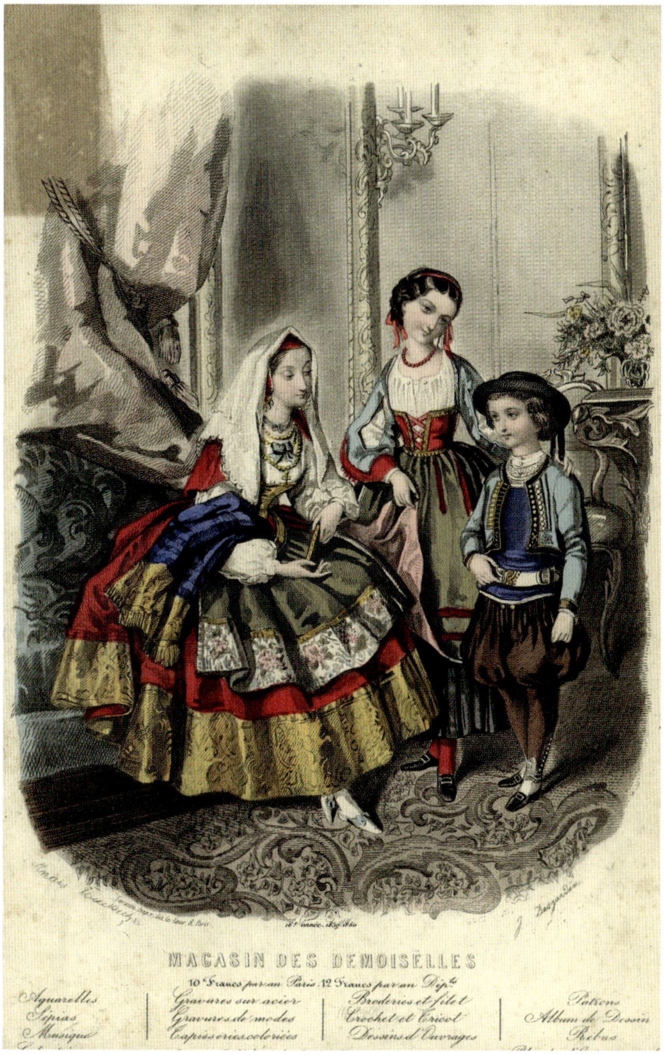

Fashion plate of children's fancy dress ball costume advertising the French shop Le Magasin Des Demoiselles, dated 1859–1860.

Fulford Place Museum, the former home of Senator George Taylor Fulford, whose fortune derived from the sale of Dr. Williams' pink pills for pale people, boasts a wonderful reproduction of a costume based on the theme of his empire. A number of other museums maintain photographic records of these Victorian fancy dress ball costumes as well.

Fashion periodicals carried fashion plate illustrations of such costumes. Seamstresses with scant imagination or modest means could purchase patterns directly from companies like Butterick and McCalls.

The Button Boom

One of the simplest and most rewarding areas of costume collecting has been the accumulation of buttons; in fact, many nineteenth-century garments are collected solely for the purpose of harvesting their buttons. Iconic of their period, buttons are easy to display and store. A carefully curated selection can even tell the story of children's costume through the decades. Kathleen Vocelle, contributor to *Bead and Button Magazine*, asserts that the popularity of children's mass-produced metal picture buttons reached its zenith c. 1880. Children's costume enthusiasts prize fairy tale subject matter and scenes pertaining to children's play. Glass buttons were also molded into a number of thematic designs, making them popular with modern collectors.

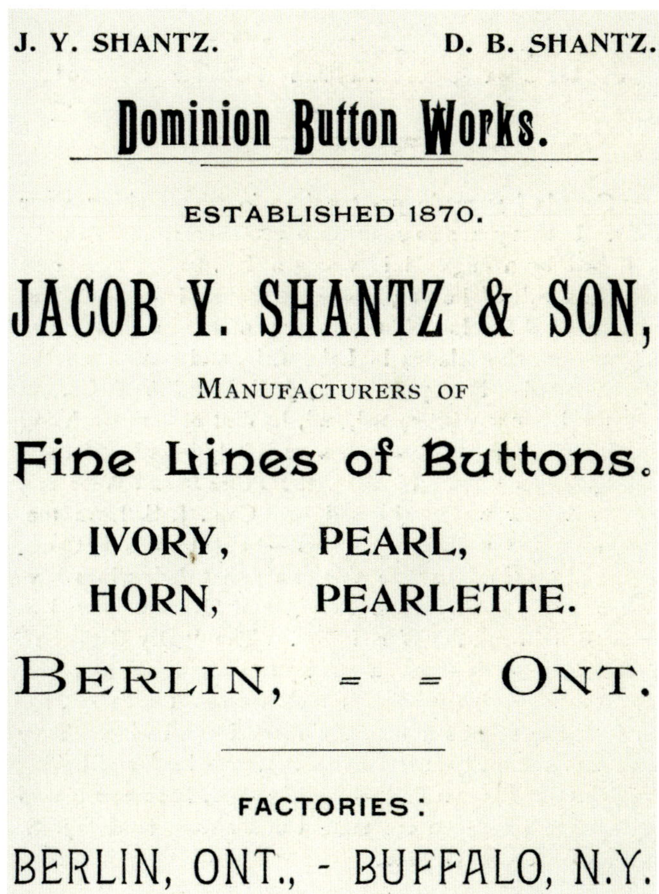

Advertisement for a button manufacturing company established in 1870. *Canada and Her Commerce*, 1894.

CHAPTER ONE

Miniature Adults
1860–1870

"Nothing is ever well done in a small household if the master and mistress are ignorant of the mode in which it is to be done."—Godey's Lady's Book, *June to December 1861*

Cultural Influences

The New York garment industry that had hitherto supplied the South with time-saving, ready-made clothing for slaves benefitted from the development of the commercially viable sewing machine. Ready-made clothing for men quickly became the norm, with custom tailoring reserved for upper-class women and children's clothing. Women of lesser means also benefitted from the mass production of Isaac Singer's machine. Its affordability and convenience allowed women at home to create clothes for themselves and their children in record time.

By the 1860s, thanks to Eli Whitney's earlier invention of the cotton gin, the American South was producing over one million tons of cotton a year, much of it exported to Britain. To meet the need for pickers, the slave trade had increased to such a degree that an estimated one in seven Americans was captive property. With Northern states wielding political and economic power and Southern states ready to secede over the abolition issue, it seems inevitable that civil war would ensue. When the conflict did develop, the New York garment industry received a further boost as it began to supply uniforms to both the Union and Confederate armies.

British and French textile industries were feeling the effects of the events of the decade before, each having participated in the Crimean War. The cardigan, the balaclava, and the nightingale cape all owe their origins to this conflict.

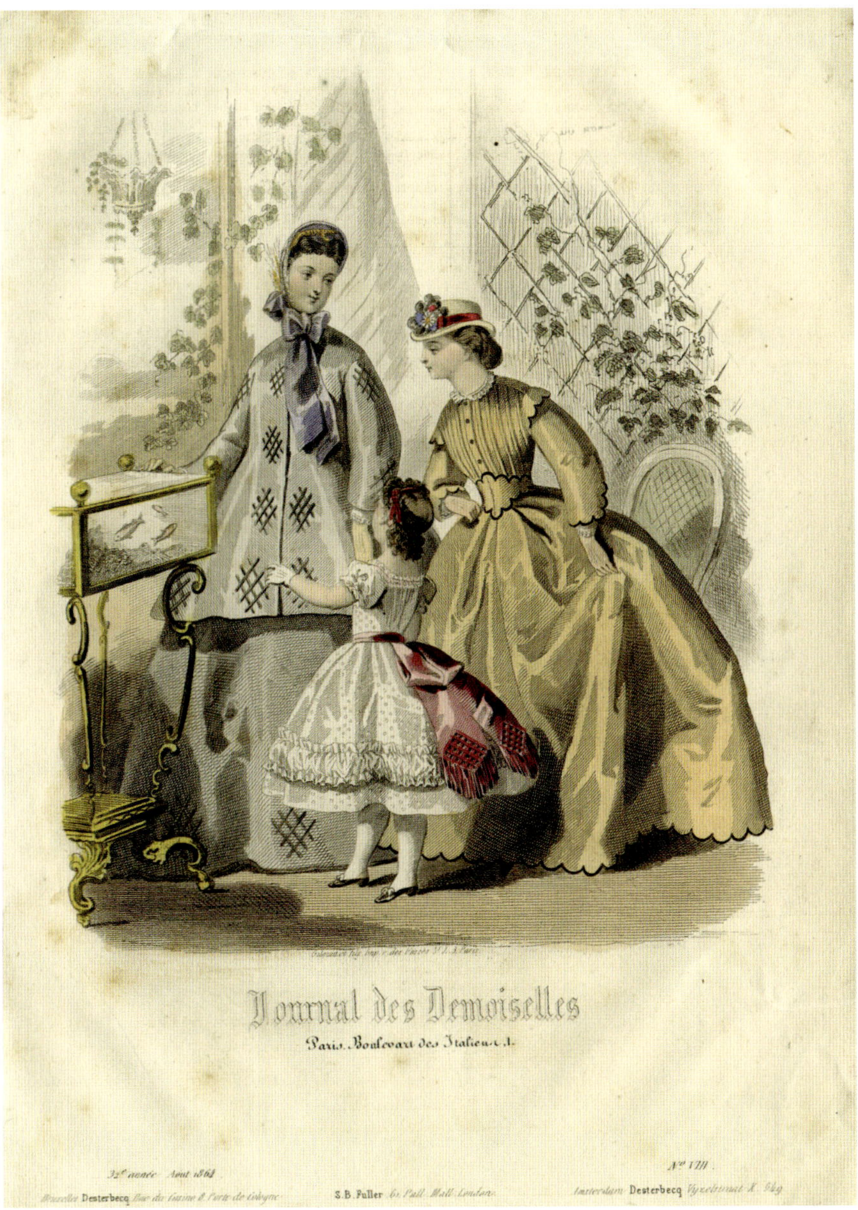

Colored fashion plate revealing a young girl's hoop-skirted dress with contrast sash and matching bonnet. *Journal Des Demoiselles*, August 1861.

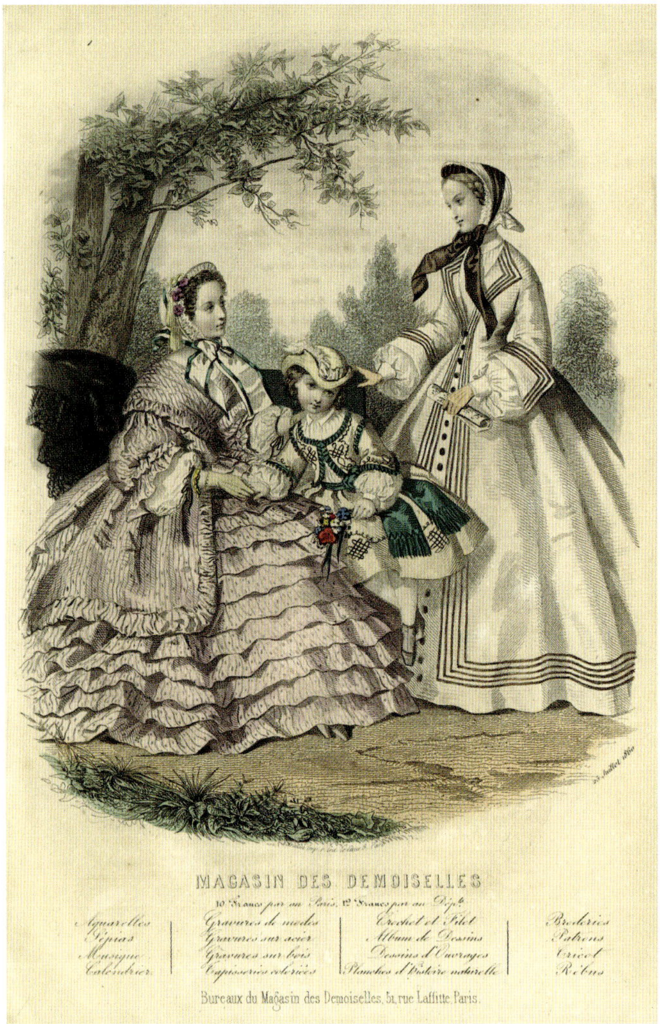

Colored fashion plate of a young girl's sashed dress with embroidered bolero and hem, full sleeves, cuffed at the wrist, and bonnet with rolled brim. Shop advertisement for Le Magasin Des Demoiselles, July 1860.

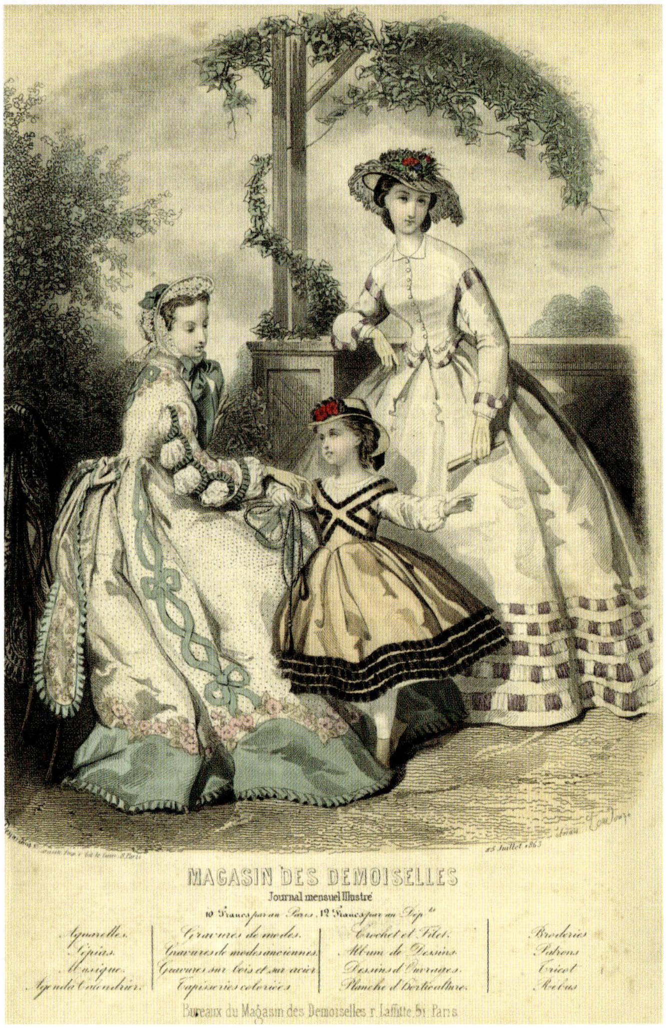

Colored fashion plate of a young girl's ruffle-trimmed dress, worn over a long-sleeved white blouse and floral-trimmed hat with asymmetric brim. Shop advertisement for Le Magasin Des Demoiselles, July 1863.

With the establishment of France's second empire and its concurrent economic prosperity, Paris dominated fashion. Wealthy women took their sartorial cues from French fashion plates, many of which were appearing in color in English publications such as *The Queen*, *The Lady's Newspaper and Court Chronicle*, and *The Englishwoman's Domestic Magazine*. Due in part to the patronage of Empress Eugenie, Englishman Charles Frederick Worth, who established his Parisian salon in 1858, was the first to be recognized for his sartorial artistry.

Socialites on both sides of the Atlantic emulated the fashions of the French court and followed closely the style choices Queen Victoria made for herself and her children. This was intensified following the death of Victoria's beloved Prince Albert, who died in 1861. Victoria set the standard for the observance of mourning through dress, which would continue until the turn of the century.

Additionally, the invention of synthetic aniline dyes (mauveine, rosaniline, alizarin) facilitated speedier and less expensive production processes for the garment industry. Being pretty in pink was a relatively new sartorial experience as textile makers produced chemically dyed fabrics in the new shades, magenta and solferino.

For home sewers, simpler, easier to construct clothing meant there was more time for hand crafted embellishments and girls as young as four years old were expected to learn the needle arts.

The importance of socially acceptable dress during this era cannot be overstated. Despite early dress reform efforts by feminist activists like Amelia Bloomer, sartorial imperatives were so ingrained in society that a woman could be jailed for wearing pants.

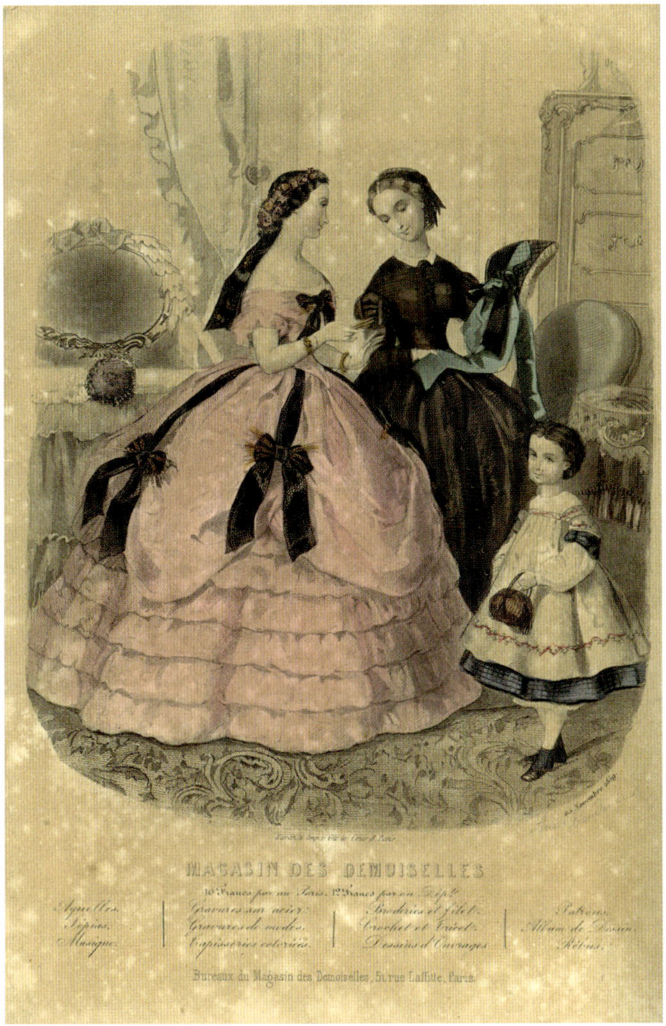

Colored fashion plate dated November 1859 showing fashions on the cusp of the new decade. The child pictured wears a layered outfit that tents out from the yoke. Frilled bloomers peek from below the hem. Shop advertisement for Le Magasin Des Demoiselles, Rue Laffitte, Paris.

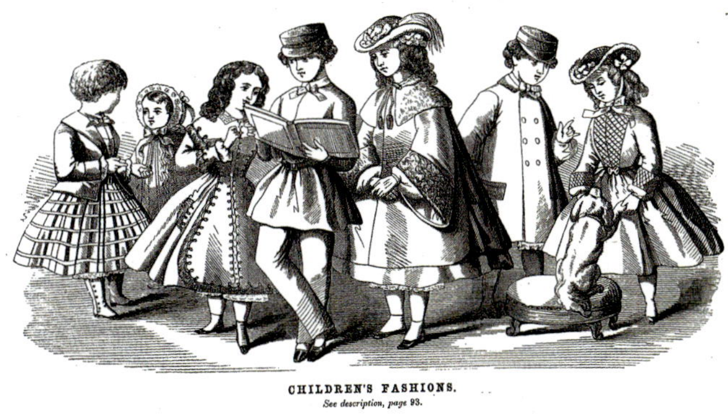

Fashion illustration of children's winter fashions including some neckties. *Godey's Lady's Book and Magazine*, January to June 1861.

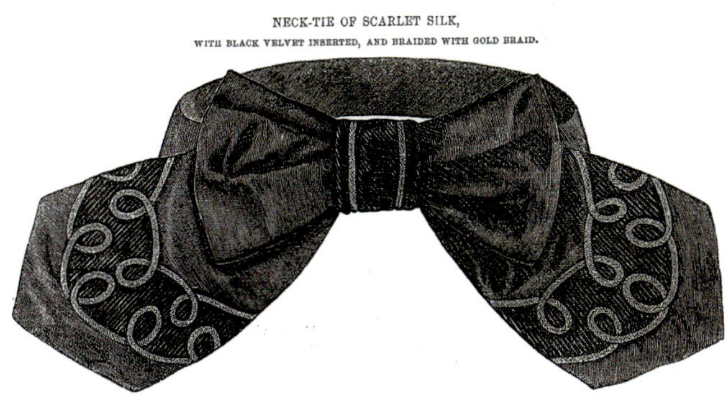

Pattern illustration for a scarlet silk necktie with black velvet and gold braid. *Godey's Lady's Book and Magazine*, July to December 1861.

Style Retrospective

> "If the wind is blowing [when skating], a veil should be worn over the face at least of ladies and children; otherwise fatal inflammation of the lungs, 'pneumonia,' may take place."—"Rules For Skating," *Godey's Lady's Book and Magazine,* February 1864

Full-skirted dresses supported by hoops, crinolines, and/or multiple petticoats ruled the day in women's fashion. Girls' dresses were similarly designed for tots as young as two years old. The skirt silhouette shifted early in the decade from a bell shape to a flat-fronted style with fullness in the hips and back. These new skirts might be adorned with lace, braid, ruffles, puffs, ribbons, and swags. It was rare or impossible to find two dresses alike due to the multitude of trims available, but standards were set for their placement. A grouping of buttons, at times even of different sizes, was made uniform by covering them with velvet. Ribbon and braid applications made the grade as long as they were applied in a slanting fashion.

Overlays appeared as the decade progressed, and *Godey's* provided a simple pattern for a buttonholed tab used to secure a skirt drawn up in festoons. Skirt length varied depending on the child's age, with young children (both boys and girls) wearing below-the-knee dresses over pantalettes.

As boys aged they switched from dresses to jacket and pants ensembles. Buttons were a particularly popular

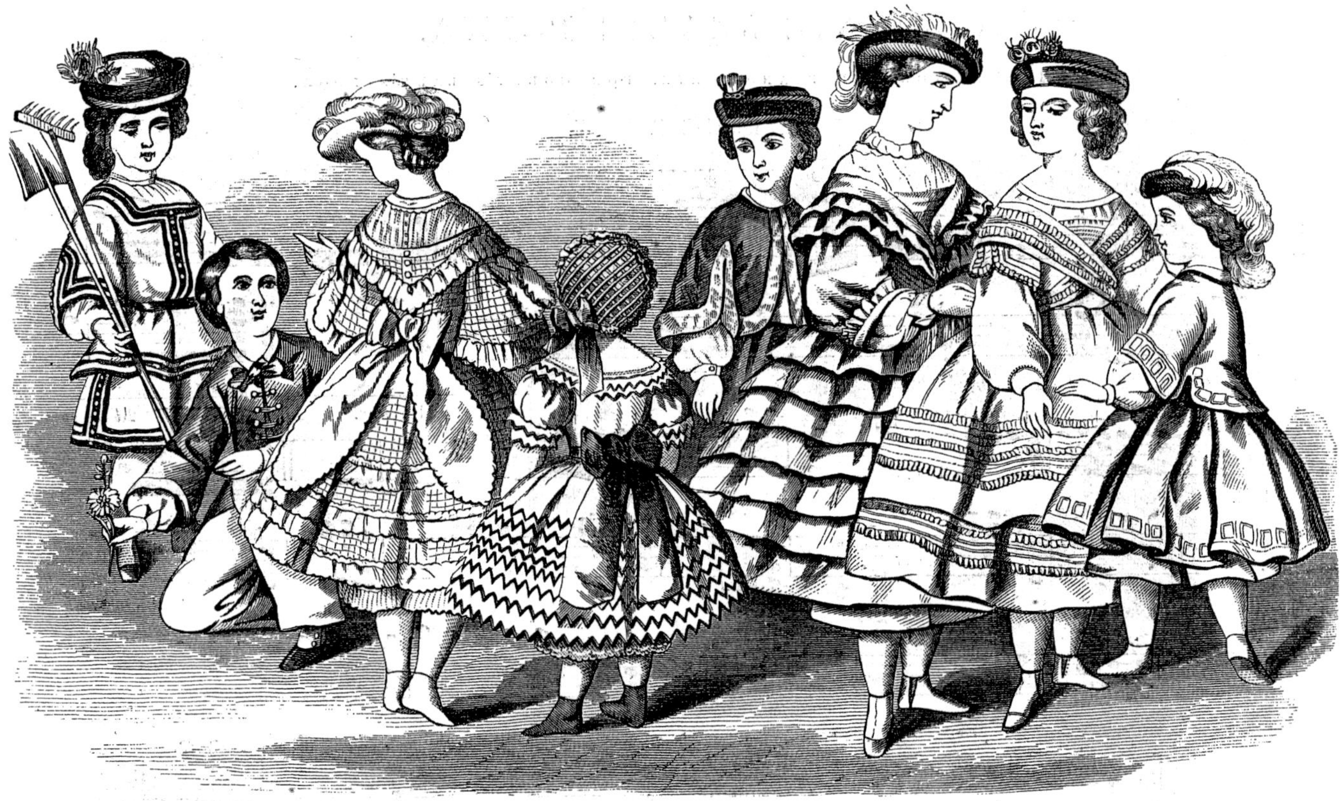

CHILDREN'S FASHIONS.—(*See description, Fashion department.*)

Fashion illustration of a variety of spring and summer styles for boys and girls c.1861. Collars and capes show prominently, as does criss-cross bodice trim. Note the plumed hats. *Godey's Lady's Book and Magazine*, Vol. LXIII, July to December 1861.

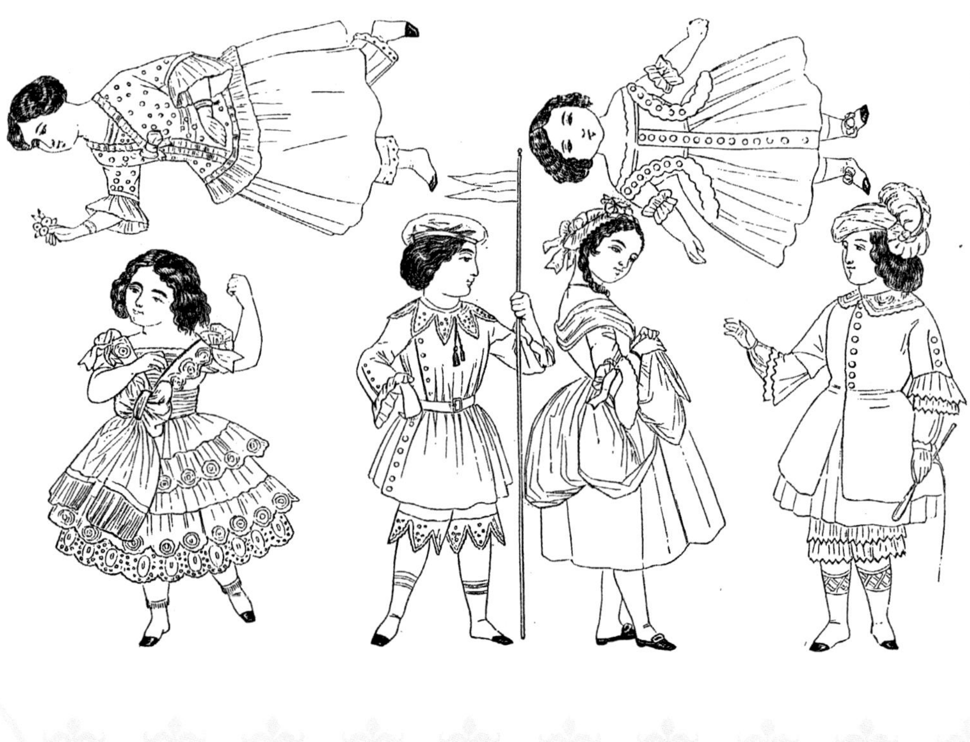

From Godey's children's page, an illustration of fashionable children's dress to color and paste onto card stock. *Godey's Lady's Book and Magazine*, Vol. LXIII, July to December 1861.

WALKING-DRESS FOR A YOUNG LADY.

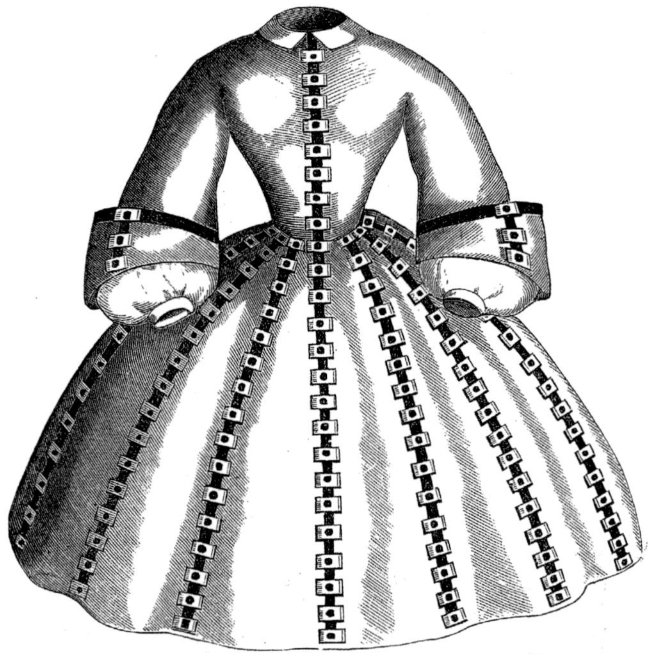

MADE of steel-colored poplin; trimmed with Magenta-colored velvet and buttons. The velvet is crossed at intervals by squares of the poplin, having a button in the centre, which makes a very stylish trimming.

Illustration of a walking dress for an older girl. Bands of poplin overlay strips of velvet ribbon to be further adorned with buttons. *Godey's Lady's Book and Magazine*, January to June 1861.

THE EVELYN.

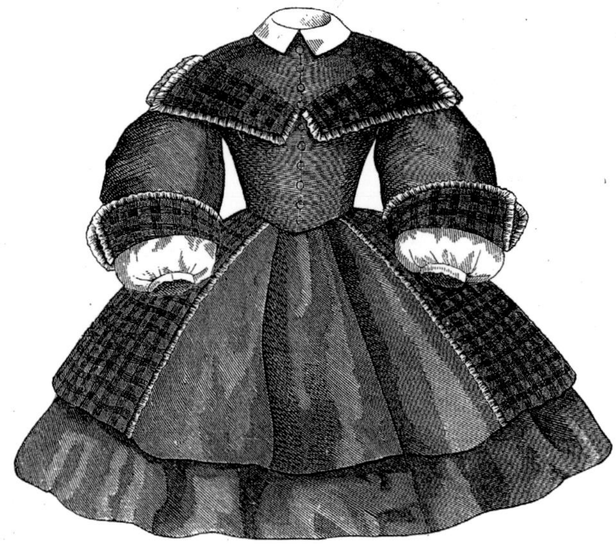

Named "The Evelyn," this girl's full-skirted winter dress is made of plain-colored merino, trimmed with bright silk or poplin. *Godey's Lady's Book and Magazine*, January to June 1861.

BASQUINE COAT FOR A LITTLE GIRL.

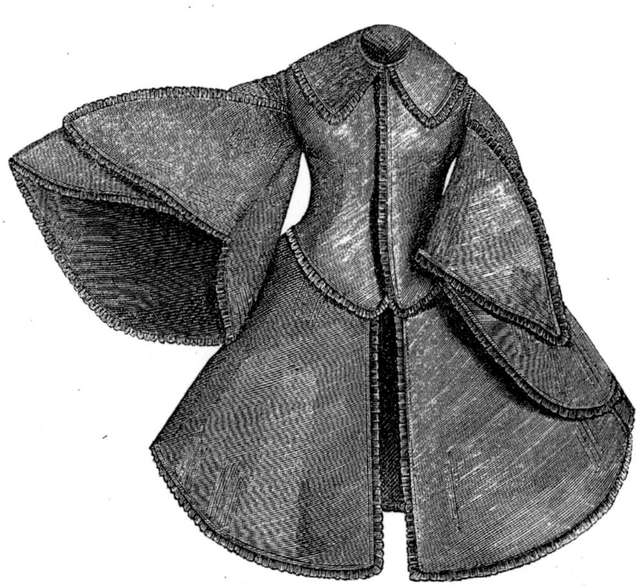

To be made of cloth, and trimmed with a ruffle of fluted cloth pinked on the edge.

Illustration of a "Basquine coat for a little girl." Enormous bell sleeves cascade from a drop-shouldered bodice. *Godey's Lady's Book and Magazine*, Vol. LXIII, July to December 1861.

embellishment for these, with a trend toward square buttons developing in the latter half of the decade.

Bodices featured pagoda sleeves, capelets, and high rounded necklines with or without lace collars. Delicate chemisettes formed a decorative contrast at open necklines and might be set in or detached.

Washable cotton pinafores protected formal dresses made from brightly colored silks, woolens, and combination textiles. Bright colors, sometimes referred to as Scottish colors, were applied to ribbons and bonnets. The Scottish influence was also felt through the adoption of plaid, as well as through the practice of drawing a scarf from the left shoulder to just below the waist at the right side. This style was featured in several magazines. By the summer of 1864 plaids were even adopted for the gauntlets of silk gloves.

Three-quarter-length capes or woolen shawls provided warmth in winter. These were often fringed with chenille, and a new taste for "Roman scarves" ensured multi-colored neck coverings for the spring of 1864.

With industrialization came innovations in the style and production of underpinnings, most notably the cage crinoline, a mass-produced contrivance of steel hoops connected to fabric tapes and worn about the waist.

THE GARIBALDI SUIT.

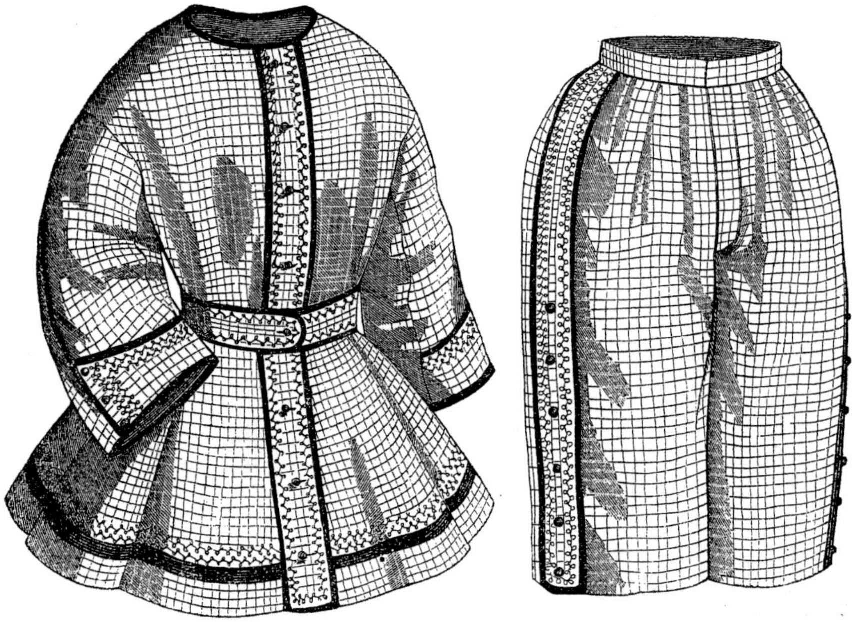

22*

Illustration of a child's Garibaldi suit in a checked fabric with buttons and braid trim. *Godey's Lady's Book and Magazine*, January to June 1861.

THE VICTOR COAT.

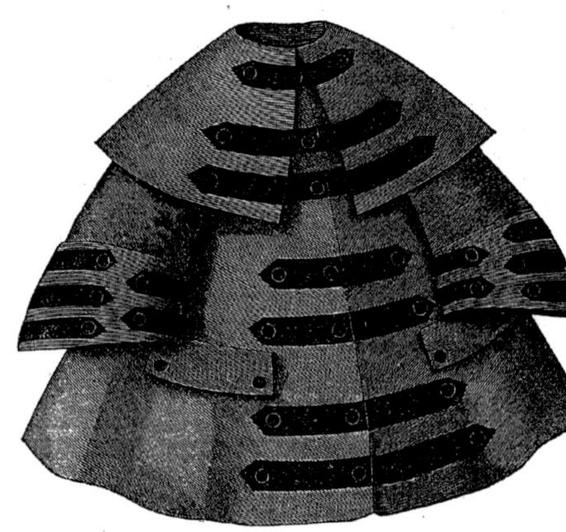

Illustration of the Victor Coat. *Godey's Lady's Book and Magazine*, January to June 1861.

CHILD'S GARIBALDI.

MADE OF VELVET CLOTH, BOUND AND TRIMMED WITH A BRIGHT COLORED SILK.

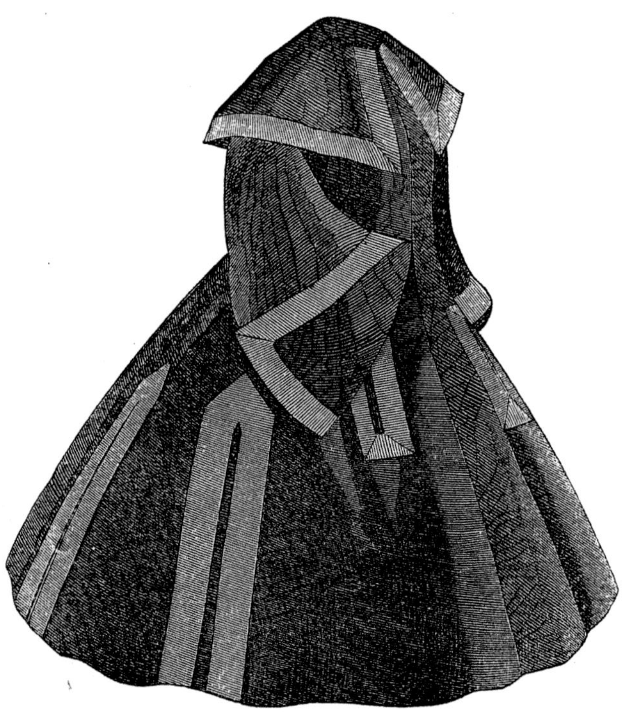

A second Garibaldi design. *Godey's Lady's Book and Magazine*, January to June 1861.

Fig. 4.

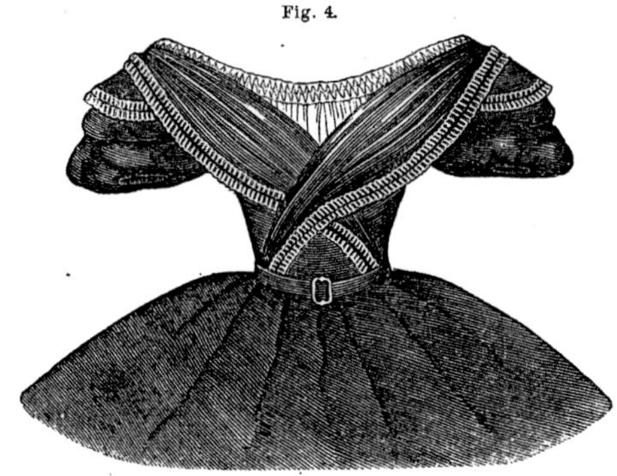

Pattern illustration for a young girl's dress with open neck and lace chemisette. *Godey's Lady's Book and Magazine*, January to June 1861.

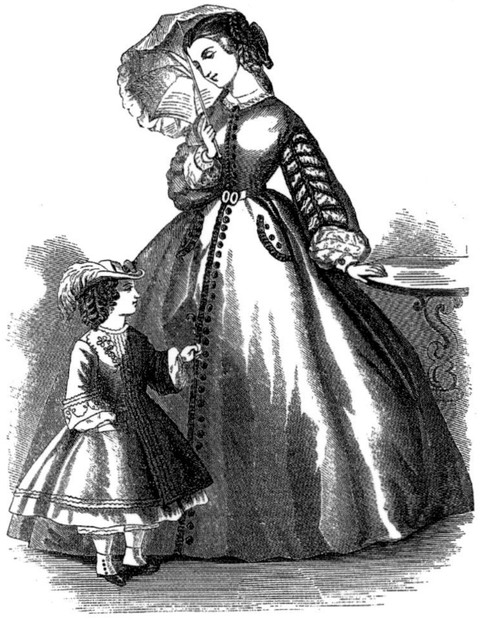

Illustration of a child's braid-trim piqué coat and white muslin dress. The child also wears gaiters and a straw hat with a white plume. *Godey's Lady's Book and Magazine*. January to June 1861.

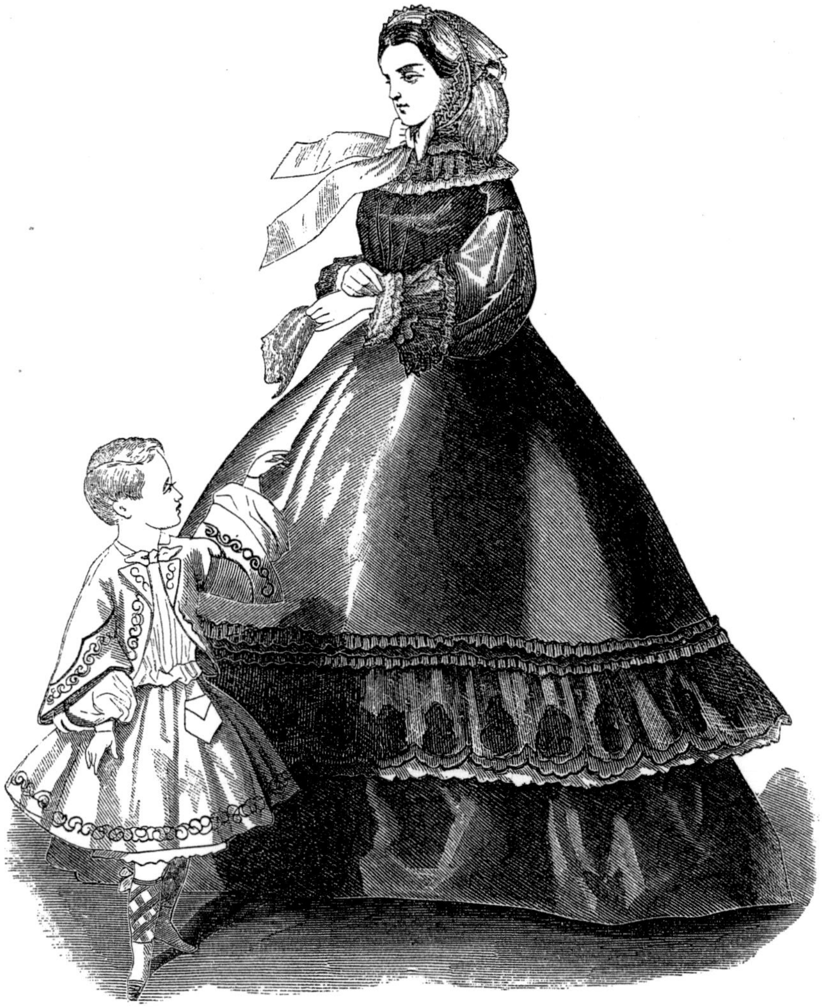

Sketch of a braided poplin Zouave suit for a young boy. Note the fullness of the skirt. *Godey's Lady's Book and Magazine*, January to June 1861.

Fig. 6.

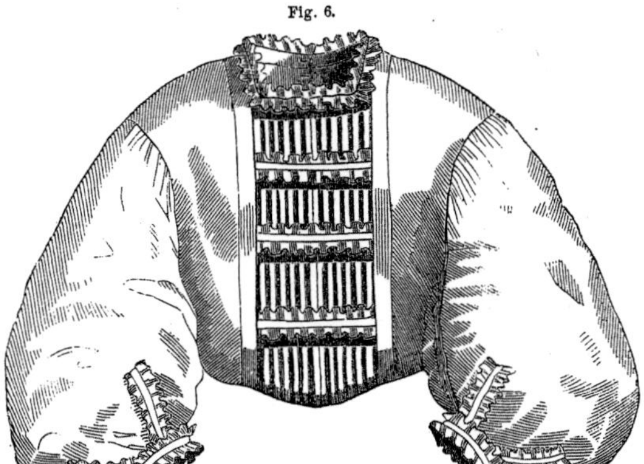

Square-necked shirt for a Zouave jacket embellished with fluted ruffles. The full sleeves fall from a drop shoulder. *Godey's Lady's Book and Magazine*, January to June 1861.

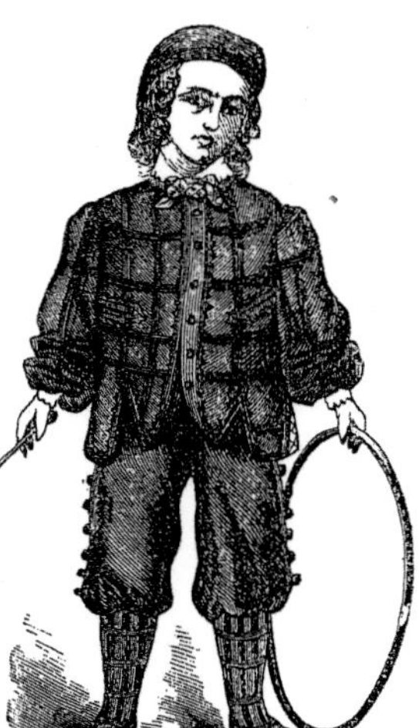

This sketch described as a Zouave suit for a boy of five years is ornamented with buttons at the wrists and down the outer leg seams of the short pants. "Plaid stockings, low black shoes, collar and plain tie complete the outfit." *Godey's Lady's Book*, July to December 1861.

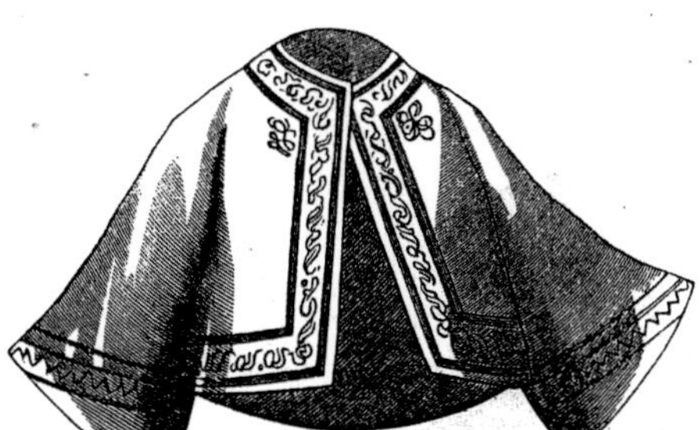

Illustration for a Zouave jacket for a little girl. *Godey's Lady's Book and Magazine*, January to June 1861.

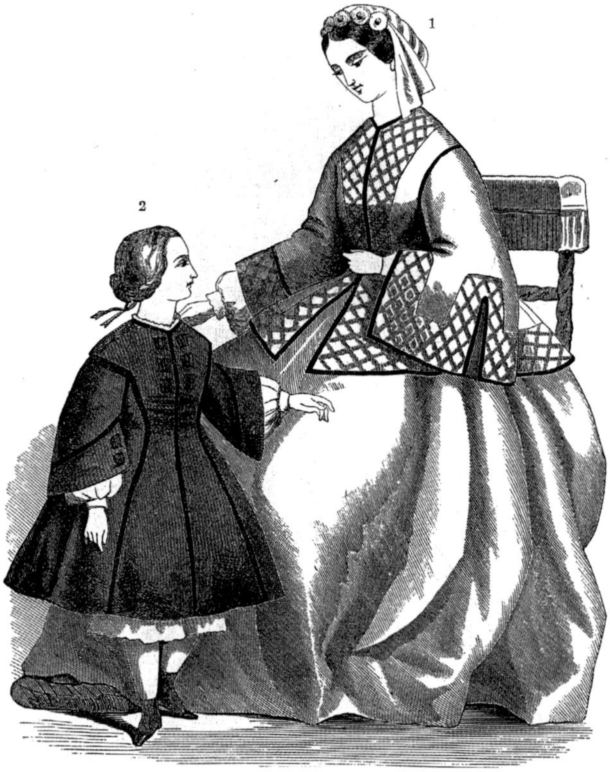

Illustration of a child's 1860s streetwear costume cut similarly to her mother's Zouave. *Godey's Lady's Book and Magazine*, Vol. LXIII, July to December 1861.

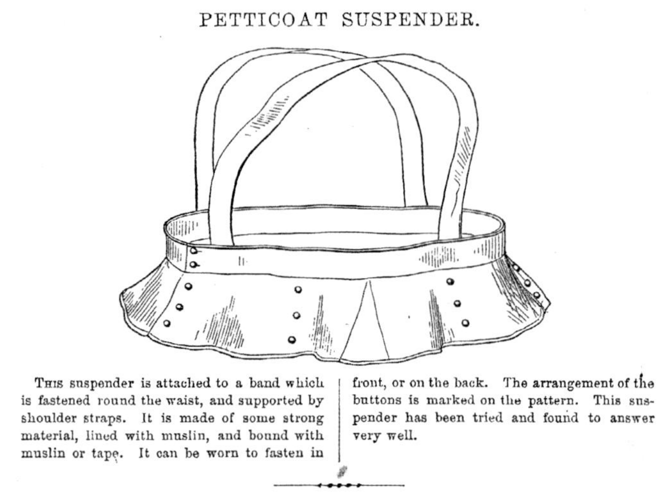

PETTICOAT SUSPENDER.

THIS suspender is attached to a band which is fastened round the waist, and supported by shoulder straps. It is made of some strong material, lined with muslin, and bound with muslin or tape. It can be worn to fasten in front, or on the back. The arrangement of the buttons is marked on the pattern. This suspender has been tried and found to answer very well.

Illustration of a petticoat suspender with graduated buttons for the attachment of several petticoats. *Godey's Lady's Book and Magazine*, July to December 1861.

By mid-decade *Godey's* announced "it is now the fashion to use butterflies for ornamenting bonnets and headdresses (July to December 1864)." Patterns for these ranged from wool wrapped around wire to intricate crochet designs. Butterflies were also embroidered on the ends of ties or neckerchiefs. Bugs, flies, and butterflies incorporated into the design of summer textiles such as calicoes and cambrics were considered eccentric but highly fashionable when first introduced in June 1864. Shoes might also be decorated with butterflies.

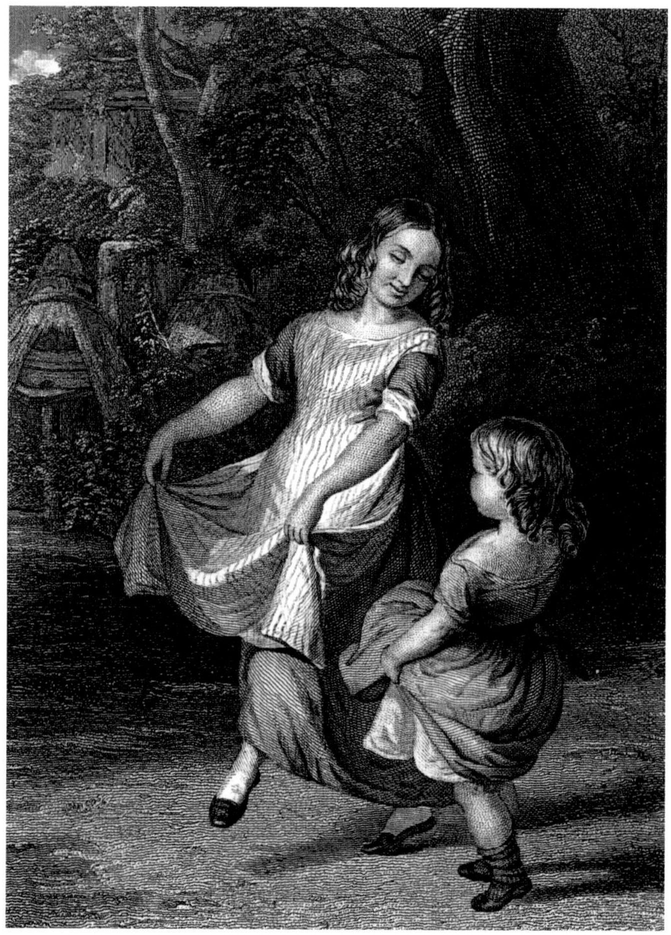

Illustration of young girls at play; the hems of their dresses differ in length according to their ages. *Godey's Lady's Book and Magazine*, Vol. LXIII, July to December 1861.

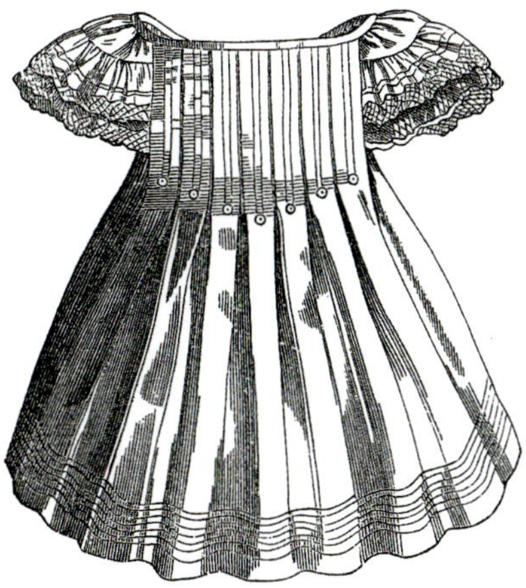

Fig. 9. A very simple style of dress, suitable for any kind of material.

Illustration of a "simple style of dress." *Godey's Lady's Book and Magazine*, Vol. LXIII, July to December, 1861.

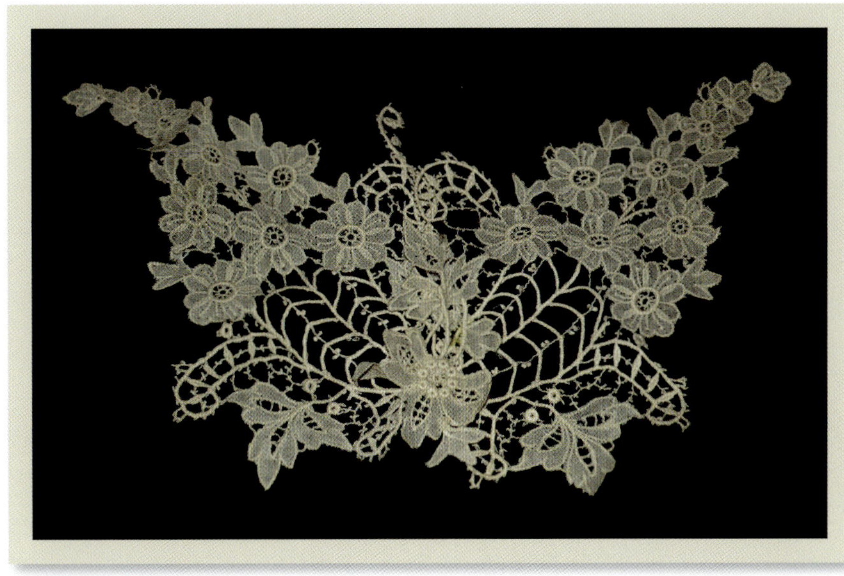

Victorian butterfly of delicate lace.

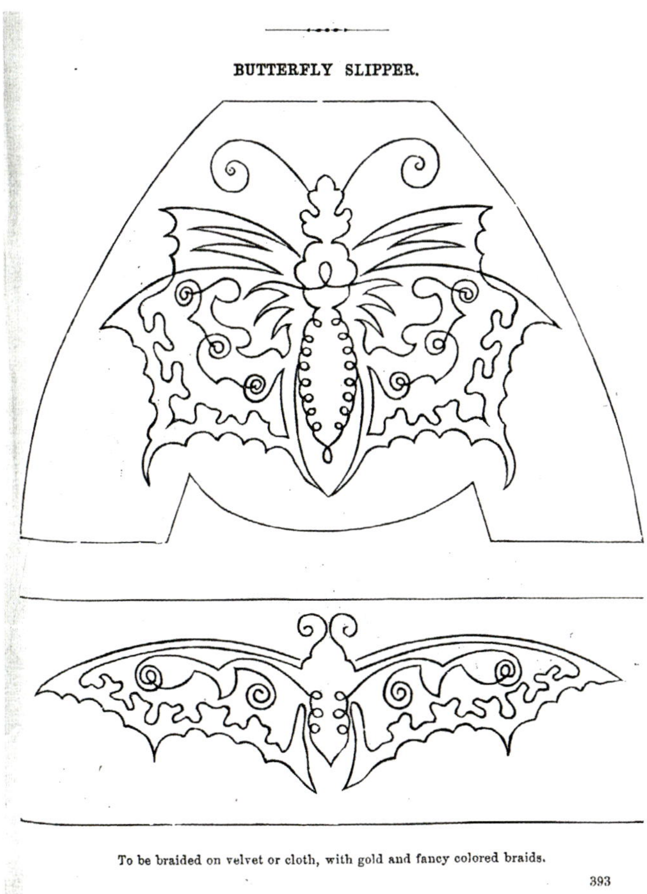

BUTTERFLY SLIPPER.

To be braided on velvet or cloth, with gold and fancy colored braids.

393

Pattern for a cloth slipper with butterfly embroidery. *Godey's Lady's Book and Magazine*, Vol. LXIII, July to December 1861.

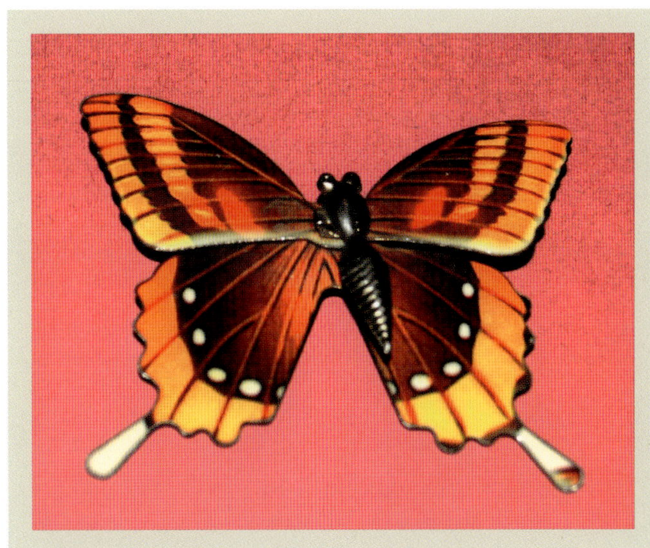

Victorian butterfly pin.

Footwear

Stockings and house shoes or morning slippers for children were commonly made at home. A sparkling number called the Cinderella slipper incorporated steel beads into its multi-colored woolen construction. *Godey's* declared, "its glittering appearance, which sparkles with every movement of the foot, has an exquisite effect (July to December 1864)." These must have been very attractive when worn with a pair of striped railway stockings popular c.1860.

To complement their ruffled and bustled dresses, girls wore low-quartered, ladder-vamped shoes of kid leather, often trimmed with one to three fabric bows. These fastened with buttons and were elevated on spool-shaped Louis heels in imitation of shoes worn by adult women. For sober occasions black patent was in order.

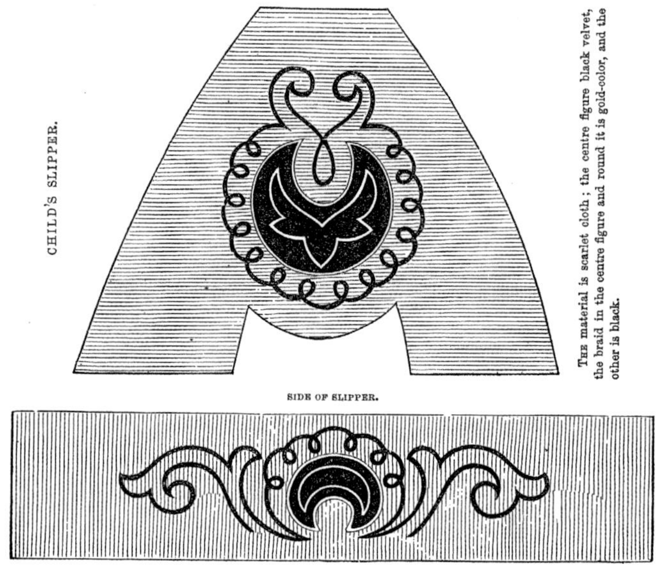

Child's slipper pattern to be made up at home. Black velvet appliquéd on scarlet cloth and embellished with gold braid is suggested. *Godey's Lady's Book and Magazine*, Vol. LXIII, July to December 1861.

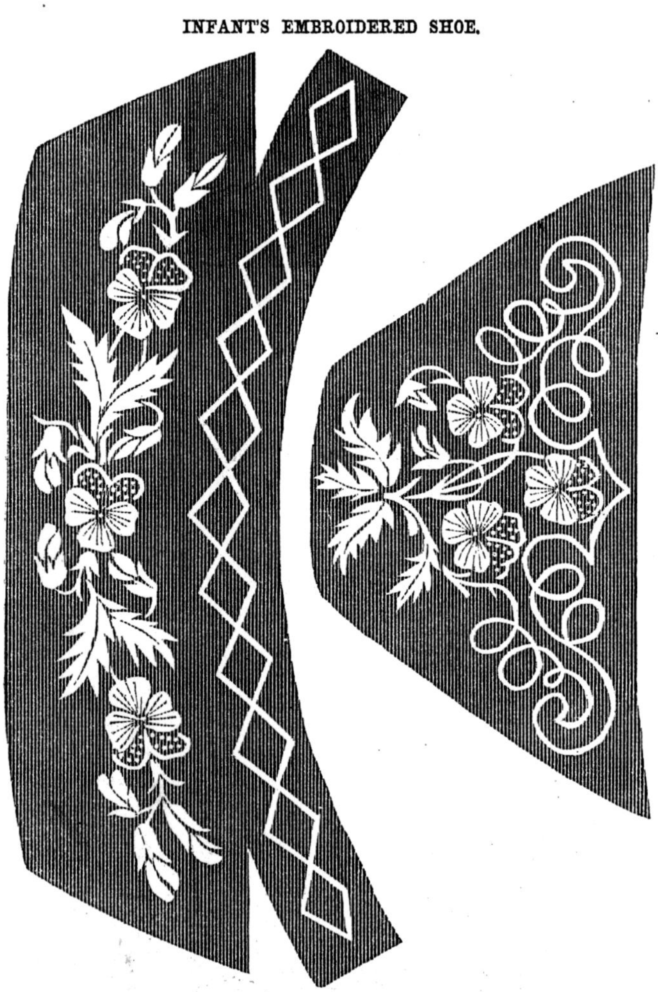

Pattern for an infant's heavily embroidered shoe.

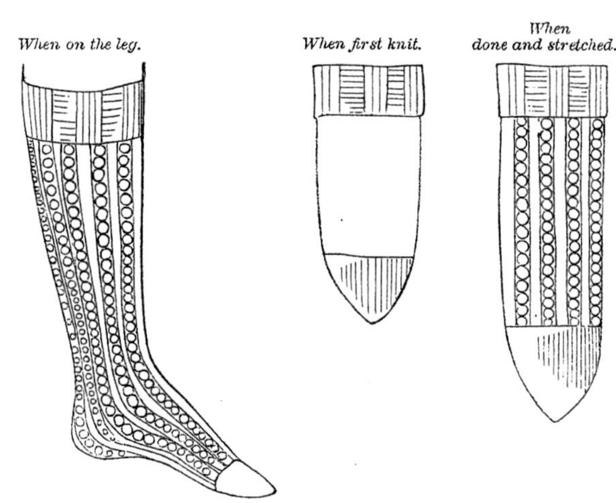

Knitting pattern illustration for ribbed railway stockings. *Godey's Lady's Book and Magazine*, January to June 1861.

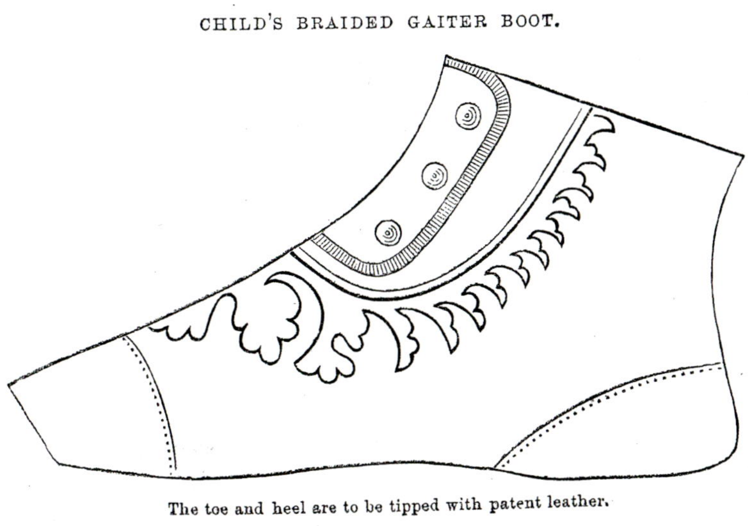

Pattern for a child's gaiter boot with placement indications for buttons and applied braid. Toe and heel to be reinforced with patent leather. *Godey's Lady's Book and Magazine*, 1861.

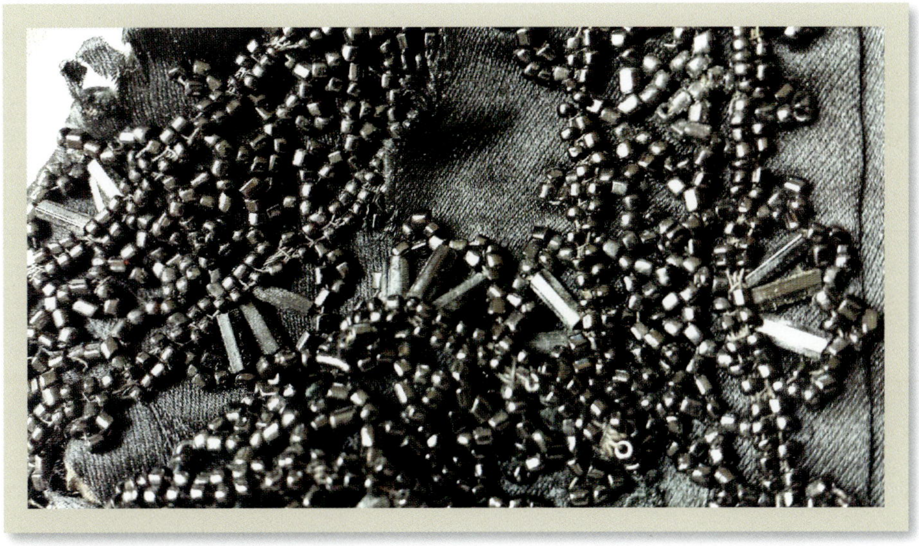

Victorian textile embellished with steel beads.

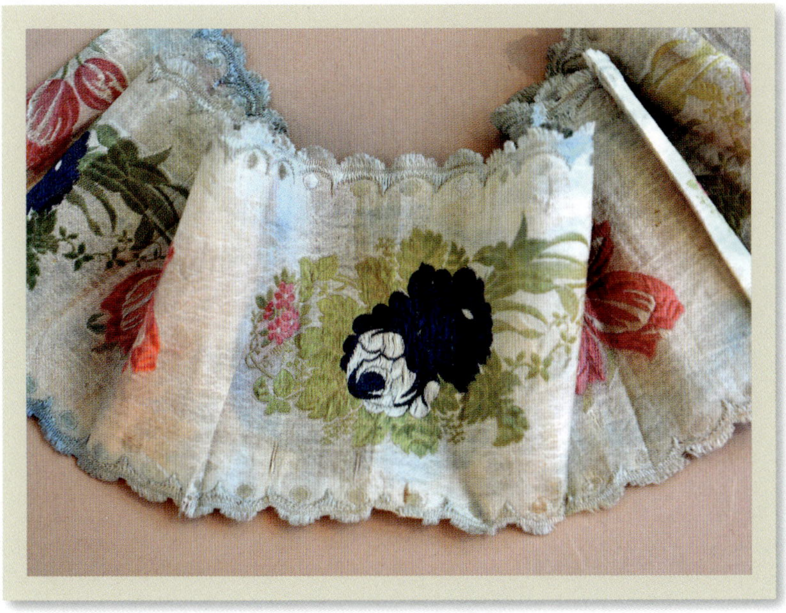

Fancy French silk ribbon with scalloped edge.

Lids

At the outset of the decade, separate, quilted hoods stood in for little girls' hats, which in summer were styled off the brow with a fabric bavolet. Summer bonnets were decorated inside and out with fabricated flowers. Ruffled tulle, delicate feathers, and or chenille tassels made a pretty contrast when set against a leghorn straw hat. Netted ribbons attached to the bonnet made a pretty casing for the hair. Richly colored ribbon ties could also be formed into a bow or left to hang. In March of 1864 *Godey's* announced that striped ribbons were a novelty, "for until now plain ribbons alone have been tolerated for bonnet strings." By the summer, fashionable straw hats were pointed at the front, flared at the sides, and turned up at the back to allow for a full cap of lace and ribbons. These "half gypsies" were an alternative to feather-trimmed silk bonnets also popular for little girls at the time. Mask veils worn close to the face and secured to the bonnet with insect pins graced the faces of older girls, while little boys made do with the ever-popular Scotch toque.

Ladies' and misses summer hats might be elaborately trimmed with peacock feathers, spun glass, or bird-of-paradise; flowers, shells, ribbons, or wheat tassels were deemed more appropriate for children's millinery. Come fall, hats and bonnets were stripped of their summer frou frou and dressed with the colors of autumn.

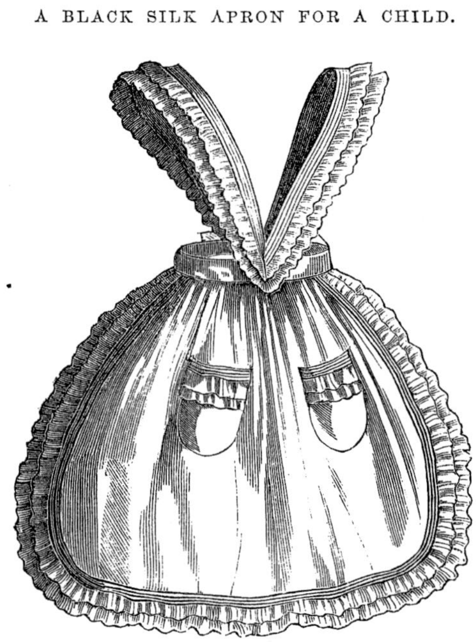

Illustration of two pinafore styled aprons, "suitable for a little party." *Godey's Lady's Book and Magazine*, July to December 1861.

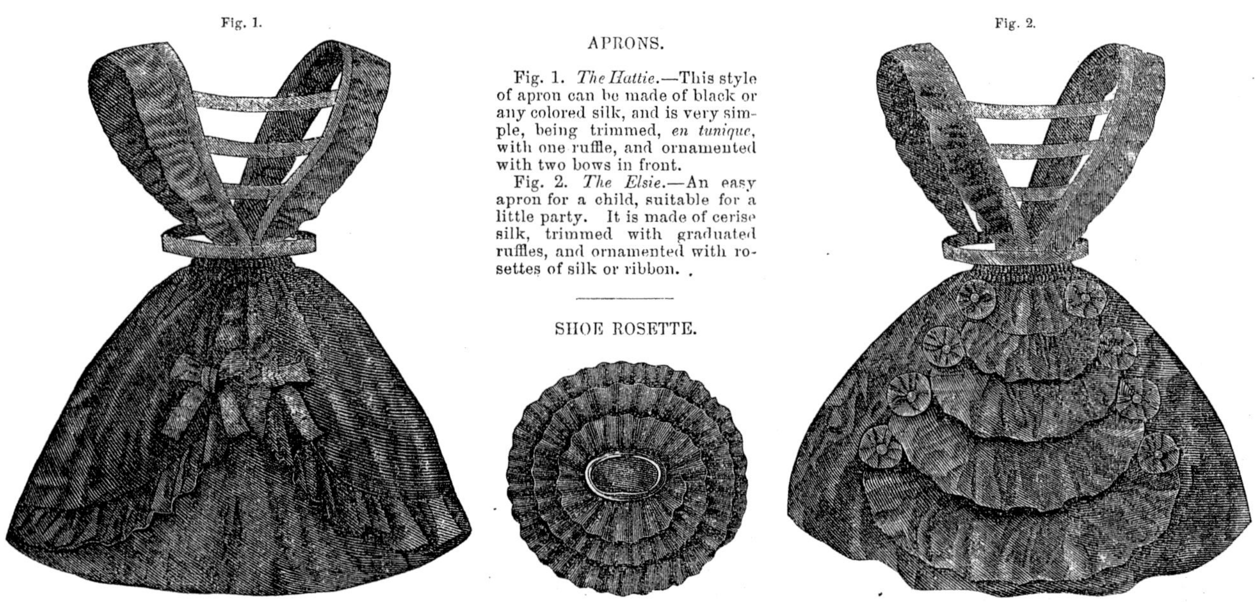

A black silk apron trimmed with ruffles and velvet ribbon. *Godey's Lady's Book and Magazine*, January to June 1861.

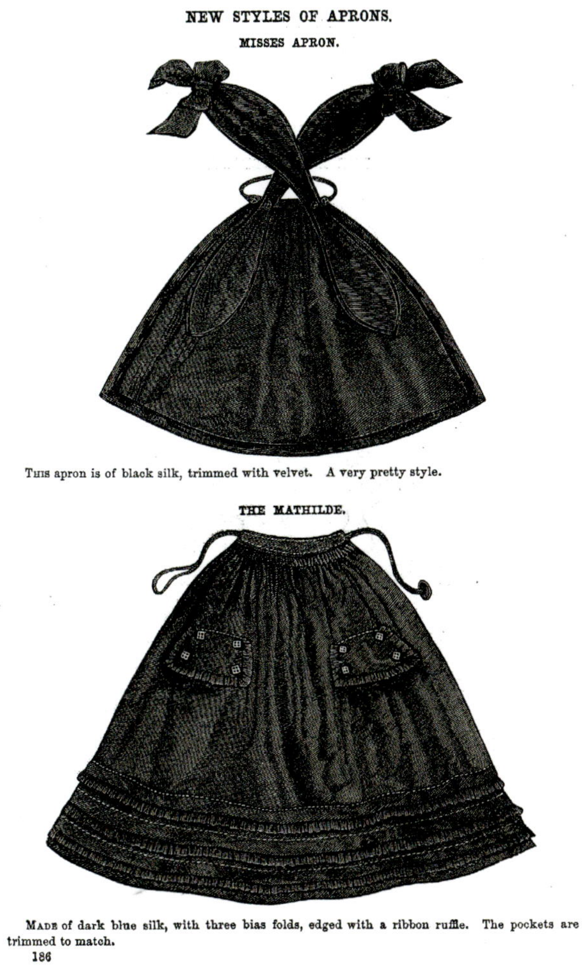

NEW STYLES OF APRONS.

MISSES APRON.

This apron is of black silk, trimmed with velvet. A very pretty style.

THE MATHILDE.

Made of dark blue silk, with three bias folds, edged with a ribbon ruffle. The pockets are trimmed to match.

186

Two formal aprons for older girls. *Godey's Lady's Book and Magazine*, 1861.

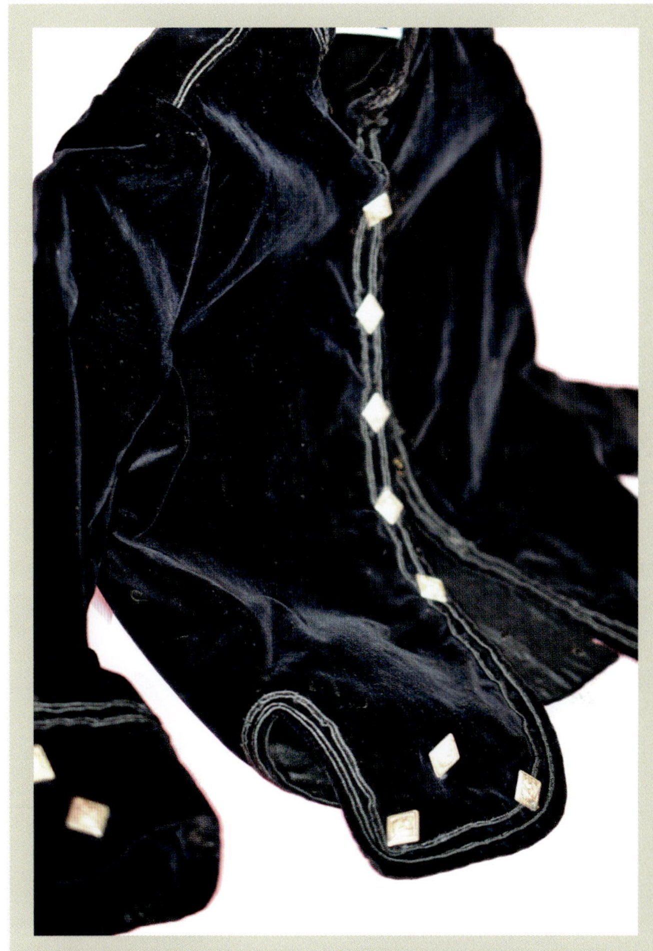

Black velvet Little Lord Fontleroy jacket.

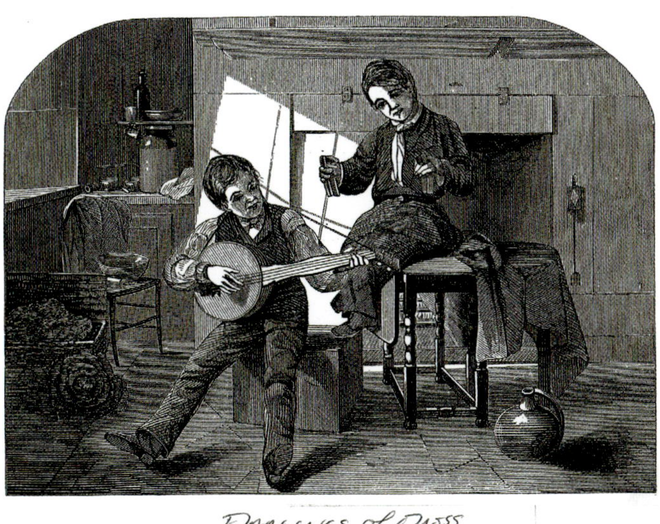

1861 *Godey's Lady's Book and Magazine* illustration of boys at play. Note the casual necktie of the boy seated on the table.

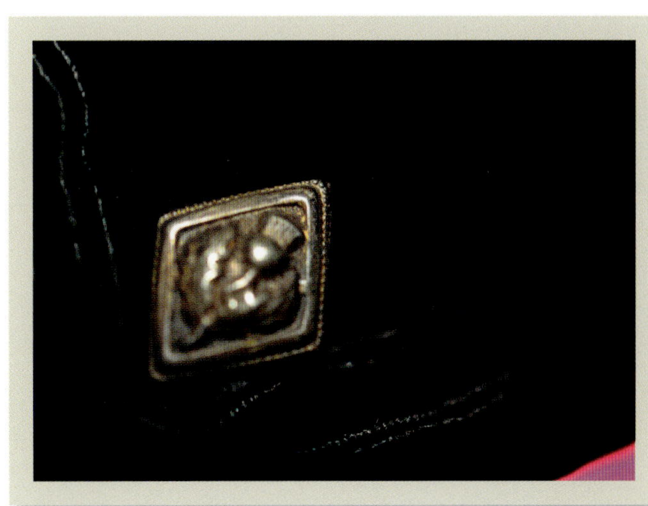

Detail: metal button with Scottish thistle motif.

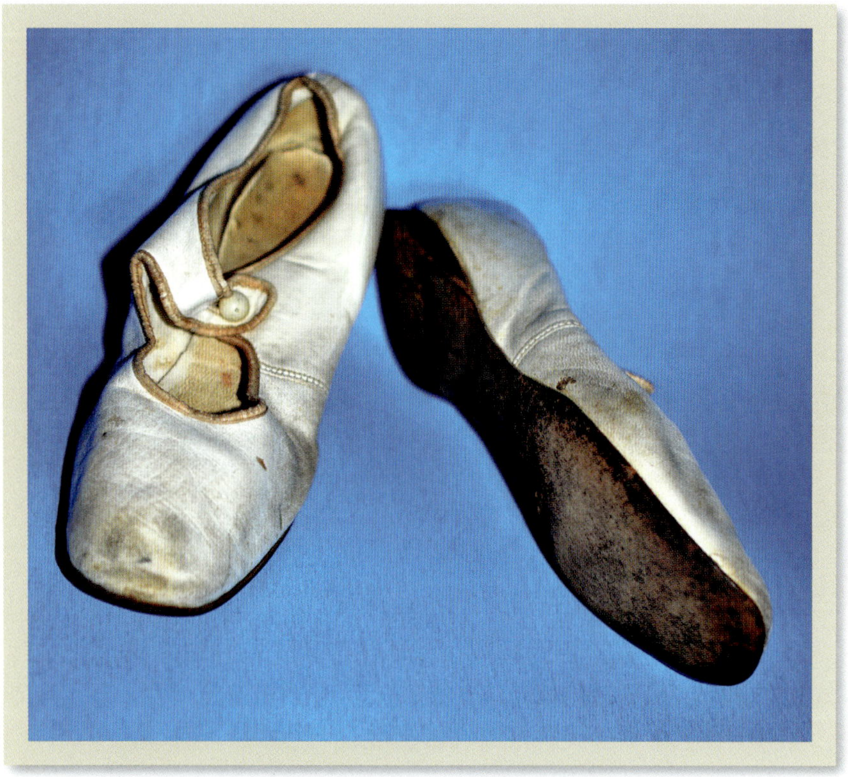

C. 1910: Young girl's white kid leather one-button shoes. 7¼" from heel to toe, ¼" heel. Label: The H. White Co., Boston.

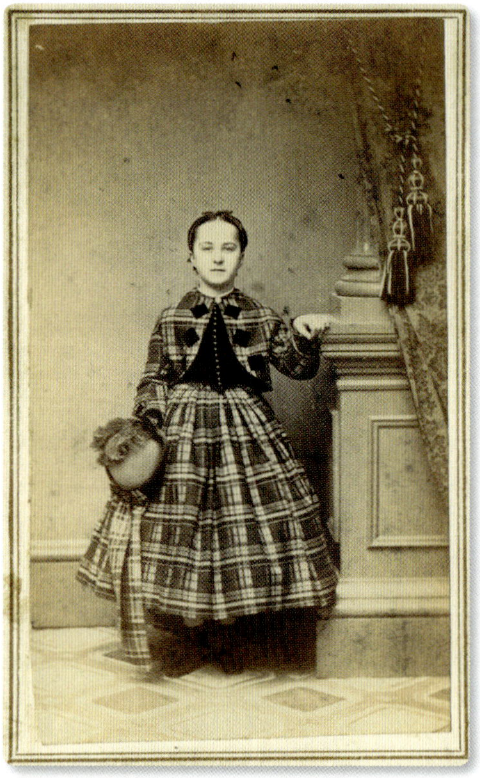

A young girl dressed in a highly fashionable 1860s tartan ensemble comprised of a vest, collarless jacket, and full crinoline-supported skirt. Tartan ribbons trail from a feather-trimmed straw hat.

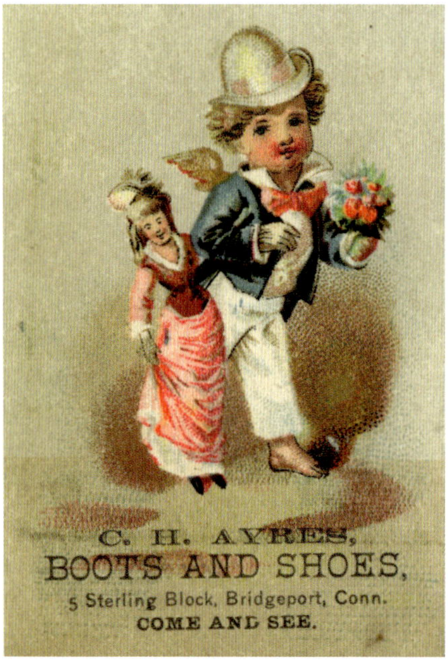

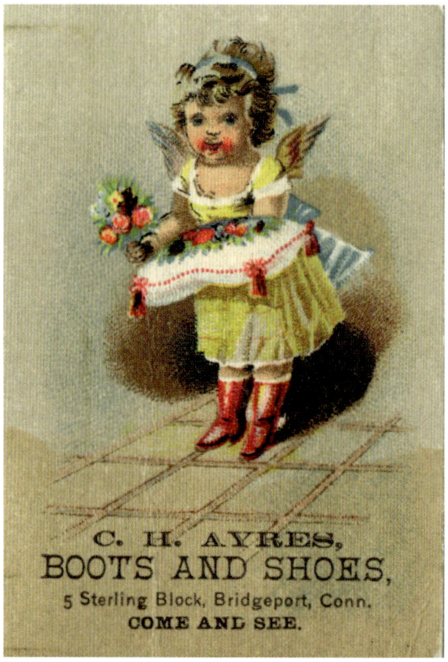

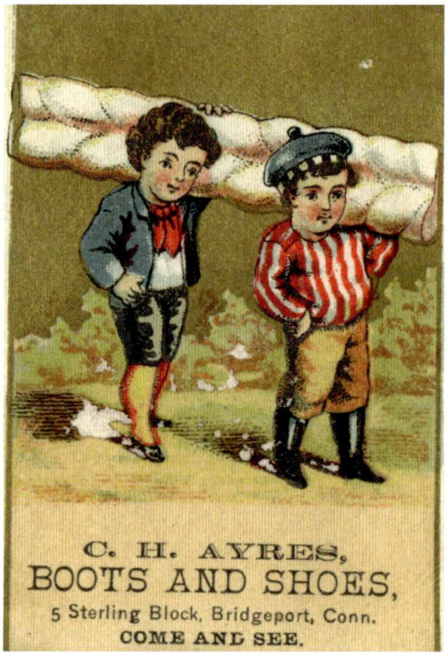

Victorian Trade Cards for C. H. Ayres Shoes, Bridgeport, Connecticut.

Play Clothes

Knitting was more than a pastime for women during the Civil War era. Knitted garments were highly fashionable and ranged from mittens, cuffs, and scarves to petticoats and close-fitting cardigans worn for warmth under dresses and jackets.

Color and Texture

During the 1860s it was not uncommon for children's clothing to be trimmed in fashionable black. Women's periodicals provided guidelines for the specific placement of black sashes, lace, quillings, buttons, ribbons, braids, and tassels on everything from dresses and neckties to hats and boots. The October 1864 issue of *Godey's* even recommended sewing three rows of black silk braids to a child's muslin petticoat. Blouses fashioned entirely of black cloth were also devised for children.

Black velvet added textural interest when set against blue poplin, salmon-colored feathers, scarlet silk, or white poplin.

1860s Textile Cleaning and Preservation Methods

• To Preserve Furs: Wrap some cloves or peppercorns with them and keep in a dry place.

• Grease Stains in Silk: A sure and safe way to remove grease stains from silks is to rub the spot quickly with brown paper; the friction will soon draw out the grease. Alternatively: Lay the silk on a table with an ironing blanket under it, the right side of the silk downwards; put a piece of brown paper on the top, and apply a flat iron just hot enough to scorch the paper.

• For Black Silk: Take one quart of soft water and put into it an old kid glove, and boil it down to one pint; then take a sponge or a soft piece of flannel, and sponge it over; then iron it on the wrong side while it is damp. It will look bright and new and will be quite stiff. (For light-colored silk, take a white glove.)

• Restoring Velvet: When plushed from pressure, hold the parts over a basin of hot water, with the lining of the dress next to the water; the pile will soon rise and resume its original beauty.

• Gold and Silver Lace: May be cleaned by sewing it in clean linen cloth, boiling it in a pint of soft water and two ounces of soap, washing it in cold water; if it be tarnished apply a little warm spirits of wine to the tarnished parts.

• To Bleach a Faded Dress: Wash well in hot suds, and boil it until the color seems to be gone, then wash and rinse, and dry it in the sun; if it is not sufficiently white, repeat the boiling.

—*Godey's Lady's Book and Magazine*, July to December 1864

CHAPTER TWO

Dressed as Never Before

1870–1880

Alex and Jane

On January 13, 1874, Alex Philip wrote to his intended, Jane Croll, who was happily working at a linen factory in Scotland. She had advised him in a previous letter that, except for being reprimanded for "the threads knotting" and having her hand "nipped" in the loom, she was making "pretty good wages now and not so hard work to do (author's private collection of letters)."

As Jane planned on joining Alex in Montreal, he scoped out employment opportunities for her and reported on them in his January letter. He expressed the certainty that she would not require his assistance in finding employment as "there is always an awful outcry for such as you, for almost any sort of work. There are no linen factories, however, but there are some new cotton factories, just finished . . . boot and shoe factories without number, and always more girls wanted that can be got."

Cultural Influences

By the 1880s most major North American cities were replete with textile mills and factories even though steamers continued to ferry clothing, novelties, and yard goods from Europe to the Americas. New York's R. H. Macy & Co. offered catalogs free of charge to urban and rural locations across the country, and promised that mail orders would be filled promptly. A number of other department stores followed suit.

The *Domestic Monthly*, a periodical that claimed devotion to the "highest interest of fashion, literature, and art," offered postage-free subscriptions to any part of the United States for $1.50 per year. An advertisement for the magazine, published in a December 1879 issue of the *Illustrated Christian Weekly*, outlined the *Domestic Monthly's* approach to fashion coverage, promising that each issue would provide a full account of "everything new, interesting, and useful in the fashion world."

The *Domestic Monthly* was one of a number of periodicals that enabled American women to follow the prevailing styles from Paris and London, whether they chose to have their garments custom-made, purchase them ready-made from a department store, or create the garments themselves.

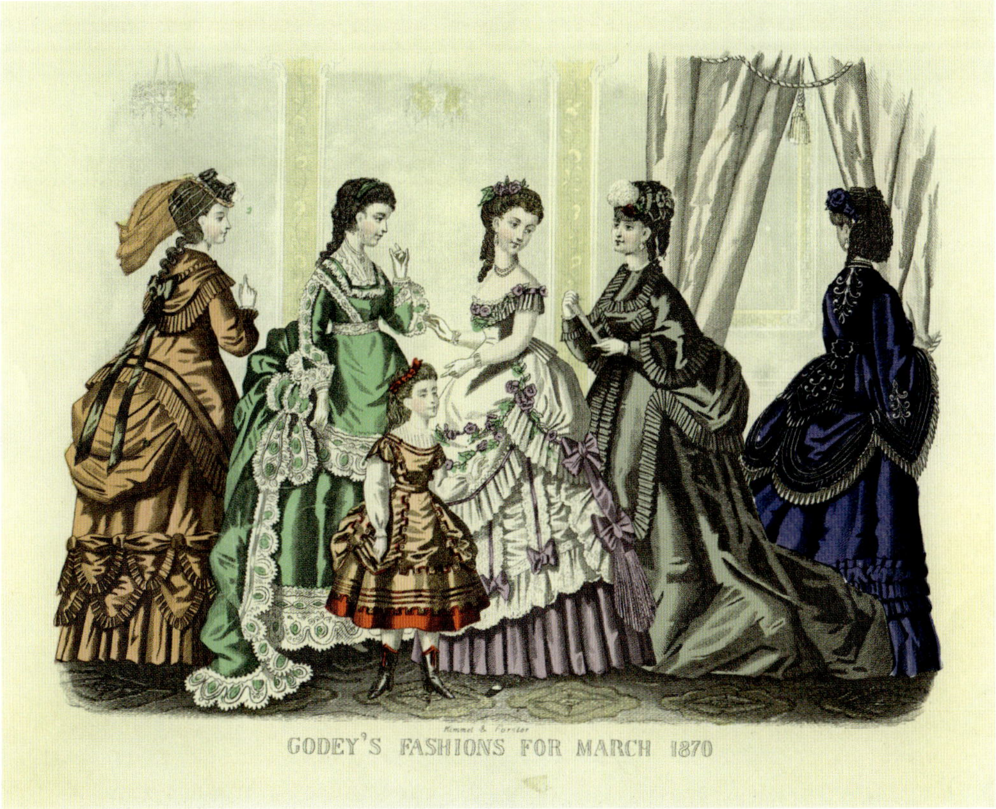

Godey's Fashion Plate showing the latest Paris fashions for spring 1870. At a glance the bronze-colored satin polonaise appears to be over-mature for the young girl; stylish boots are accented with crimson to match the trimmings on her dress, but the effect is tempered by the addition of the crisp white undersleeves and neck frill.

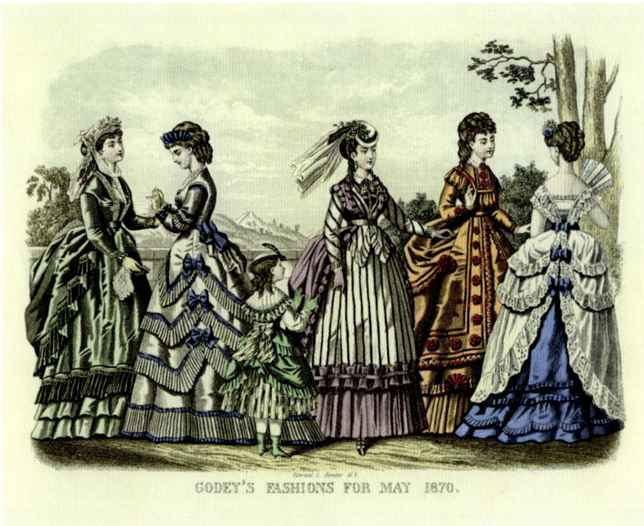
GODEY'S FASHIONS FOR MAY 1870.

Godey's Fashion Plate showing the latest Paris fashions for summer 1870. The child's back is turned, revealing the tiered effect of her collar, overskirts, and self-fabric bow, all designed to mimic the bustle silhouette favored by the adult women of the era. Her shallow topper is adorned with a single green plume to match her dress and leather boots.

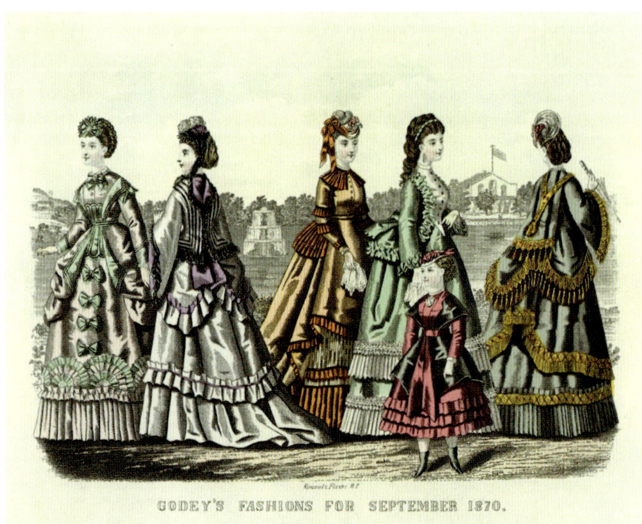
GODEY'S FASHIONS FOR SEPTEMBER 1870.

Godey's Fashion Plate showing the latest Paris fashions for autumn 1870. Except for the shortness of the hem, the young girl's ensemble is almost identical in form to those worn by women, as evidenced by the high waist, slope-shouldered cut of the bodice, and ruffled hem of the bell-shaped skirt. The fabric-trimmed saucer of a hat, which slopes forward over the brow, flatters the child's hairstyle, which is drawn up and away from the face.

With the widespread use of sewing machines in the home, children of the 1870s could be dressed as never before. The industrial revolution had enabled the lower class to replicate the costume of the wealthiest individuals since sewing machines eliminated the high cost in time and labor of producing heavily embellished garments. The fortuneless felt privileged to be able to obtain or produce clothing imitative of the finest textile creations that money could buy and eagerly sought out patterns in the pages of the Butterick pattern publication, *The Delineator.*

Mothers took inspiration from the richly colored fashion plates that were beginning to show children outfitted in the same chemically produced, jewel-toned color combinations available to themselves: gold, bronze, and apricot might be paired with white, crimson, or burgundy; red could be used to set off teal, steel gray, or deep green; emerald could be combined with plum, lavender, or aubergine, all to good effect. And with styles for children as elaborate as those for adult women, all that stood in the way of uniquely personalized dress was a seamstress's imagination.

Fashion plates, those detailed artist's representations of the latest European fashions displayed on mannequins or paraded on live models, represented seasonal alterations in cut and embellishment. The hand-colored illustrations were eagerly anticipated by housewives, tailors, and shop keepers alike.

In December 1879, *Domestic Monthly* boasted of its periodical that, "The latest styles for Ladies and Children's Costumes and Garments are always to be found in it; and its handsome colored plates give accurate representations of the latest and most stylish of prevailing costumes." As propriety was a Victorian preoccupation, the *Domestic* boasted of its mission "to teach a correct taste, and to promote neatness and economy in matters of dress."

American women also relied on *Godey's Lady's Book, Peterson's Magazine, The Standard Designer, The Ladies' Gazette of Fashion, Harper's Bazaar*, and others to instruct them on fashion trends and innovations. *Harper's Bazaar*, first published in 1867, holds the distinction of being the oldest continuously published fashion magazine.

Instructions and detailed measurements were outlined in these publications with yardage requirements spelled out according to the age of the child. Five to six yards of the fabric forming the principal component of a typical 1870s fireman's cape, for example, would be required for a girl of six to eight years. Additional yardages were quoted for contrast overskirts, linings, and velvet bindings and such trimmings as belts, bows, piping, and ribbon.

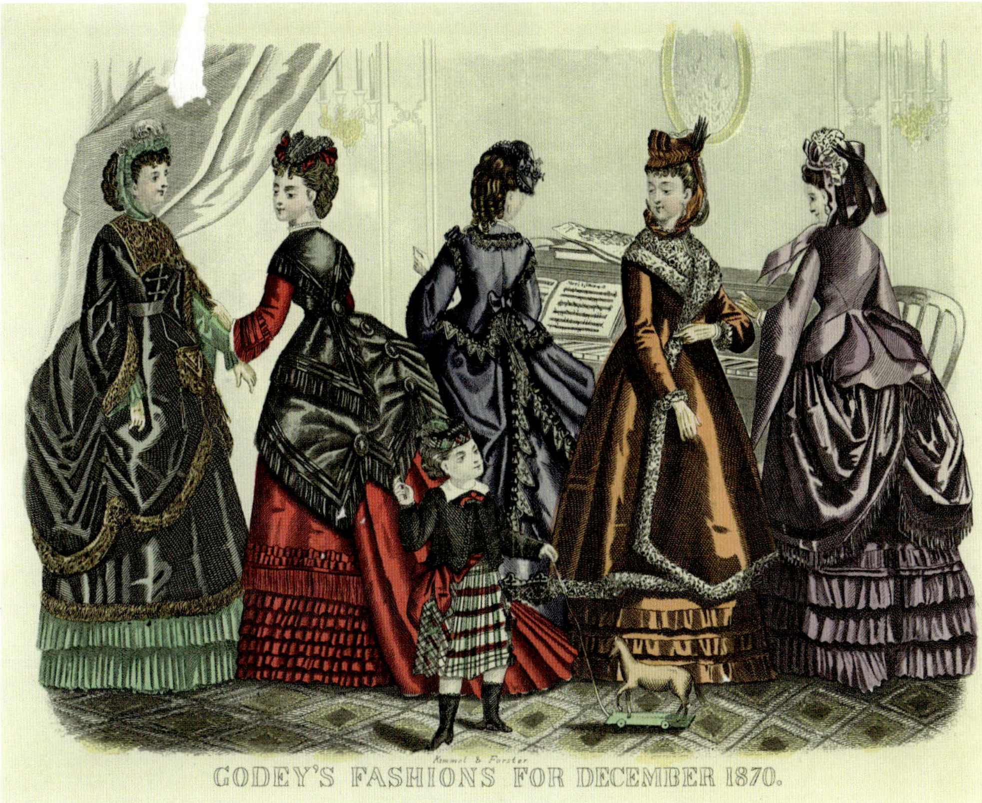

Godey's Fashion Plate showing the latest Paris fashions for winter 1870. Note the tartan kilt and tam in brilliant white, claret, and emerald. The swath of claret that drapes from the waist to the back of the ensemble appears to provide a cushion for the derriere.

Style Retrospective

Children's clothing of the period were not designed for comfort or ease of movement, but for adherence to the prevailing influence of artistic taste.

Throughout the Victorian period, basic silhouettes prevailed for lengthy periods, with major changes in contour appearing only with the arrival of each new decade. Female children of the 1870s were dressed to delineate a form similar to that of their mothers. At the outset of the decade, high, tight bodices with sloping shoulders and tight-fitting sleeves hinted at feminine helplessness, while basques, high-sashed waists culminating in backside bows, scalloped jacket hems, and Van Dyke points drew attention to the derriere. Skirts fell to a few inches below the knee and were supported by numerous petticoats as the bustle replaced the cage crinoline. The horizontally trimmed hems of the voluminous skirts served to punctuate the sleekness of the lower legs in their stockinged splendor and ankle-hugging leather boots.

A fashion plate from the *Revue de la Mode* in 1872 featured a quintet of children attired in uniquely different elegant costume: the young boy in a purple jacket with black collar, three girls in variously colored dresses (red and dove, blue, green, and white), and a younger girl in a pink jumper style with black yoke and white sleeves. Bows and contrast banding feature prominently in the embellishments and are repeated in March of the following year.

Collarless dresses prevailed, adorned with buttons, bows, ruffles, and capelets, and no discrimination was shown to boys when it came to clothing children in colorful and fashionably trimmed garments. Crimson, navy blue, and olive green were popular choices even for outerwear, according to illustrations in the February 1875 issue of *Peterson's Magazine*.

Vests trimmed with broad military braid and buttoned diagonally created visual interest when seen beneath jackets cut in front for that purpose. Chinchilla trim, black and white striped stockings, and/or knee-length pants coordinated with the variously styled suit jackets of older boys, while little ones enjoyed the comfort and visual appeal of crimson-with-gray cashmere.

The 1874 issue of *Queen Magazine* presented a colored fashion plate of a trio of spring fashions for girls, one of which was heavily embellished with lace, from collar to overskirt to parasol. Another blue-on-blue, button-trimmed number featured intricate braid embellishment on the pockets and hem, while a third ensemble shown in reddish-brown and gray displayed a less fussy, leaner aesthetic. A similar palette for children's formal attire was revealed in *Le Moniteur de la*

Mode, 1877, but the garments were decidedly more streamlined. The straight silhouette was emphasized with bold vertical buttons and balanced with sleeve cuff ornamentation.

The late 1870s princess silhouette emerged gradually, characterized by a long, slim bodice, narrow skirt, and tight-fitting sleeves. The hip-length boned cuirass bodice was similarly constructed for older girls. The long, lean lines of the princess dress were emphasized in front through the use of vertical stripes or buttons. Back interest was retained but flattened. Wide, flat, low-slung sashes for girls or boys and swags and draped vertical panels for older girls replaced the bustles and puffed bows seen earlier in the decade atop full skirts supported by crinolines.

In summer, young hands enjoyed gloves of fine cotton, leather, or lace in colors selected to match their outfits. Fur muffs served both fashion and function in winter, as did hats and capes.

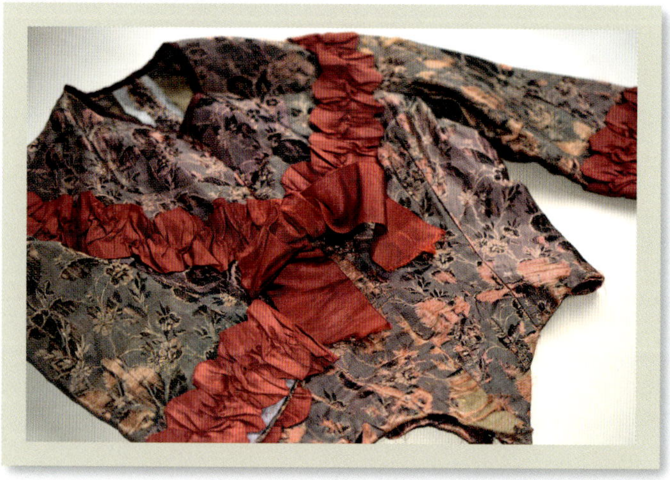

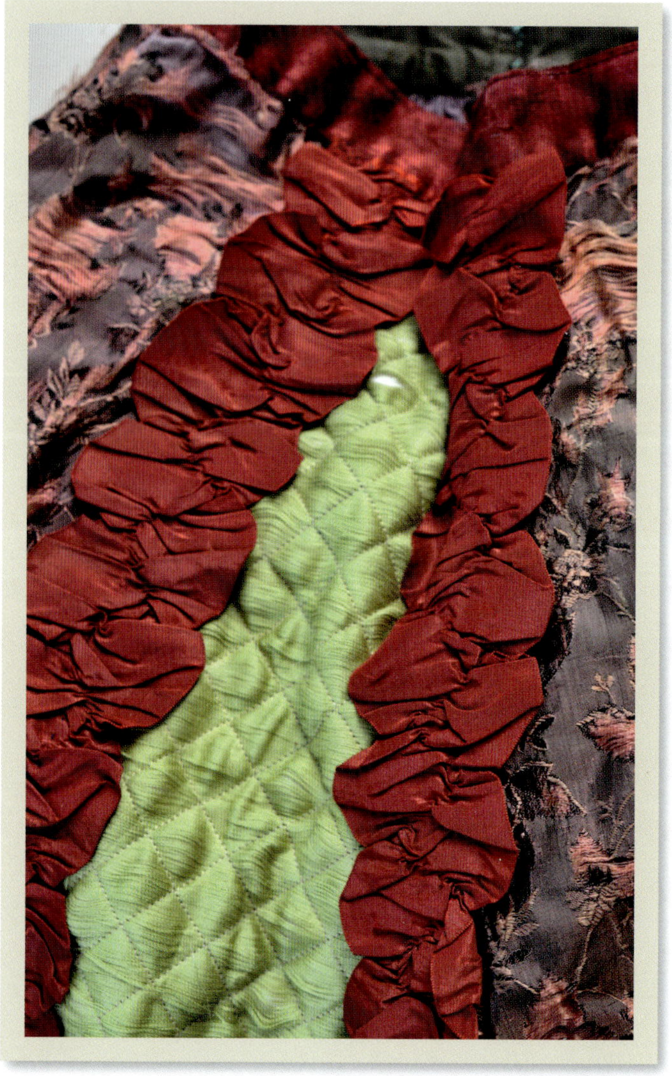

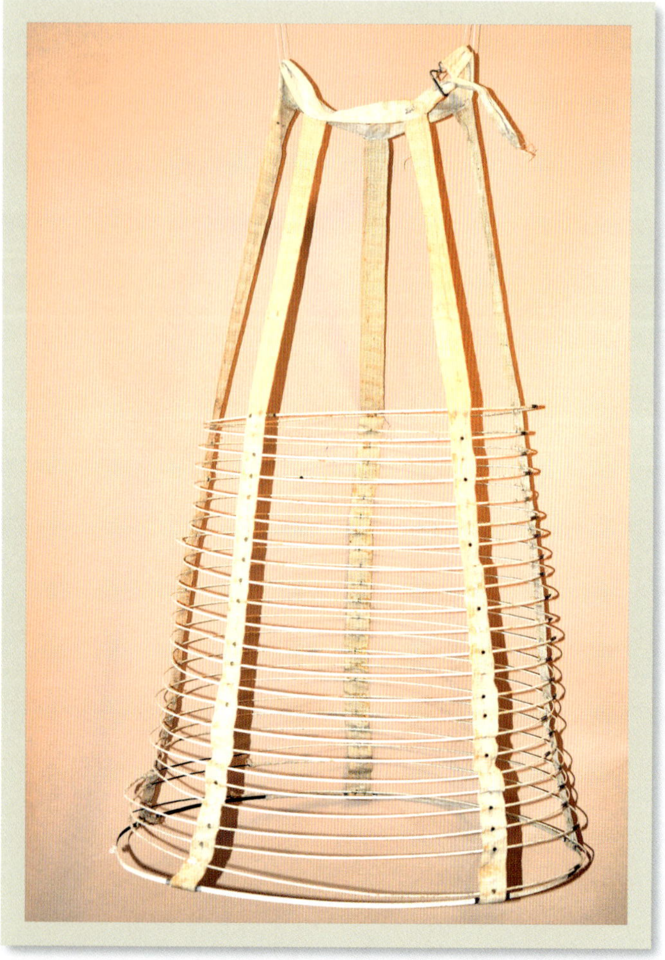

Cage crinoline comprised of wire loops strapped together with canvas tape.

Victorian silk bodice and bustle skirt ensemble for a ten-year-old girl.

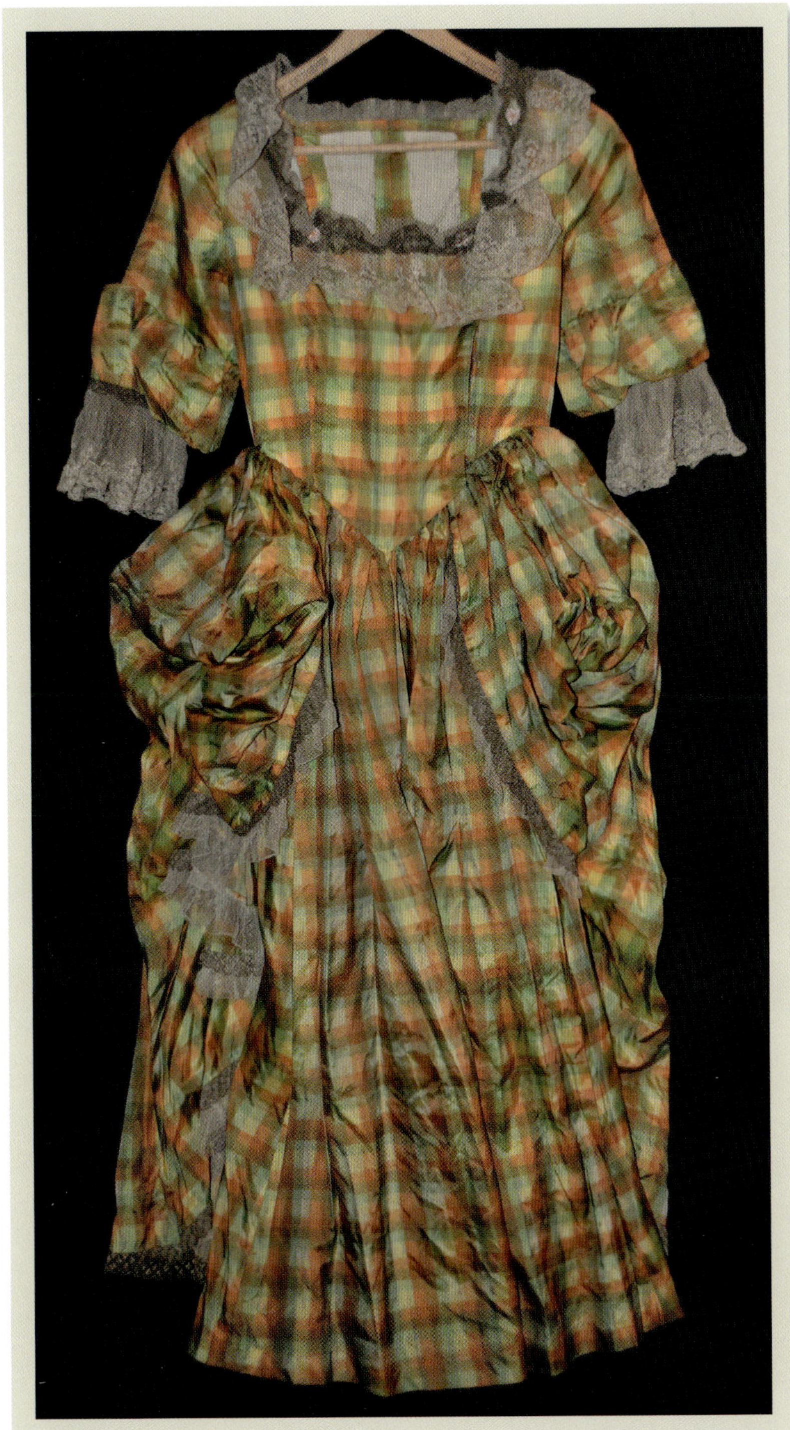

Young girl's polonaise in tartan silk, trimmed with gold metallic lace, hand-made silk lace, and tiny fabric flowers. Very Little Bo Peep.

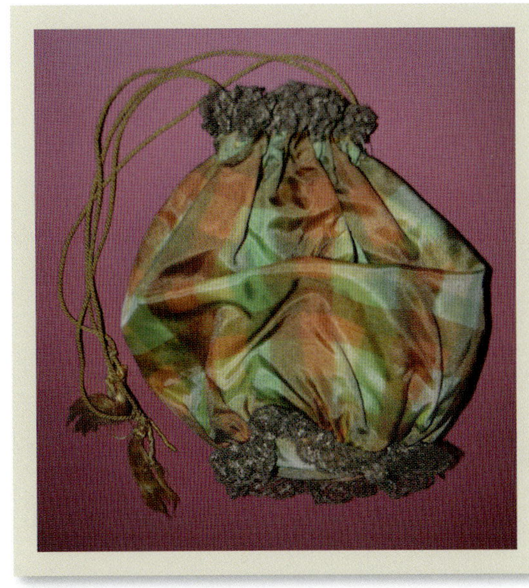

Matching drawstring reticule.

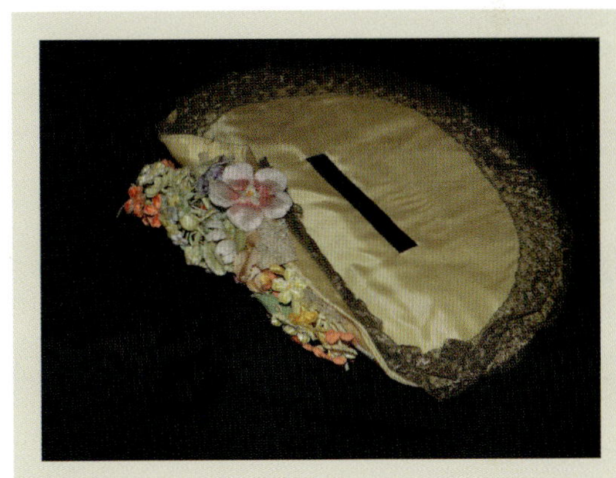

Matching Dolly Varden hat of yellow satin with black velvet ribbon ties.

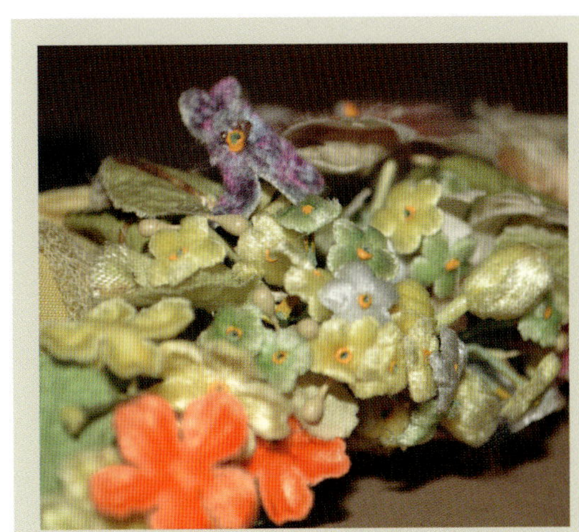

Detail: fabric flowers.

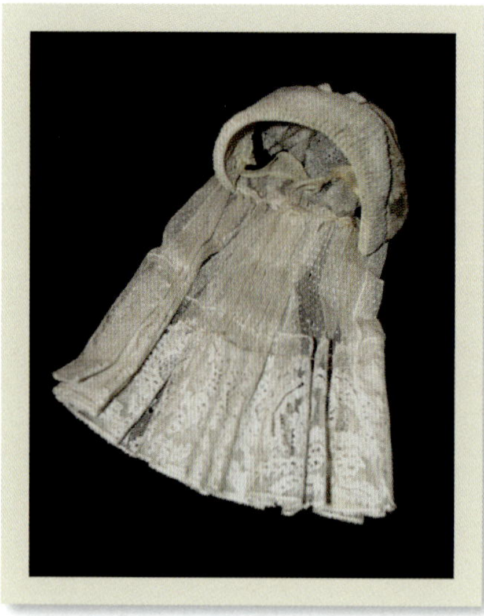

Interior view.

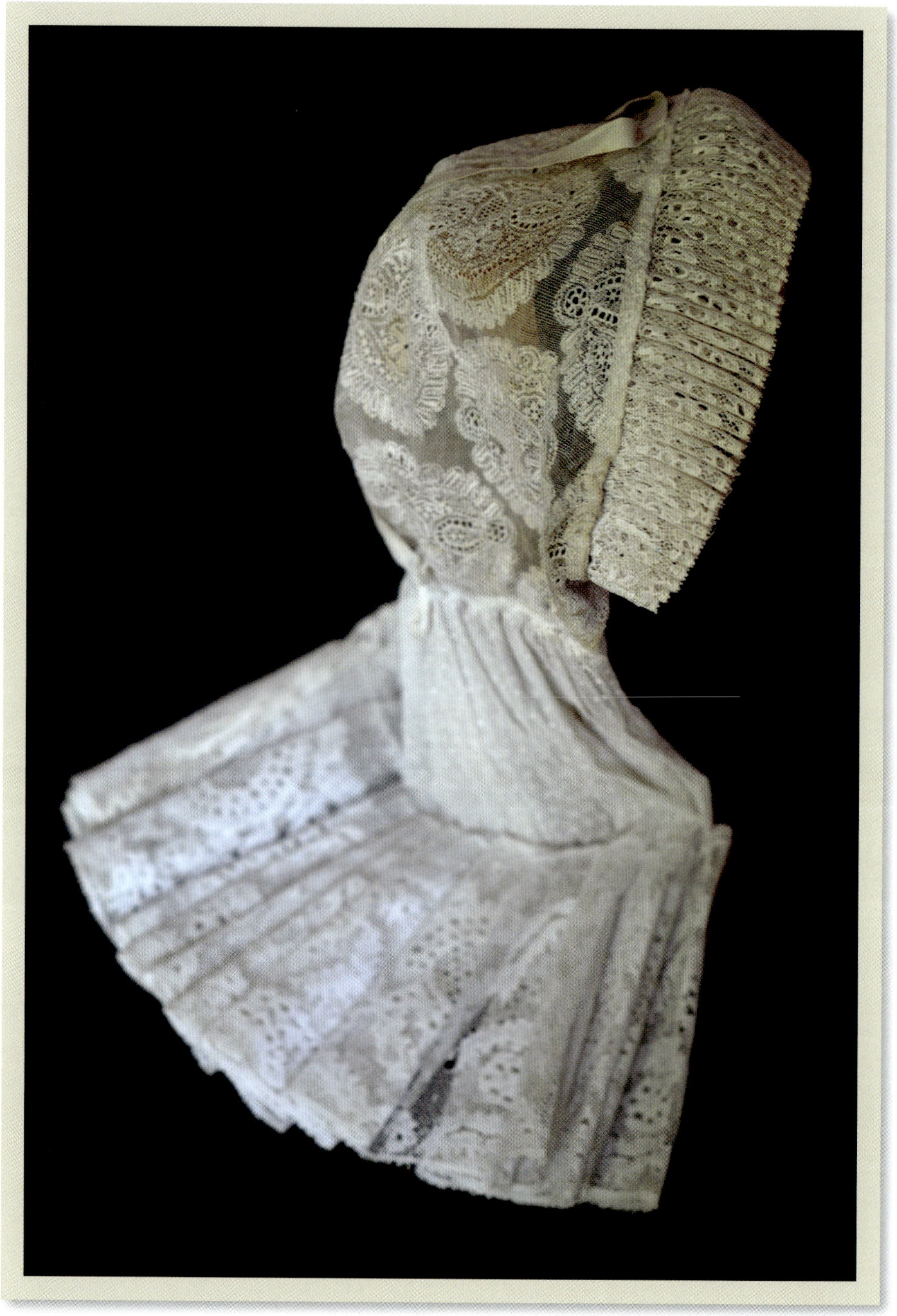

C.1870s: Child's lace bonnet with pleated bavolet.

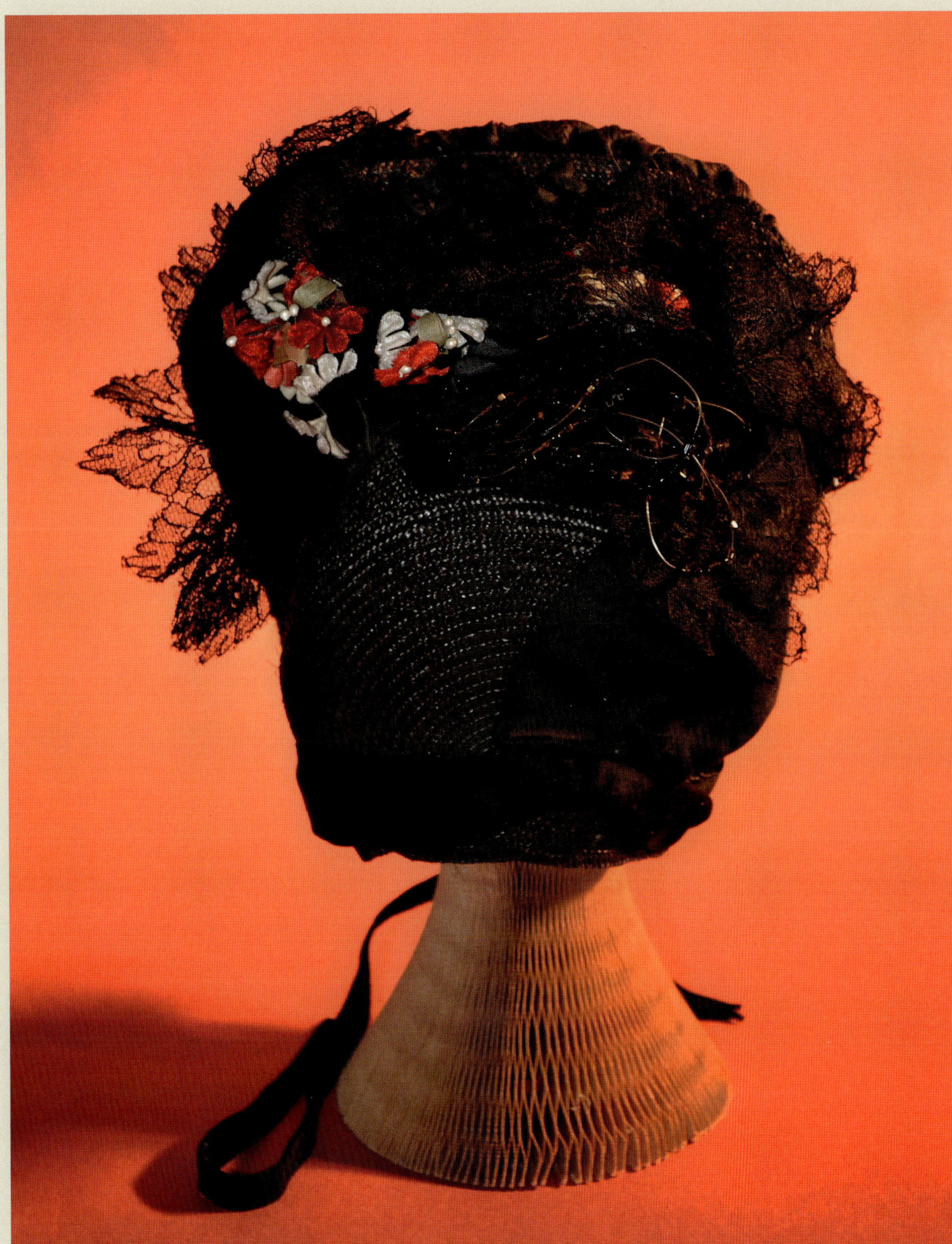

Child's black straw bonnet with lace and fabric flower adornment.
Fabric ties.

Infant's flowing cotton gown. Long sleeves, self-fabric ties.

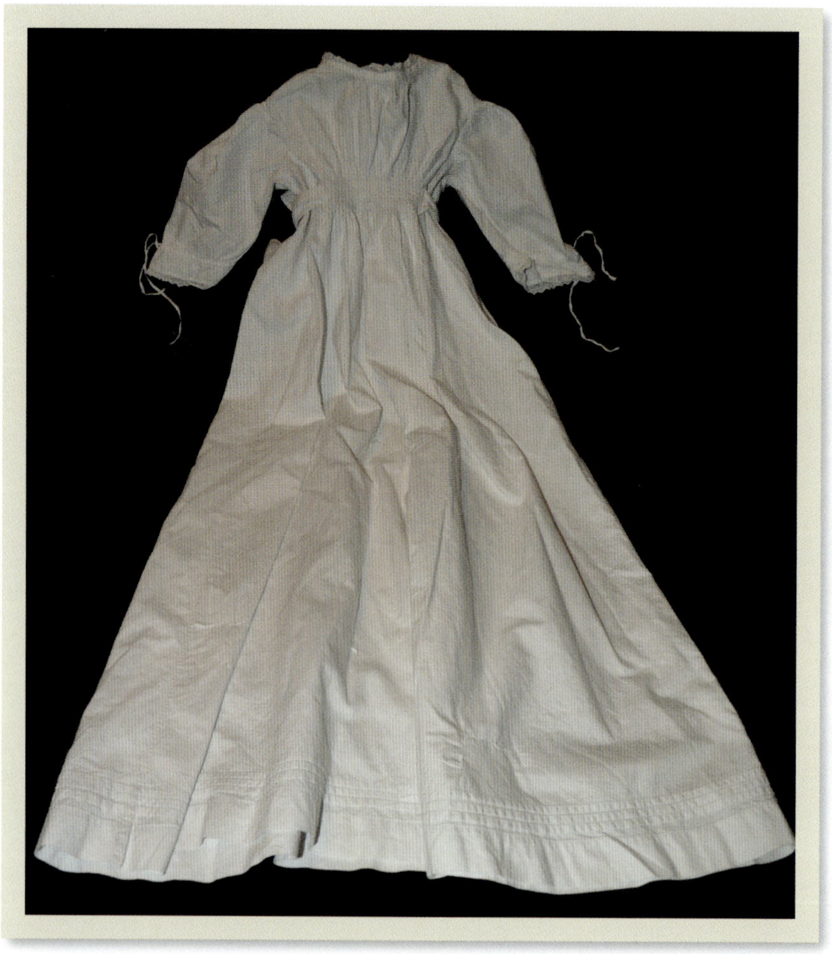

Back view.

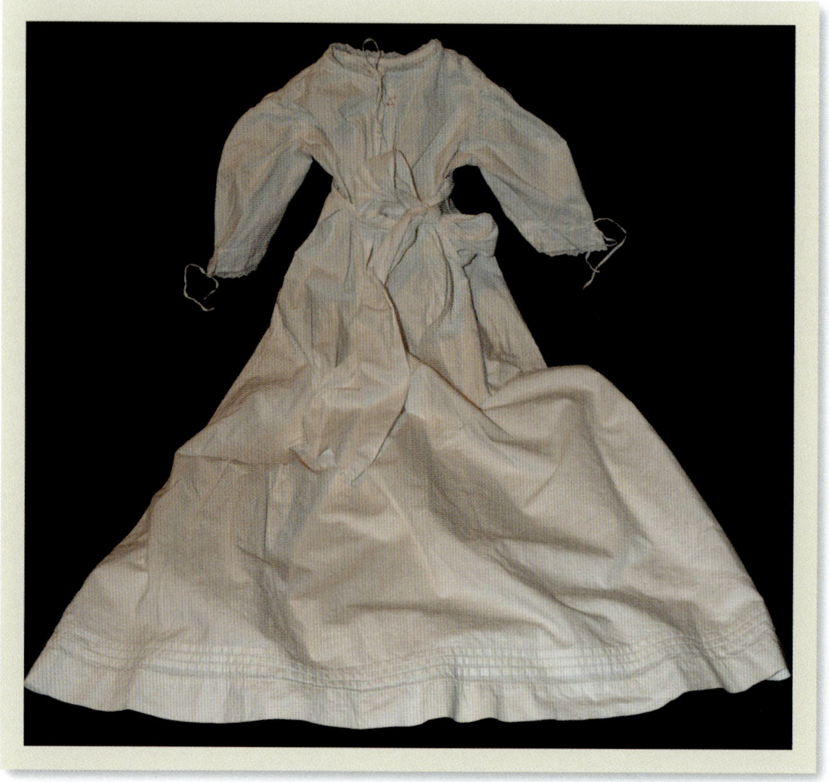

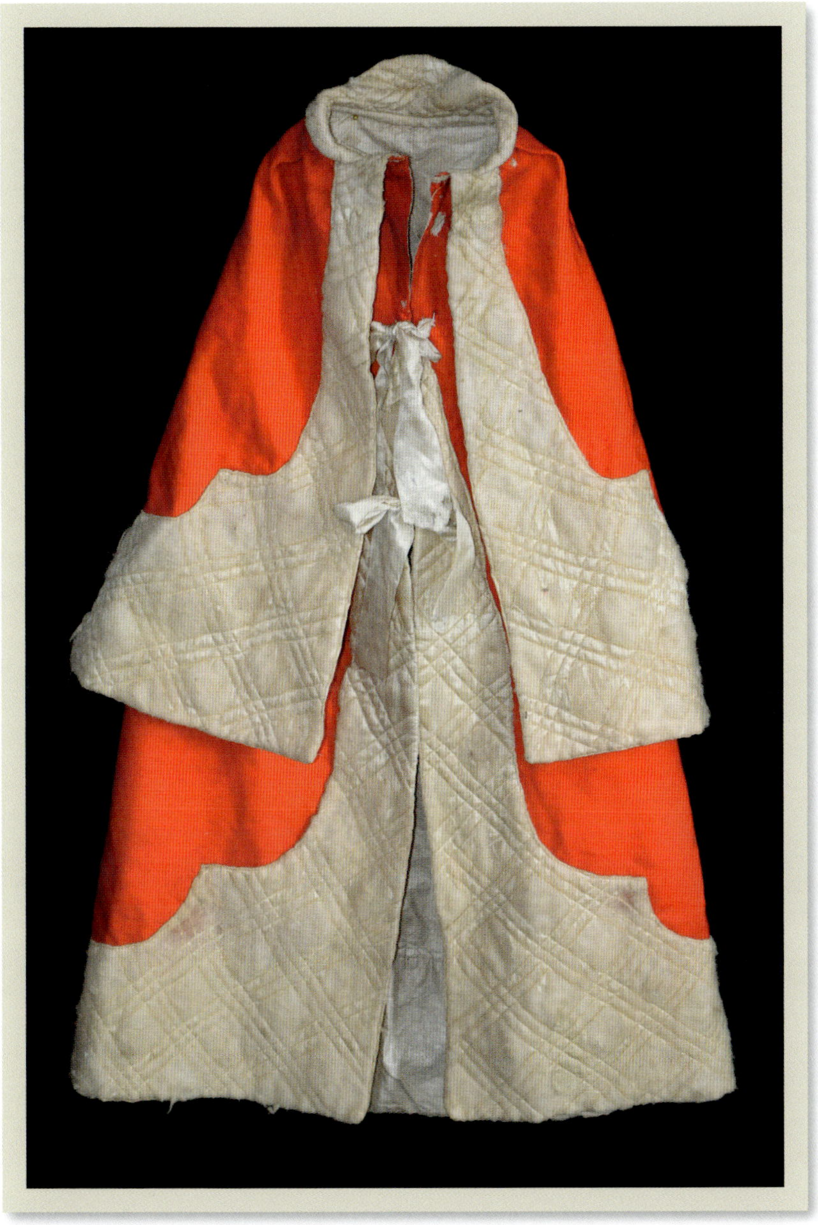

Infant's tiered "tie-down" cloak of red wool banded in quilted, cream-colored silk. Satin ribbon ties.

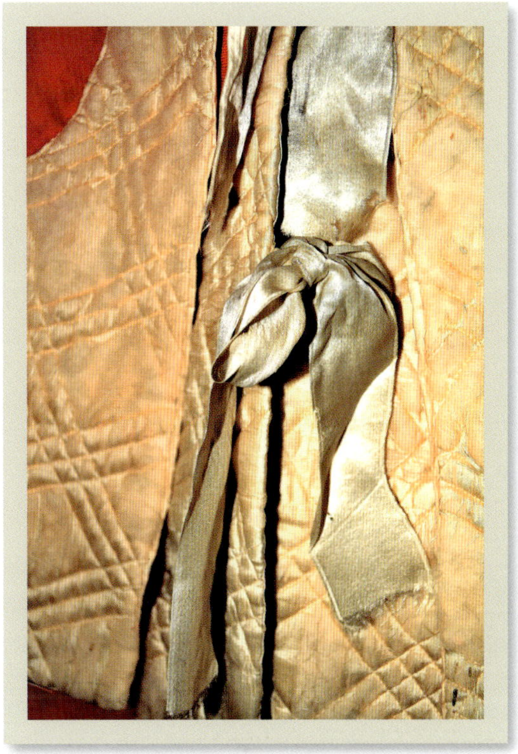

Detail.

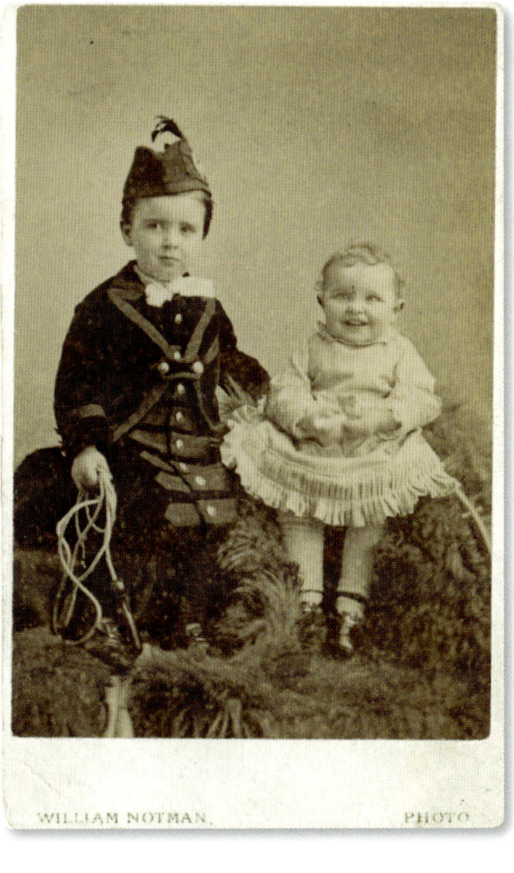

Who says dressing boys can't be fun? Award-winning photographer William Notman captured this wonderful example of a boy outfitted in late Victorian highland dress: Glengarry cap, brass buttons, white necktie, and close-fitting bolero. Notman posed the younger child to display the accordion-pleated ruffle that hems her special-occasion dress.

CHAPTER THREE

Dressed to See and Be Seen

1880–1890

Cultural Influences

By the 1880s, the aesthetic dress movement had infiltrated the mainstream and decorative touches were simplified. Dresses with flowing lines featured hand embroidery and self-fabric sashes and bows, particularly toward the end of the decade when delineated waistlines had all but disappeared. Small botanical prints in earth tone colors of brown, green, or blue satisfied the cultural desire for organic themes and motifs. Sunbonnets found favor with both genders, as did round collars and large, circular hats.

Steam-powered industrial sewing machines and the development of specialized button sewing machines enabled the mass production of ankle and high-button boots suitable for riding and for the Victorian custom of long-distance walking.

Britain's Princess Alexandra set a trend for neck chokers and lace-trimmed collars because of a scar she liked to hide.

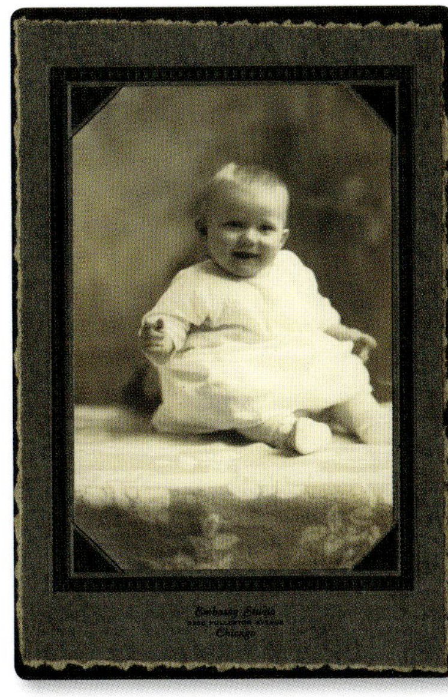

Short dress c. 1886. This happy tot is dressed for her formal portrait in a crisp white, pin-tucked cotton dress worn over a long-sleeved undershirt, white woolen stockings, and white leather booties. Cabinet card photograph by Embassy Studios, Fullerton Avenue, Chicago.

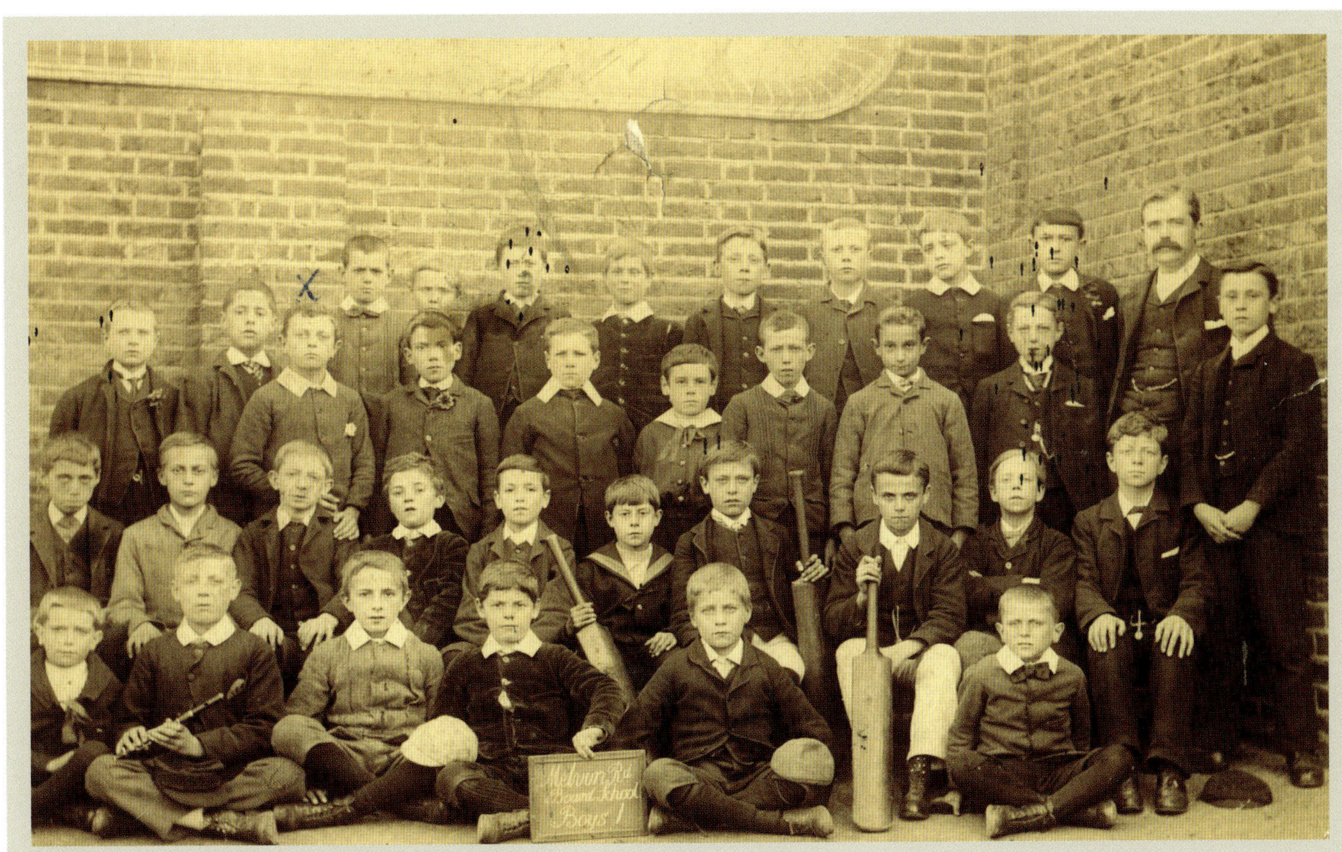

A class photograph of London, England school boys c.1885. Though all are dressed formally in the prevailing style for men, some variety is achieved in their attire.

A Rural Mother's Efforts to Obtain Fashionable Clothing for Her Children c. 1890

By 1886, Jane Croll had emigrated to Canada, married Alex, and produced two daughters, Kate and Maggie. After Jane died giving birth, Alex married Christina Ferguson. By 1890, Christina was nursing her firstborn and raising Alex's two other children in a rural cabin some forty or fifty miles from Montreal, while Alex sought employment in Portland, Maine. In a letter to Alex dated May 13, 1890, Christina brings her husband up to date on her efforts to clothe herself and the girls on their limited budget. "Mary came home last Wednesday and she brought me everything I wanted (for making the children's clothing). I don't admire some of her taste, but one thing that is just what I wanted is my own dress, a pretty brown cashmere." The older girls were provided with cashmere stockings and the baby was the recipient of a new dress.

Christina thanks her husband for the money he sent and explains the difficulties involved in obtaining proper attire for the children. "Do not fear, I will get what we need, but it is hard to manage things when you have to get others to buy it for you. The boots Mary brought the girls would do for here, but I will have to go to Sandies and get them stronger ones that will do them nice for Sunday boots when we go away." (Christina and the children planned to join Alex in Portland.)

Christina mentions the children's clothing needs again in a letter to Alex dated August 19 of the same year. She has done so much sewing that she can say with pride, "I think I have for the children all I will need for a year. Except boots." Christina also mentions having had her hat dyed and trimmed when her relative shopped in the city for her. Since they were planning a trip to Portland, it is likely that hats were among the items that Christina had ordered for the girls, while she herself made do with a refurbishing.

When Christina eventually moved with Alex to Chicago from her rural Quebec home she had five young daughters to clothe. In addition to Kate and Maggie, three—Jane, Ella, and Mildred—were born to her in the 1880s. Two boys, Edward and Fergus, would follow. As the girls grew into women they never forgot their shopping trips with "Mother" in Chicago, often remarking on the fun they had, and how they were dressed to ride streetcars, gaze at skyscrapers, and shop the downtown stores: blanketed in fur collars and muffs in winter, protected from the sun by straw hats and parasols in summer.

Maggie was not yet ten years old when she received her first fashionable fur, a birthday gift from her Uncle Jim. In another letter to her husband, Christina writes, "Maggie got a fur cape which is old enough for myself, and a string of black beads that resemble horse bells." (Sources from author's private collection of letters.)

Style Retrospective

The 1880s silhouette shifted to a more S-shaped figure, for both women and girls. Emphasis on the derriere remained, with skirts falling in a slimmer line at the front and sides to present a more prominent uplifted posterior. Dresses were often constructed of a separate bodice with attached draping for the overskirt and a separate underskirt. Undergarments, key to supporting such a contour, consisted of various types of bustle pads attached to a band worn around the waist or pocketed into the skirt itself.

By February 1883, *Peterson's Magazine* was showing girls' cutaway basque coats and tunics designed to accentuate the waist and expose coordinating ruffled and/or box pleated underskirts. Brandebourg fasteners secured the close-fitting outer garments. A fashion plate from the same periodical shows a boy's knickerbocker trouser suit with sacque coat belted low and secured with a buckle. Fur collar, cuffs, and hem add panache to the smart winter costume.

Necklines rose and straight inset sleeves with fullness at the shoulders allowed for greater movement. Waistlines dropped to the midsection and bodices slackened, falling away from the body by mid-decade in a loose A-line delineation, or presenting a blouson effect when joined to a skirt. Skirts billowed out to just above the ankle in the case of young children.

Infant wear did not change much over the final decades of the nineteenth century. Babies continued to be clothed in gender-neutral white cotton dresses, and mothers dressed their active youngsters in natural fiber "washables" for obvious reasons. Some textiles treated with arsenic-containing fabric dyes were throught to be harmful, if not poisonous, to the skin. Presumably, stains from non-colorfast fabrics occasionally appeared on the undergarments of sweaty little bodies.

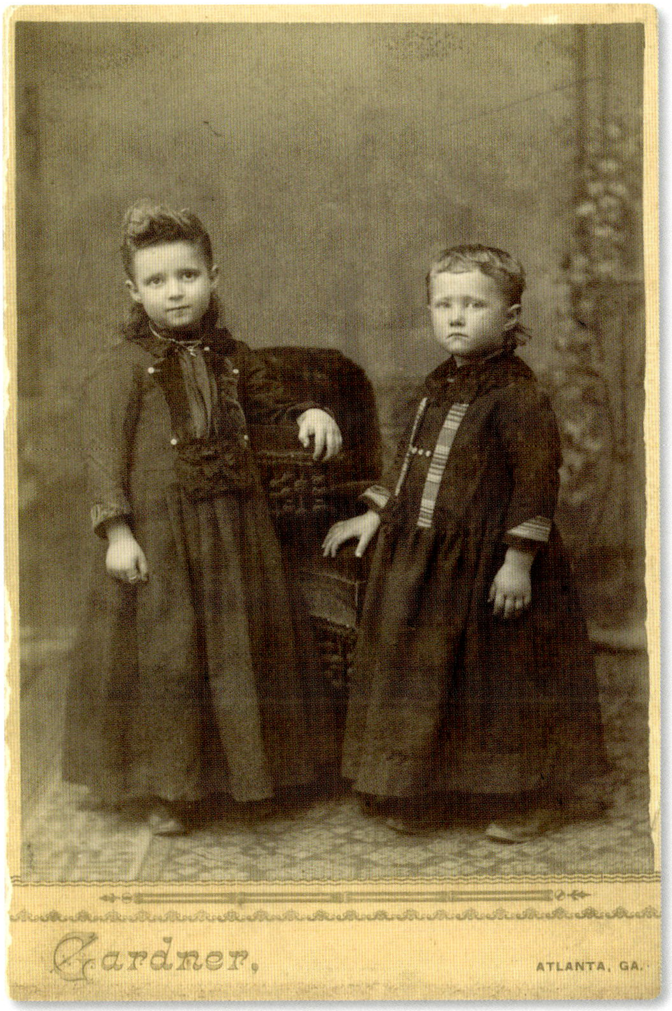

Two Atlanta tots in crinoline-supported, deep-toned dresses with elaborate front bodice embellishment. Cabinet card of H. Gardner, Atlanta, Georgia.

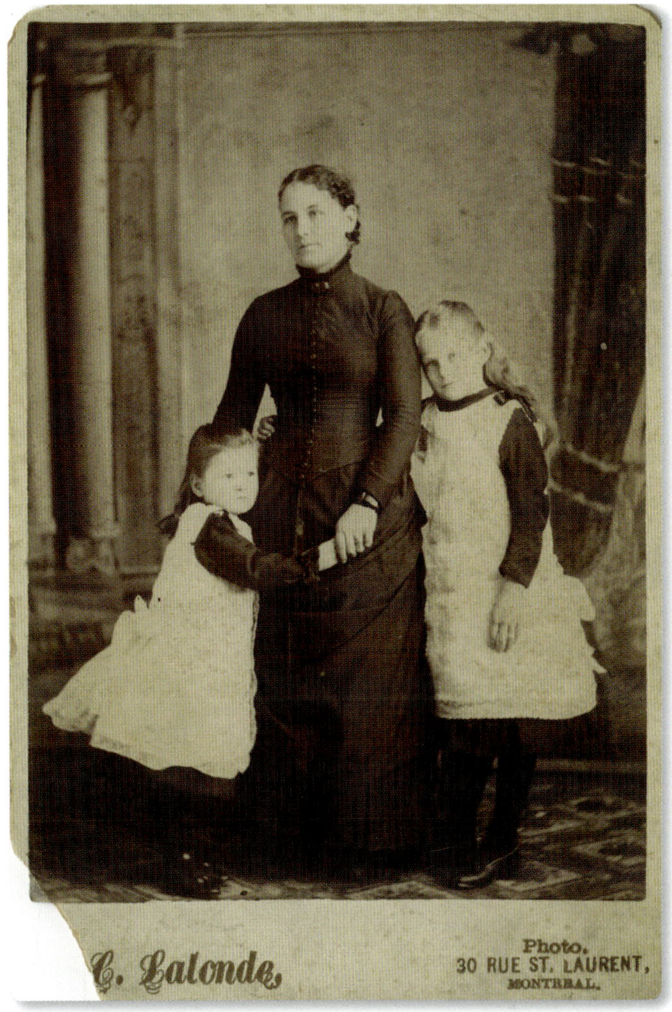

April 1886. Four-year-old Katie and ten-year-old Maggie are dressed in matching outfits for a studio portrait with their Auntie Maggie. Each wears a frothy lace pinafore over a dark bustled dress with satin ribbon bows at the shoulders. Dark woolen stockings and black leather shoes complete the outfits. Cabinet card photographed at Studio Lalonde, 30 Rue St. Laurent, Montreal.

Hats and Bonnets

During the 1880s, the number of pages devoted to children's millinery in Canadian and American mail order catalogs attests to the fact that hats took pride of place in every child's wardrobe. And no child need go without if mother was able to call on the services of one of the many custom milliners who plied their trade in every city, town, and village throughout North America.

Millinery styles changed with the seasons and were designed to complement the prevailing costume silhouette. Fashion plates, millinery shop windows, and department store catalogs showed the latest styles and trimmings. Most children's hats were presented as women's hats in miniature, with some even "warranted to wash" (*Ladies' Home Journal*, April 1898).

Footwear

Unadorned, low-rise slip-on shoes became trendy for indoor wear. Silk ribbons were employed to lace open-fronted kid leather boots for both women and girls.

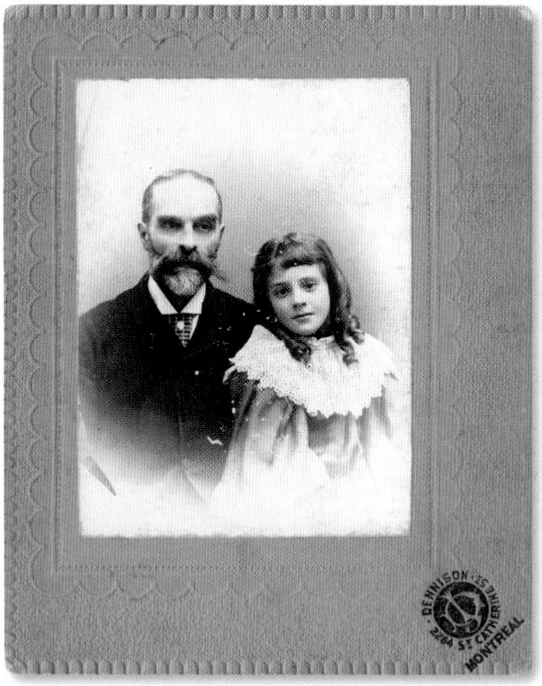

Late Victorian studio portrait of a young girl named Pearl in a dress with very full sleeves. Pearl's detachable white eyelet Bertha collar forms a romantic backdrop for her ringlets. Studio portrait by Dennison, St. Catherine St., Montreal.

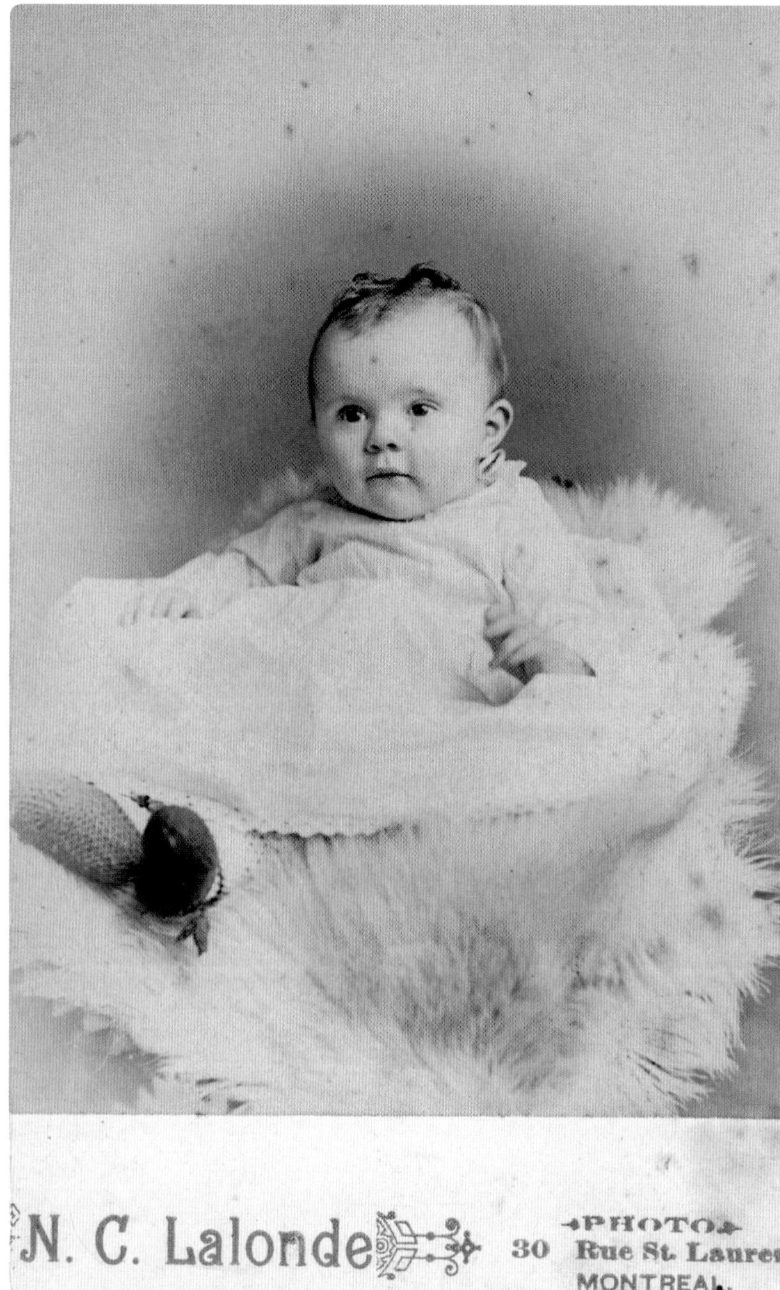

The author's grandmother, ten-month-old Jane Christina Philip, is photographed on March 20, 1889, in a white cotton dress trimmed at the hem with lace. Dark woolen hand-knit booties complete the outfit. Cabinet card photograph by N. C. Lalonde, Rue St. Laurent, Montreal.

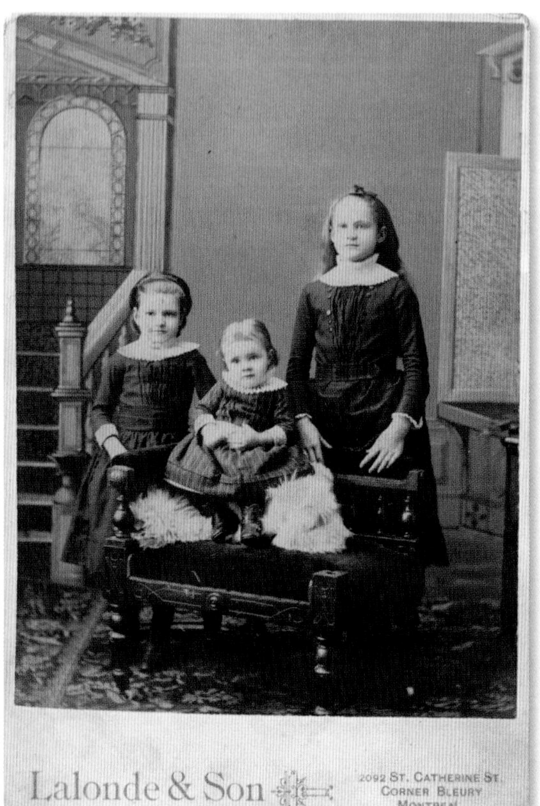

Sisters Margaret, Jen, and Kate Philip in round neck dresses with detachable collars and trimmed cuffs c.1890. The full skirts are gathered onto the bodices at the natural waist. The dresses are possibly red in color. Cabinet card photo by Lalonde & Son, St. Catherine St., Montreal.

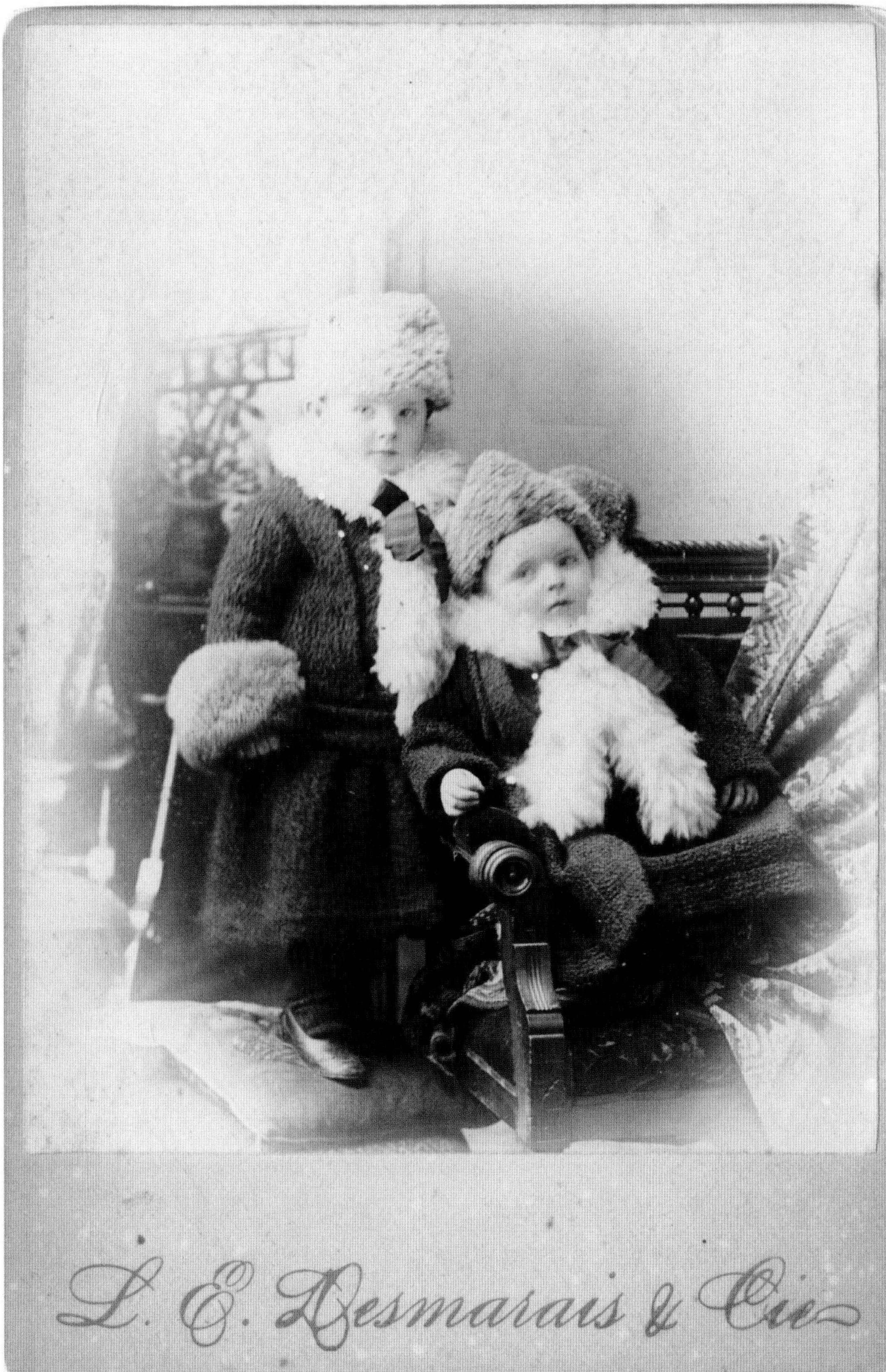

Jane and Alexander Philip's daughters, Maggie and Katie, in woolly winter coats, fur neck pieces, and astrakhan hats c. 1882. Cabinet card photo by L. E. Desmarais, 17 St. Laurent, Montreal.

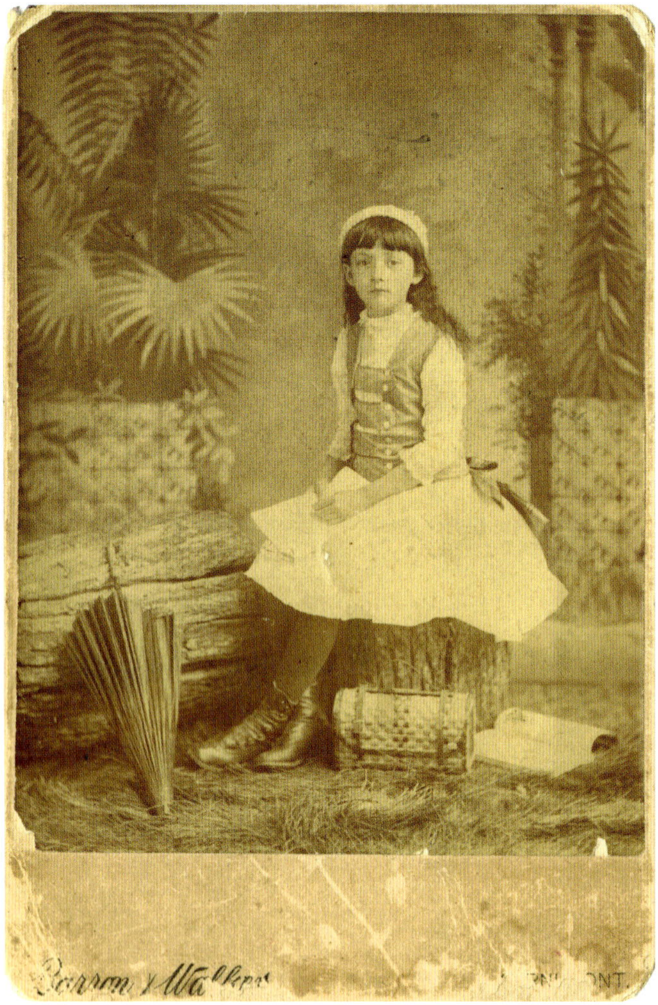

Cabinet card image of a young girl in a white dress with three-quarter sleeve and tiered skirt. A button-trimmed vest is finished in the back with a giant self-fabric bow. The parasol and bag may be studio props.

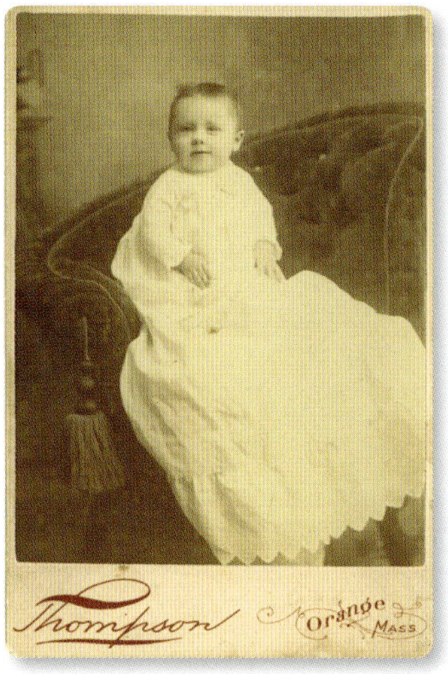

It is difficult to tell where the baby stops and the dress continues, but these enormous white-work cotton gowns were popular for infant christenings c.1900. This may have been a family treasure or even a studio prop. Cabinet card by Thompson Art Studio, Orange, Massachusetts.

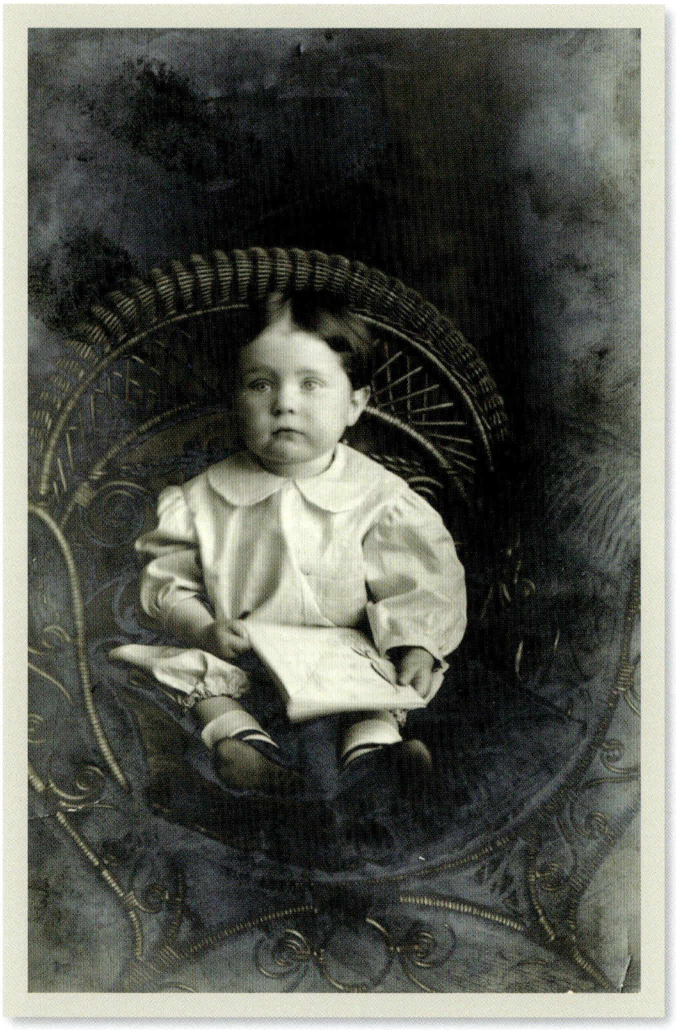

Victorian postcard image of toddler James Hunter in a unisex romper with giant sleeves, rounded Buster Brown collar, and elastic casing at the hem.

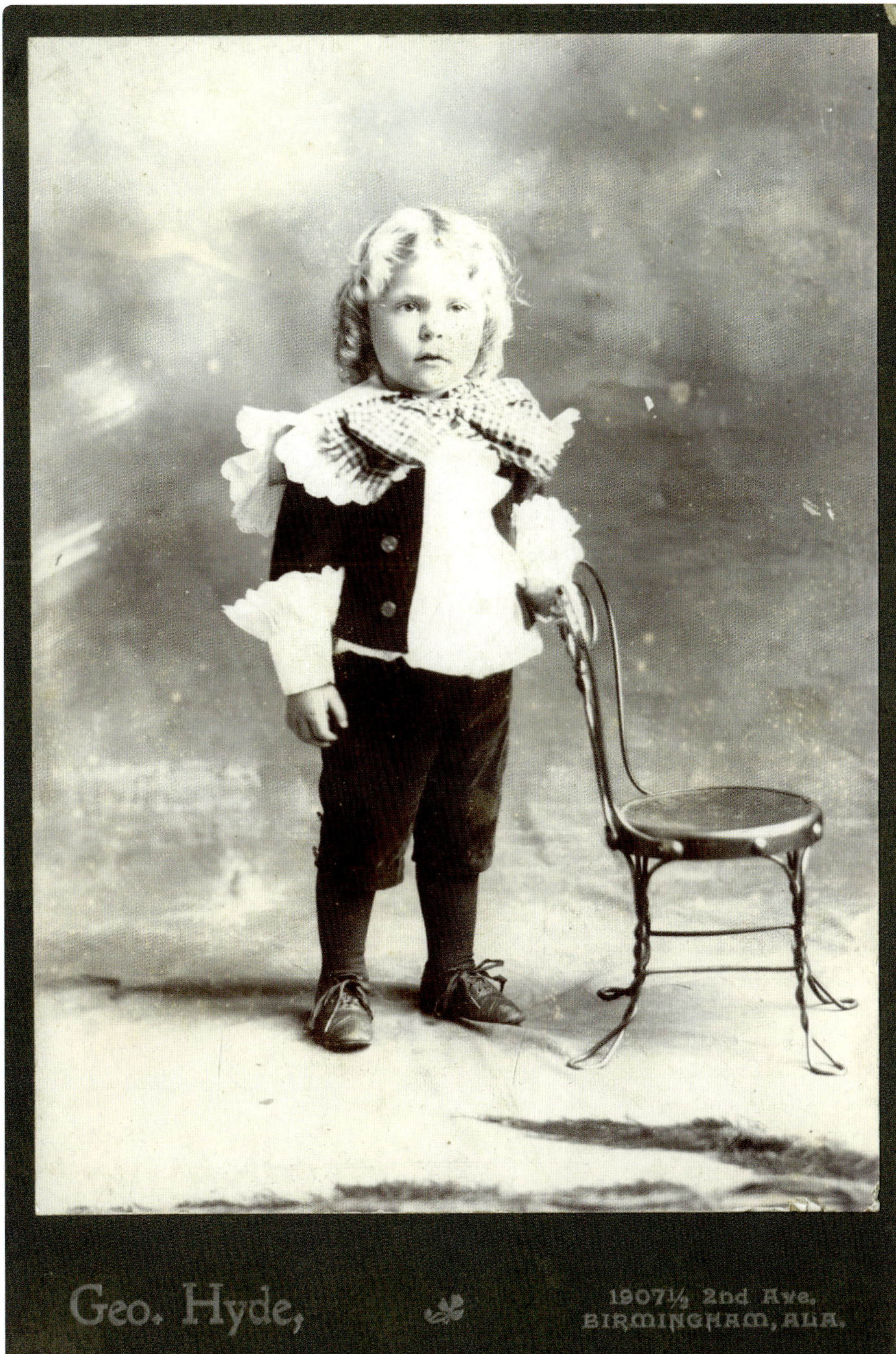

A young gentleman dressed in a Fontleroy ensemble. The layered collar features wide lace trim and a self-fabric neck bow.

This black and white studio portrait does not do justice to what must be a very colorful winter ensemble. The young boy is attired in a kilt and elaborate sweater. A white lace collar frames the boy's face.

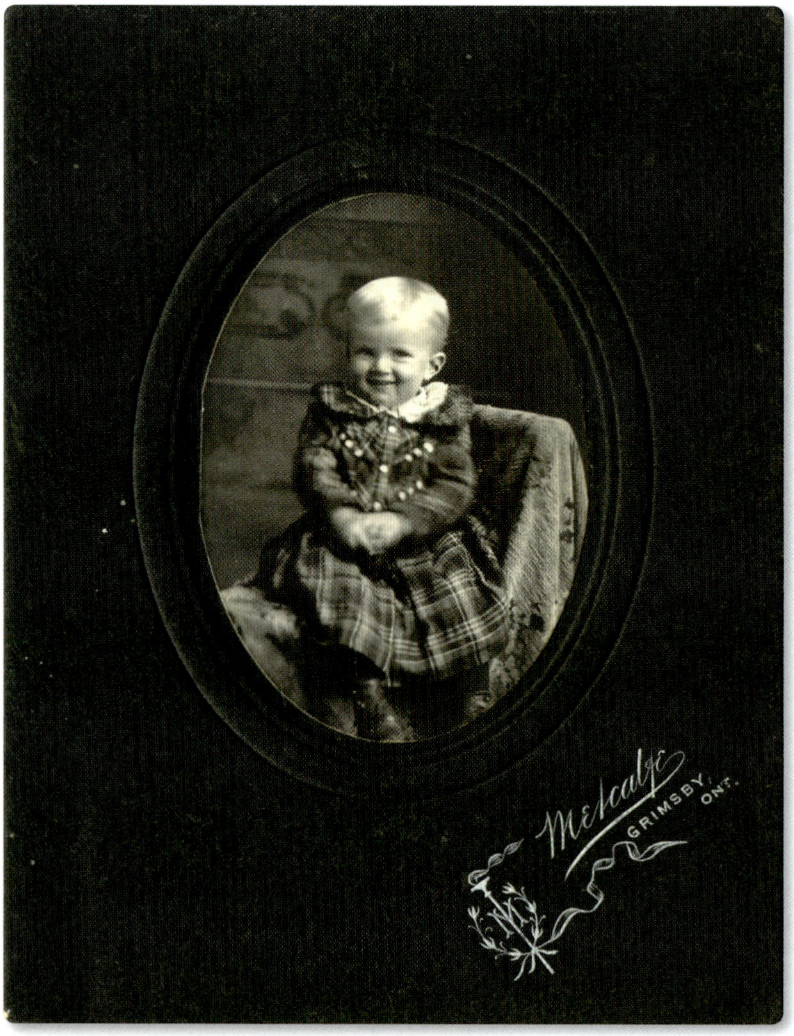

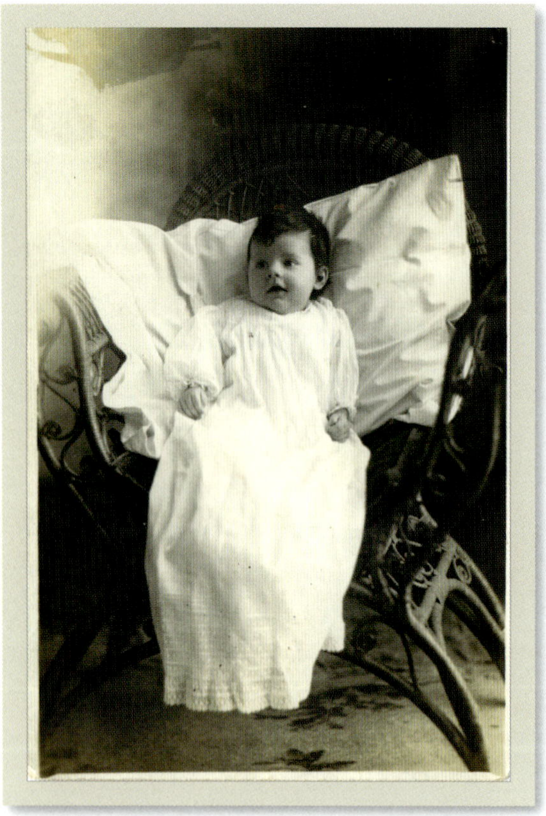

A bright-eyed baby in a long white gown with pin-tucked yoke and lacy hem relaxes against a down-filled pillow. Victorian infants wore these long gowns until they were able to crawl.

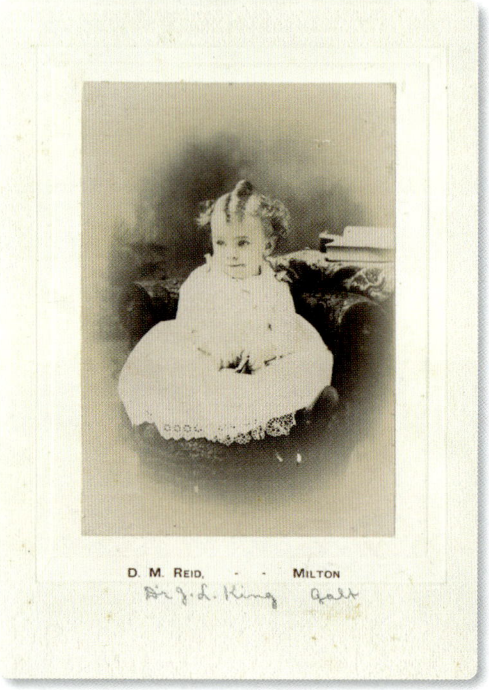

One of several petticoats is visible below the hem of this young child's white gown. Fashionable sausage curls add to her charm.

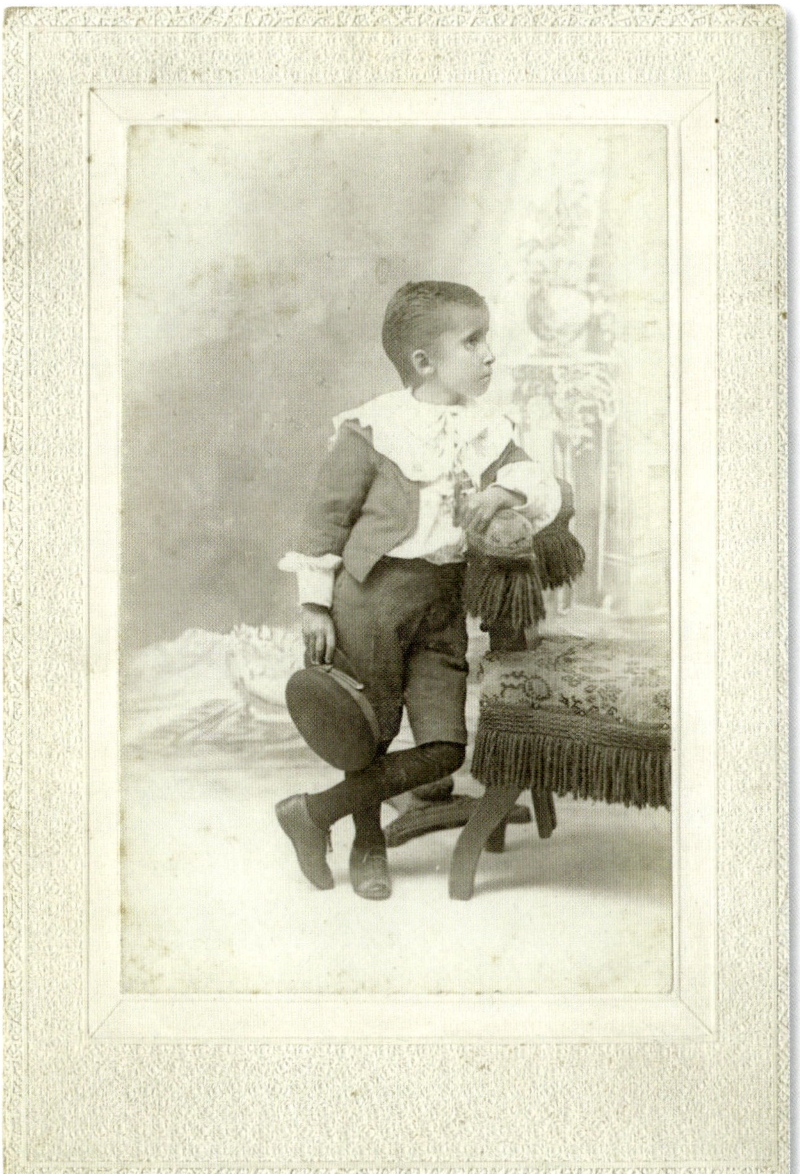

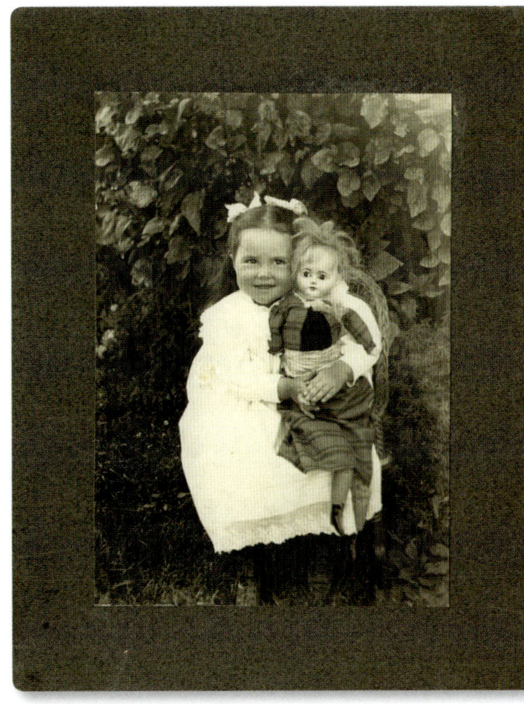

Little Alice Hunter hugs her dolly, who is as fashionably dressed as herself. The lace hem of Alice's long-sleeved white cotton dress contrasts sharply with her black, lace-up leather boots.

The cap and closely cropped hair lend this Little Lord Fauntleroy suit a military air.

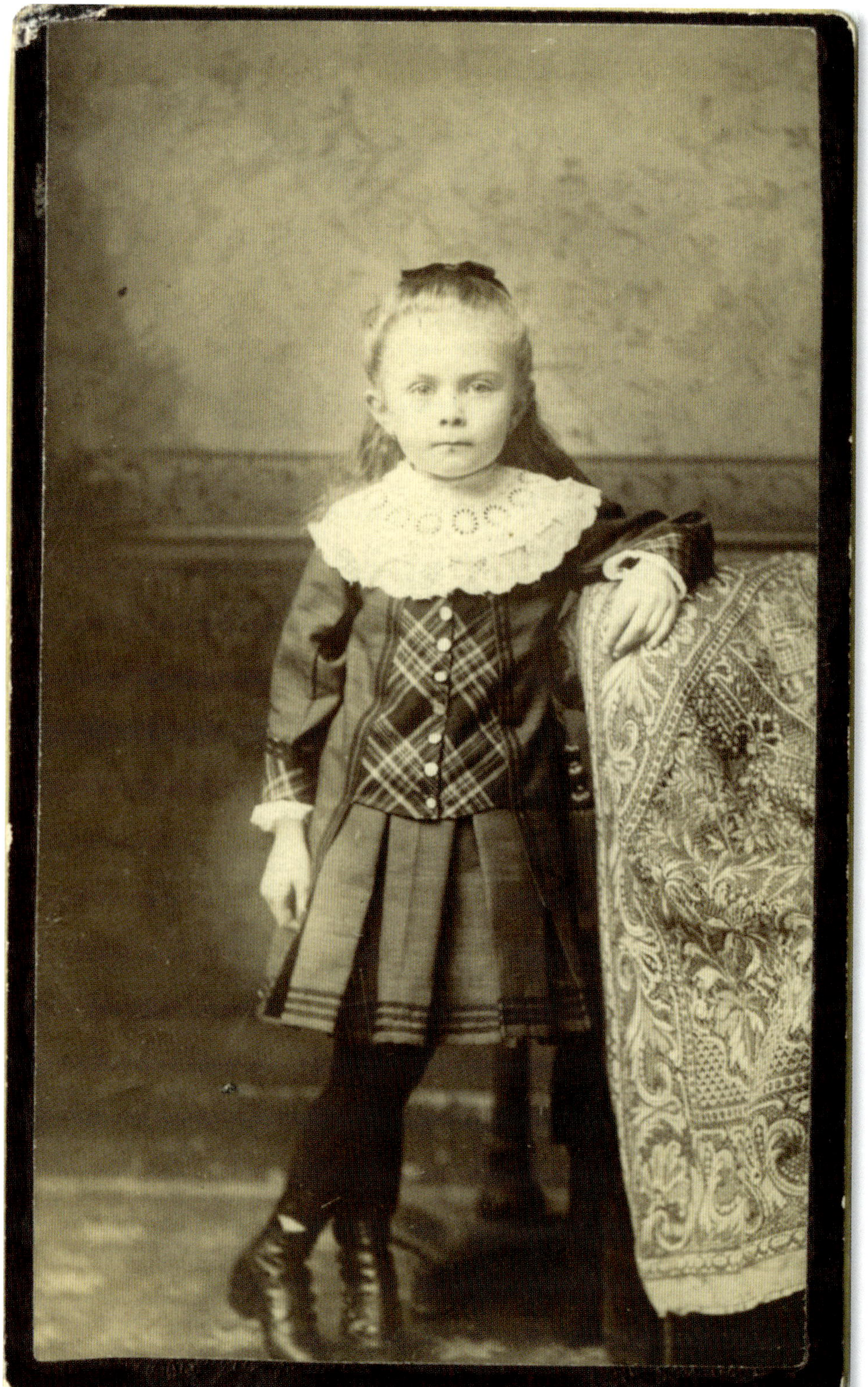

A touch of tartan and an intricate lace collar gives this Victorian youngster the confidence to pose so casually for her portrait. The tartan and lace is repeated at the cuffs. Wouldn't it be nice to know the original colors of this outfit?

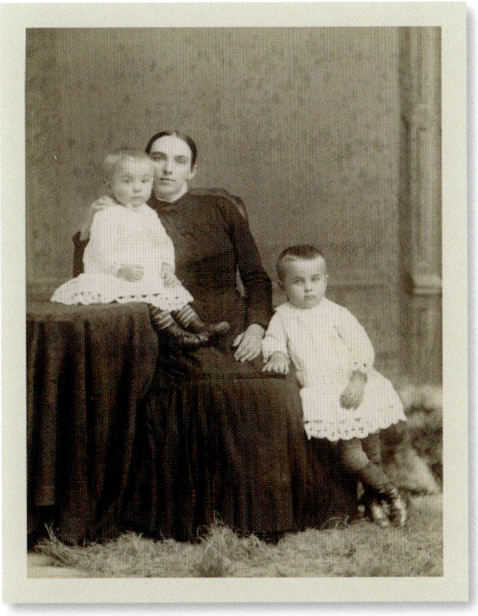

Except for the stockings, this young mother has dressed her children in identical lacy white dresses. Are they boys or girls...who can tell? Image by J. Pollard's Photographic Studio.

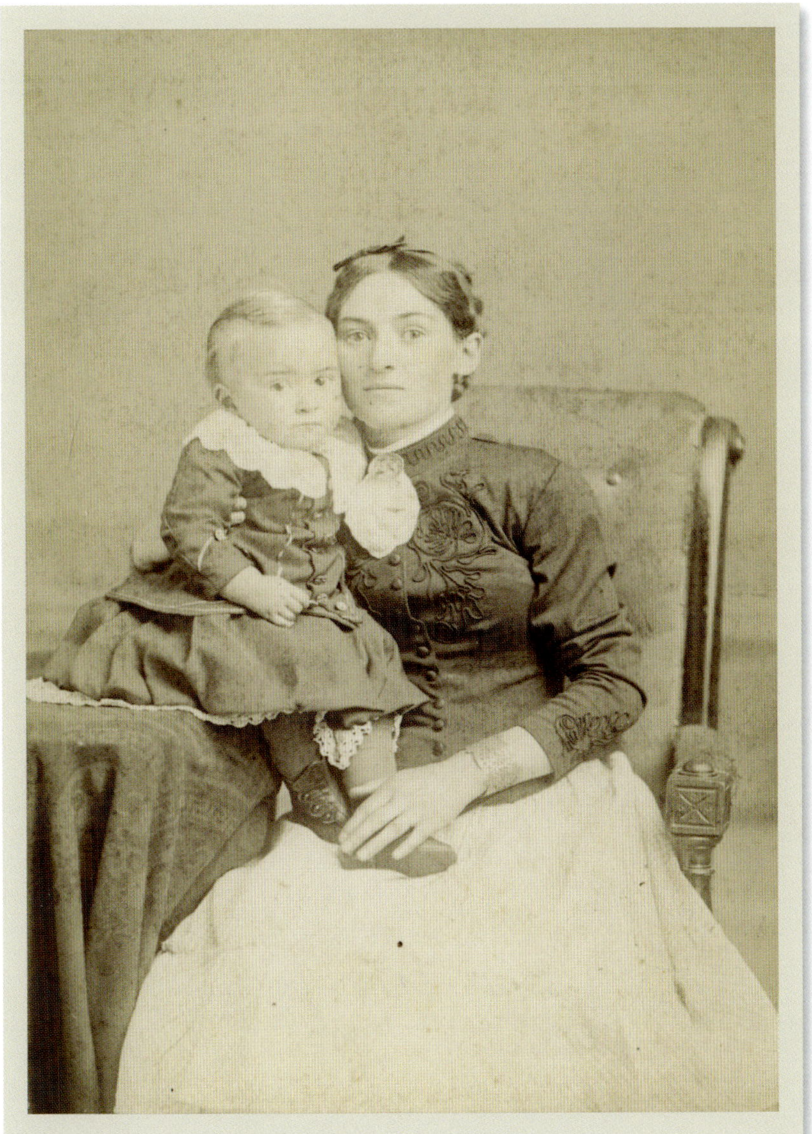

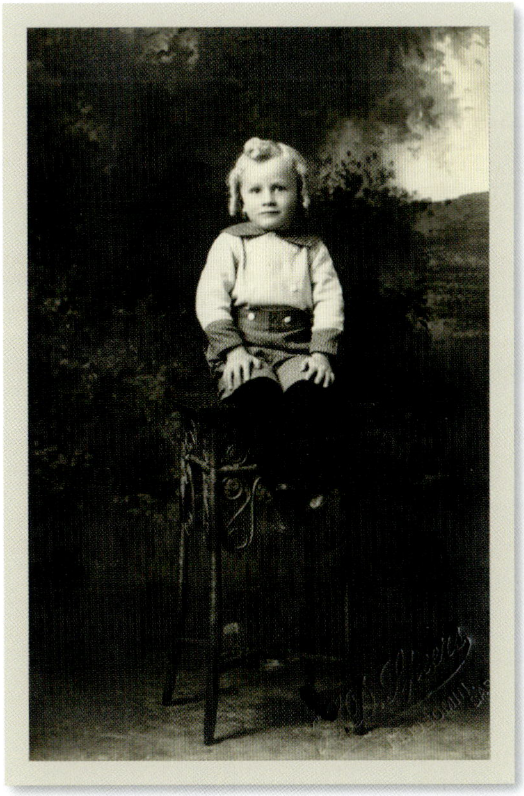

This boy, c. 1885, likely went to bed the night before this photograph with his hair tied in strips of cotton to produce the ringlet curls so popular at the time. His suit, in contrasting colors, appears to be made of wool.

What an elaborate dress for such a young child! Note the volume of skirt fabric that has been pleated to create a bustle effect at the back.

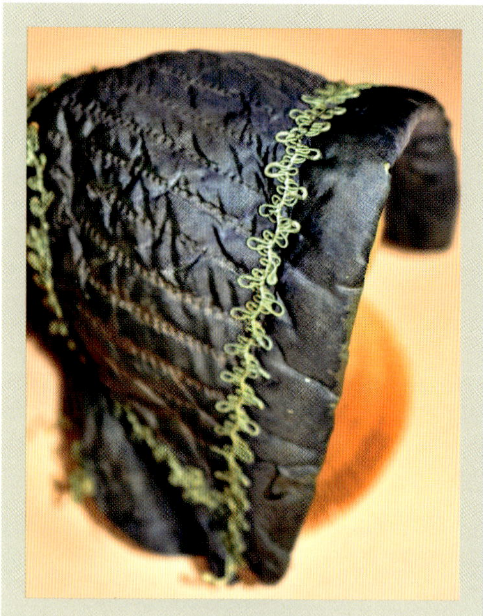

Young child's hand-quilted winter bonnet, purple faded to green with grass-green braid trim.

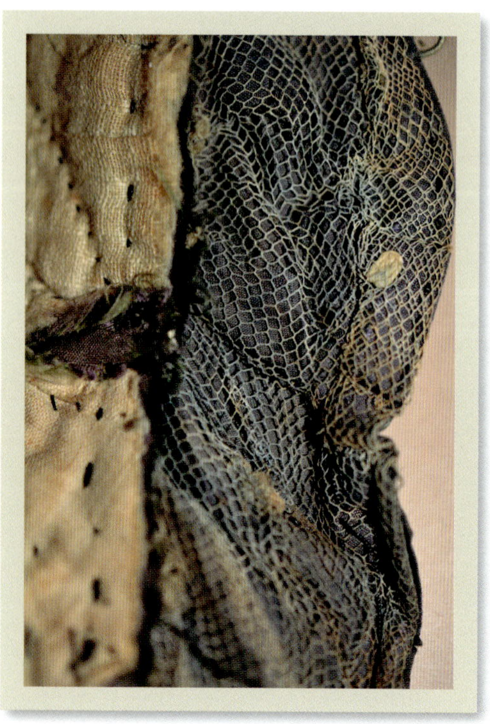

Interior, showing net-lined bavolet.

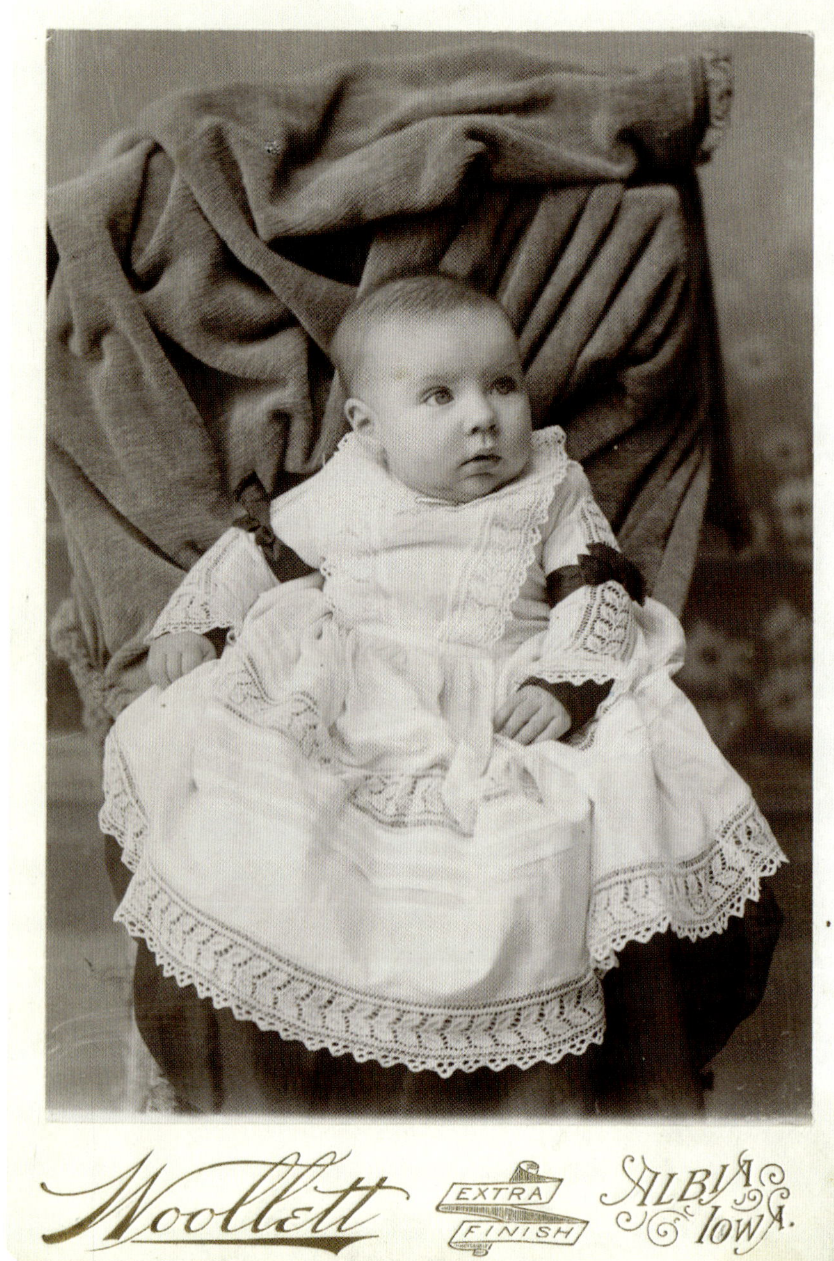

This little tyke, in white dress with black ribbon arm bands, is dressed appropriately for Victorian mourning. Photo by Woollett Studio of Albia, Iowa.

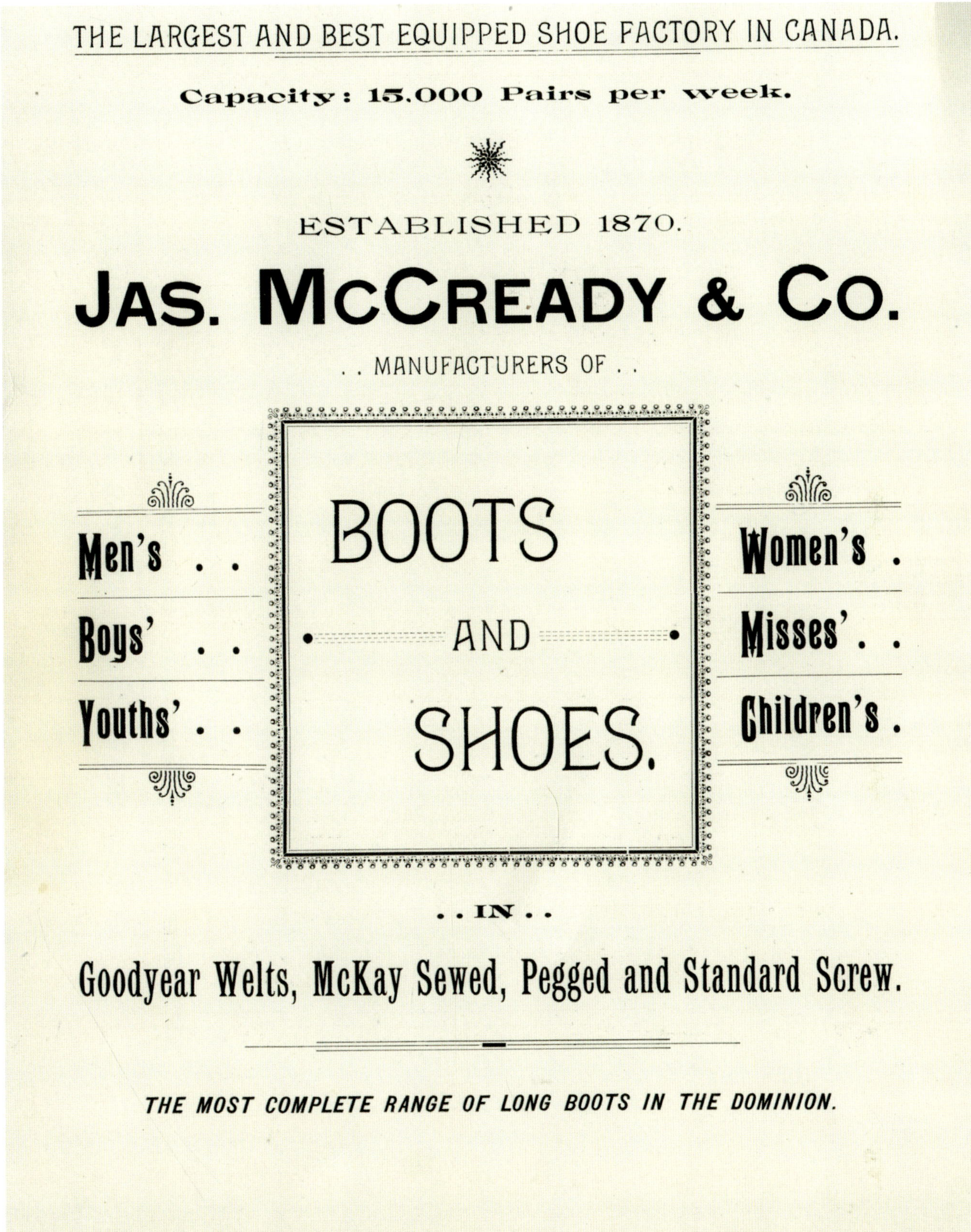

A Canadian shoe manufacturer's advertisement for the Jas. McCready & Co. firm established in 1870. *Canada and Her Commerce*, 1894.

CHAPTER FOUR

Dress Reform
1890–1900

"Of course, clothing fashions have always been impractical, except in Tahiti."—Jacques Barzun, cultural historian

"It is from the shoulders, and from the shoulders only, that all garments should be hung.—Oscar Wilde, author and poet

Cultural Influences

"There is no reason in the world why a little girl may not be dressed comfortably, and at the same time prettily. The frocks of today are quite loose enough to allow the little women to run and romp and have as much exercise as seems necessary, and those are unwise mothers who do not look out for the comfort of their little people with each change of the weather."—Isabel A. Mallon, *Ladies' Home Journal*, October 1894

Clothing as it related to the health of infants and children was of concern to late nineteenth-century society, and public lectures were held with experts espousing various theories. The Rational Dress Society, founded in London in 1881, was dedicated to the considerations of comfort, health, and freedom of movement as it related to dress, particularly for women and children. Improper clothing was blamed for everything from illness to poor posture. Proponents of the movement, including Wilde's wife, Constance Holland, held that children's clothing should be close fitting but not binding, and that children should be dressed more warmly than adults. This was achieved through the layering of garments. Simply constructed gowns that could be tied alternately down the front or the back meant that babies would not need to be turned as they were dressed.

"Corsets should never be worn by a growing girl." So wrote *Ladies' Home Journal* columnist Elizabeth Robinson Scovil in April 1898. Adding her voice to the growing number of dress reform advocates, Scovil advised mothers to select instead a corded waist. "Even this should not fit tightly," she advised, as "it is necessary that undue pressure should not be applied." To illustrate the dangers of tight corsetry, it is interesting to note that persons with a twenty-four-inch waist were advised to purchase and wear a twenty-one-inch corset.

Though invented and patented in 1850, the mercerization of cotton, (a process of chemical treatment that strengthened cotton fibers and produced a sheen) was not adopted by the cotton textile industry until forty years later, when it became an overnight success. The number of new lustrous and colorfast yard goods available to the garment industry in the last decade of the nineteenth century allowed for inexpensive garments that were lustrous, durable, and easily laundered, thus enabling a shift toward more practical dressing.

Flannel-lined leather leggings were one of the garments originally designed for boys that influential *Ladies' Home Journal* columnist Elizabeth Scovil pronounced suitable for girls. Dress reform was finally being put into practice.

The invention of the bicycle was one of the most important cultural influences of 1890s fashion. When Charlotte Brontë's character, Jane Eyre, decides to post a letter, having no access to a carriage, she sets out on a mandatory walk, returning to Lowood Institute hours later, wet and weary. Similarly, when my own great-great grandmother wanted to petition her local government for access to a road, she set out on a trek to the capitol, knitting a pair of socks on the day's journey there and back. The invention of the bicycle has long been associated with the liberation of women, so much so that it is difficult to imagine life before its invention. But along with the novel conveyance came new attitudes regarding suitable activities for women and new considerations about the practicality of dress. This, of course, also applied to children. By 1896, over 10 million men, women, and children had adopted the habit of cycling, and special cycling costume was developed for wheelwomen and girls whose lengthy skirts risked being caught up in bicycle chains. Canvas shoes also appeared, along with divided skirts and bloomers.

Style Retrospective

"Dresses for children of two or three years are worn shorter than they have been, reaching about two inches below the knees. Madras, gingham, lawn percale, and chambray are the materials used. A pretty design has a deep yoke of embroidery, coming to a sharp point in front and behind. This is edged with insertion and there is a deep frill of embroidery over each shoulder."—Elizabeth Robinson Scovil, *Ladies' Home Journal*, September 1898

"Spots can sometimes be removed from clothing by rubbing them hard with a scrap of the material. This method can always be tried first, as it does no harm if it is ineffectual. Benzine will remove grease spots but has been known to leave a mark on fabrics especially of a delicate color, showing the limit to which the liquid spreads."—Elizabeth Robinson Scovil, "Suggestions for Mothers," *Ladies' Home Journal*, October 1894

By the last decade of the century, many children's garments were fashioned of washable fabrics, lessoning the need to freshen heavier winter fabrics with dangerous chemicals like ammonia, benzene, and naptha. Instead, easily laundered

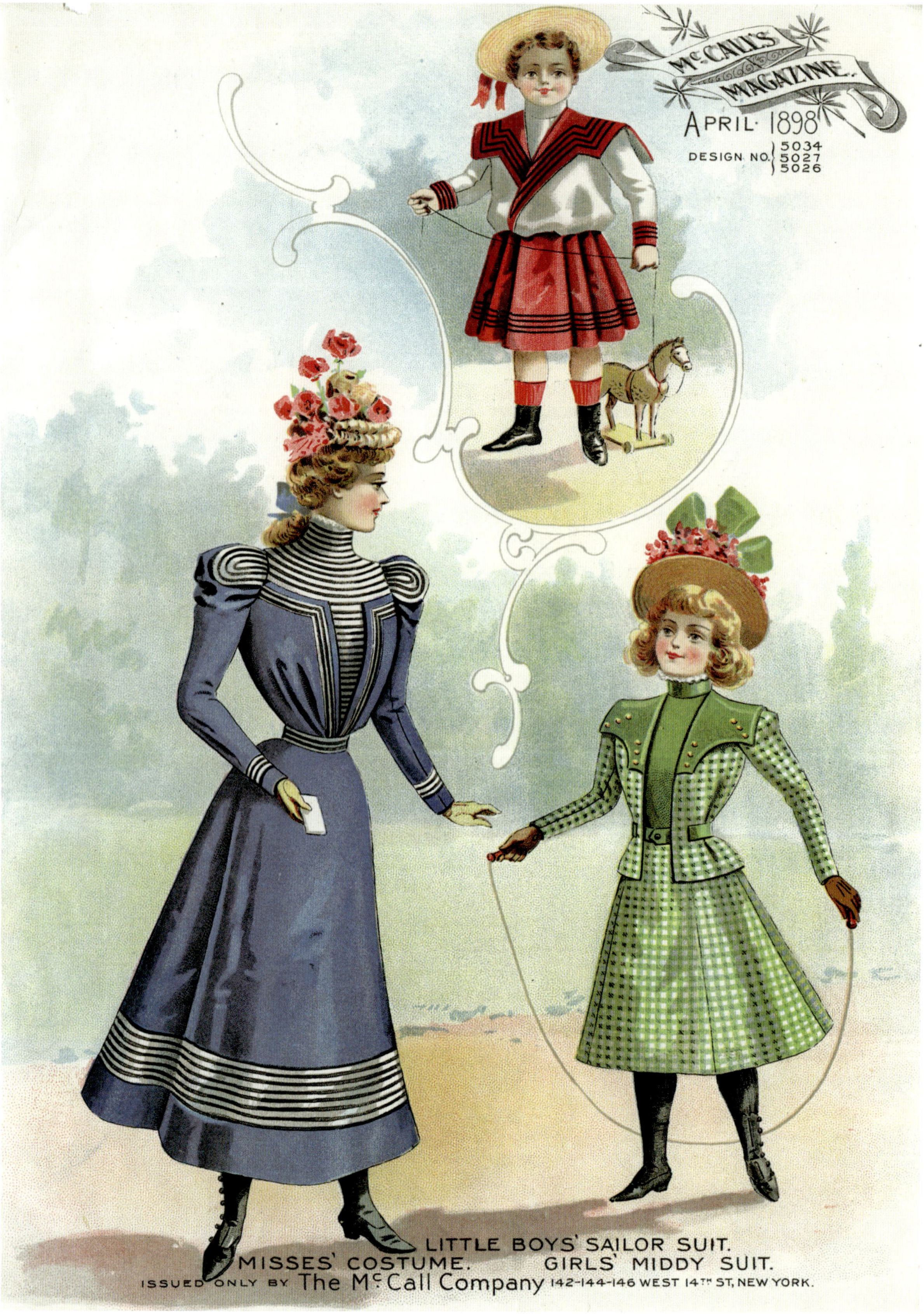

April 1898 fashion plate from the McCall Company featuring a selection of spring styles for boys, girls, and misses.

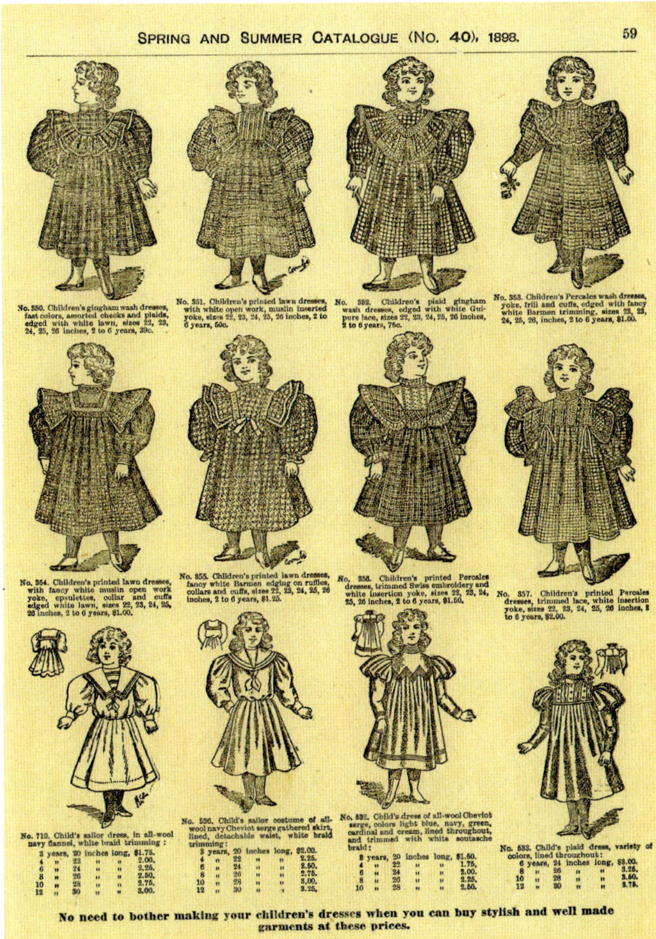
SPRING AND SUMMER CATALOGUE (No. 40), 1898.
59
No need to bother making your children's dresses when you can buy stylish and well made garments at these prices.

This page from the 1898 Eaton's mail order catalog shows a variety of gingham, percale, cheviot serge, and cotton lawn children's dresses, the billowing skirts of which emanate from ruffled epaulettes above giant puffy sleeves. Puffy-sleeved sailor dresses are also on display. *Eaton's Spring and Summer Catalogue*, 1898.

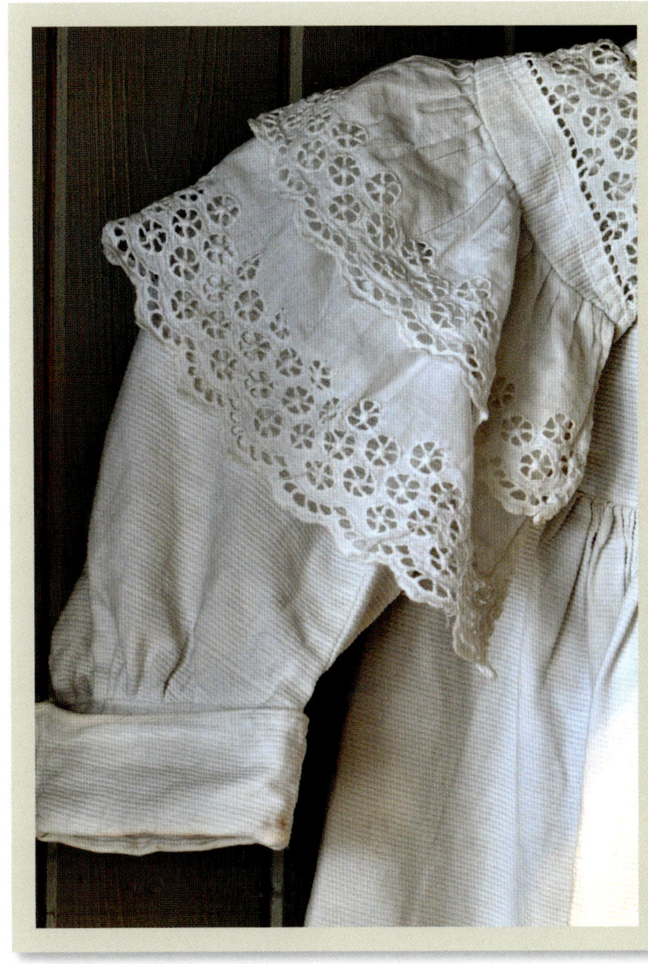

This ribbed cotton coat with mother-of-pearl buttons features beautifully embellished puffed sleeves. It hangs in a vintage shop window over a century after it was first worn.

outfits of linen, cotton piqué, or a lustrous galatea were worn over woolen undergarments. Considered a novelty at the time, linen crash fabrics were particularly suited to children's clothing, as they could be obtained in stripes or plains. These lent themselves nicely to the application of embroidery, particularly cross-stitch.

Visual interest was achieved through a contrast of textures and colors: tobacco-colored crash with red and black cross-stitching, crisp white collars and turn-back cuffs against pastel blue or green galatea, soft creamy cashmere or flannel paired with open mesh linen or rustling taffetas. With the addition of embroidery and buttons, the opportunities to personalize a garment were endless.

It was a time to see and be seen in weighty textiles—rich velvets, brocades, and cashmeres in plush white, buff, chocolate brown. Combinations such as yellow with blue, and black with red, were popular for both genders, as were pale yellows, blues, and pinks trimmed with white or cream.

Cloaks in children's and misses' sizes were often indistinguishable from those designed for grown women. Detachable cape versions came in a number of styles, including Albany, Cambridge, and Mable, a back-pleated number with circular cape. Rubber-lined 'waterproofs' also made the scene.

Toward the end of the 1890s, as women's fashion shifted its focus from the skirt to the bodice, elevating sleeve-heads, fashioning stand-up collars, widening sleeves, and narrowing skirt silhouettes, so too did children's fashion succeed in drawing the eye to the head and shoulders, relying on large neck bows, square collars, and loose, jacketed blouses in the case of boys' wear.

Through the use of underpads, lace ruffles, gathering stitches, or all three, dressmakers were able to achieve the look

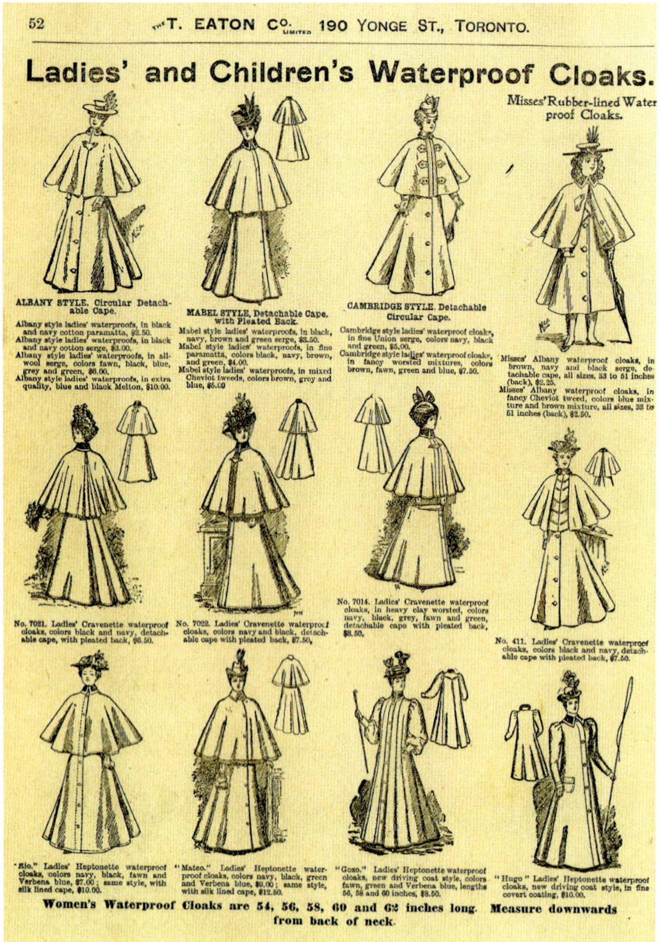

Children's and misses' warm weather cloaks shown with identical styles for ladies. *Eaton's Spring and Summer Catalogue*, 1898.

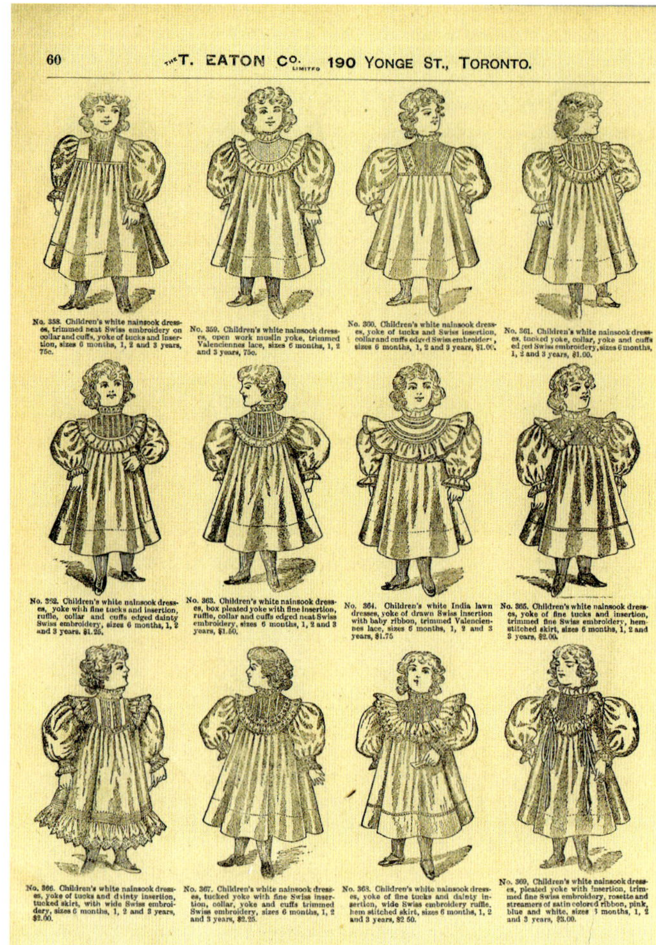

Twelve carefully drawn sketches from the 1898 Eaton's catalog advertising yoked and billowing children's dresses, all of Nainsook. *Eaton's Spring and Summer Catalogue*, 1898.

of a heightened or broadened shoulder while maintaining a narrow sleeve. And what was fashionable for mother was *de rigeur* for young girls. Reefer jackets in red, cardinal, fawn, tan, green, or navy box cloth dramatized the shoulders and sleeve caps. Exaggerated collars extending beyond the sleeve caps were further enhanced with parallel rows of braid trim, creating a power shoulder not seen in fashion again until the 1980s.

Elizabeth Robinson Scovil, writing for the *Ladies' Home Journal* in September 1898, reported on the popularity of sailor collars on shirtwaists for girls from six to fourteen years of age, advising they could be cut in square tabs or points in front and trimmed with ruffles or lace insertion. She suggested they be fashioned from Persian lawn, pink or blue chambray, brown linen, white piqué, white, pink or blue dimity, or fine gingham.

Skirt lengths were strictly prescribed for girls of various ages, with queries on the subject often addressed in correspondence columns. "The skirts of a girl of thirteen would reach to her ankles," wrote advice columnist Isabel A. Mallon in the October 1894 issue of the *Ladies' Home Journal.* For girls eight to twelve years old, skirt lengths began halfway between the ankle and the knee, gradually falling to the ankle as the child matured.

Boys' breeches appeared short and boxy, as did their jackets, which, consistent with styles for women, were decorated with buttons and applied braid in contrast colors. A few brave young souls also wore the fashionably large-shouldered knicker suits.

Sturdy, high-top leather boots were *de rigeur* for young boys of this period. Fashioned from black leather and buttoning up the side, they differed very little from styles designed for adult men.

Outerwear cloaks for both genders were fashioned from wool, cashmere, or silk, depending upon the season. Durable fabrics such as krimmer, serge, corduroy, and tweed were favored in winter.

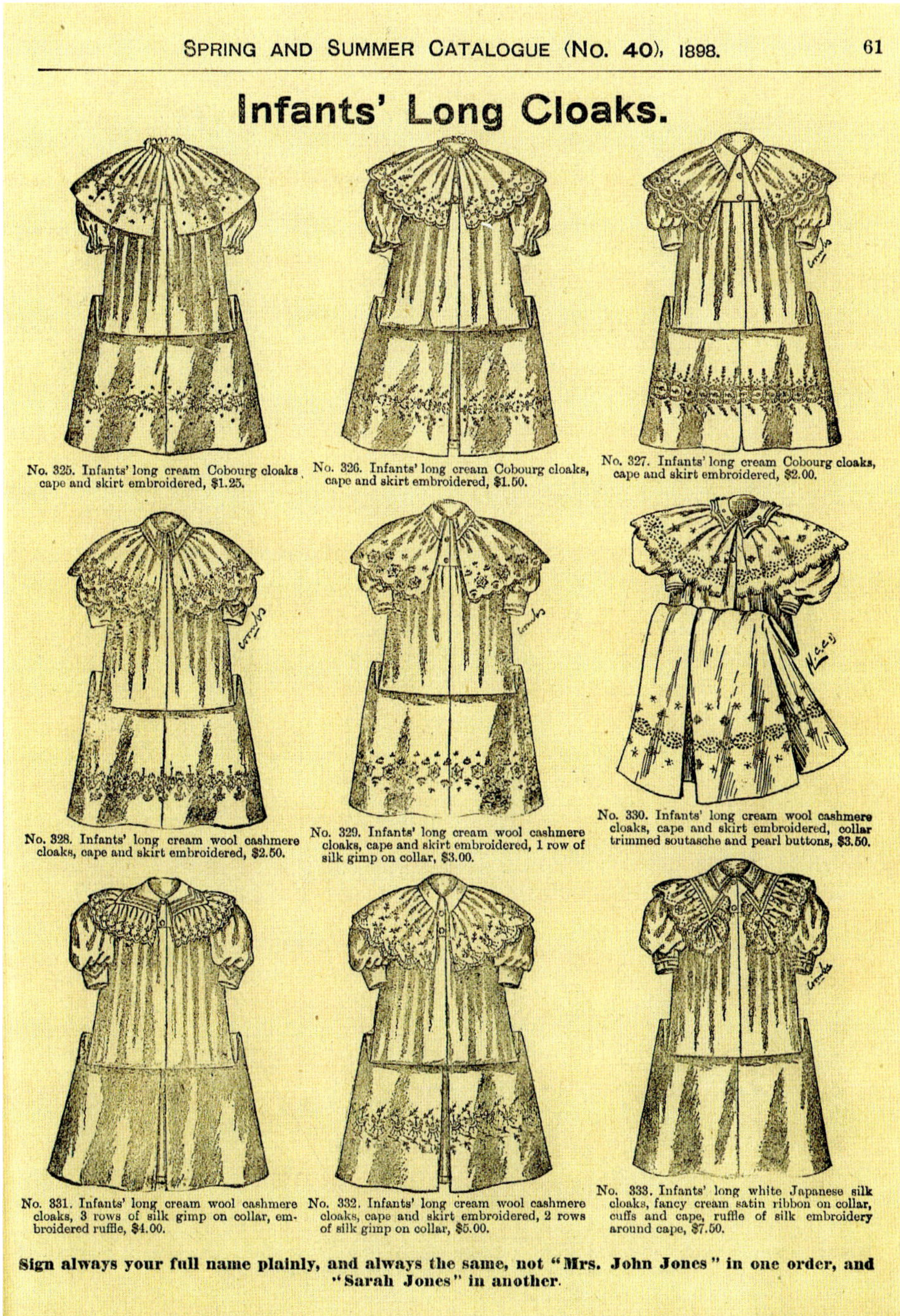

SPRING AND SUMMER CATALOGUE (NO. 40), 1898. 61

Infants' Long Cloaks.

No. 325. Infants' long cream Cobourg cloaks, cape and skirt embroidered, $1.25.

No. 326. Infants' long cream Cobourg cloaks, cape and skirt embroidered, $1.50.

No. 327. Infants' long cream Cobourg cloaks, cape and skirt embroidered, $2.00.

No. 328. Infants' long cream wool cashmere cloaks, cape and skirt embroidered, $2.50.

No. 329. Infants' long cream wool cashmere cloaks, cape and skirt embroidered, 1 row of silk gimp on collar, $3.00.

No. 330. Infants' long cream wool cashmere cloaks, cape and skirt embroidered, collar trimmed soutasche and pearl buttons, $3.50.

No. 331. Infants' long cream wool cashmere cloaks, 3 rows of silk gimp on collar, embroidered ruffle, $4.00.

No. 332. Infants' long cream wool cashmere cloaks, cape and skirt embroidered, 2 rows of silk gimp on collar, $5.00.

No. 333. Infants' long white Japanese silk cloaks, fancy cream satin ribbon on collar, cuffs and cape, ruffle of silk embroidery around cape, $7.50.

Sign always your full name plainly, and always the same, not "Mrs. John Jones" in one order, and "Sarah Jones" in another.

A selection of infants' silk and cashmere cloaks with various embroidery patterns and lace trims.

In 1898, the fashion for all-in-one caped cloaks had Canadian mothers turning to *Eaton's* catalog for inspiration. Though the general form was the same, individual examples were distinguished from one another through the decorative treatments applied to them, be they ruffles, embroidery, ribbon, or button detail. School girls kept their long hair tied in ribbons to match either their dress or its trimmings.

A young girl's clothing might be made at home of the same fabric as that chosen for her mother or for some household item, but dresses purchased from a retailer might be patterned with figurals of animals, or even children playing. Whatever the motif, the style elements mimicked that of fashionable women's wear (i.e., leg-o-mutton sleeves, self-fabric collars with contrast lace trim, empire waistlines, and delicate mother-of-pearl buttons).

Lace, ribbon banding, satin bows, heart-shaped pockets, smocking, and/or double ruffle sleeve hems added distinction to party dresses; but as in previous years, an ensemble was not complete without its coordinating hat.

Children's Reefer Jackets.

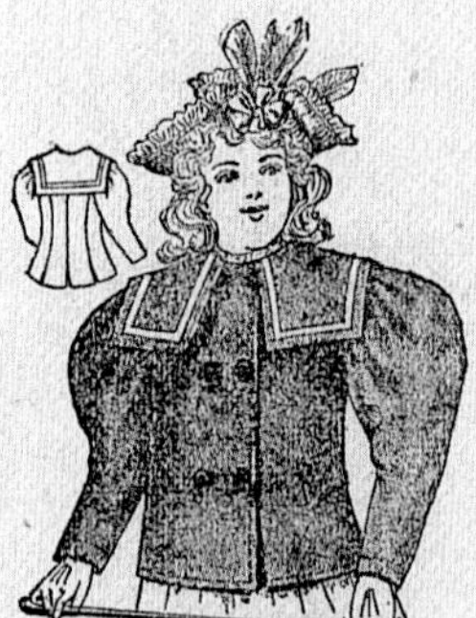

No. 300. Children's reefers of navy union serge, sailor collar, trimmed with white braid, sizes 2 to 6 years, $1.00.

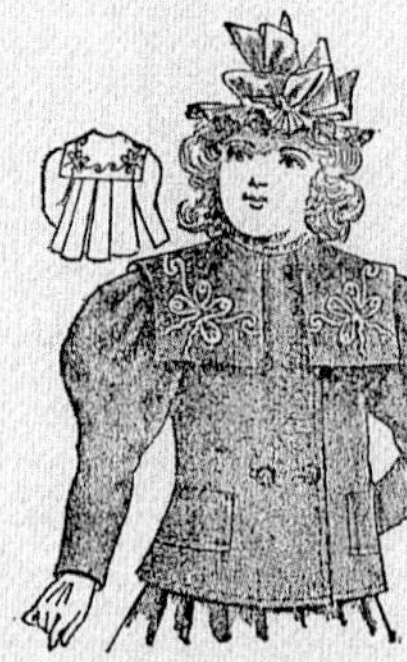

No. 301. **Children's all-wool** cloth reefers, in navy, red and cadet, sailor collar, white braid embroidered, Empire back, sizes 2 to 6 years, $1.25.

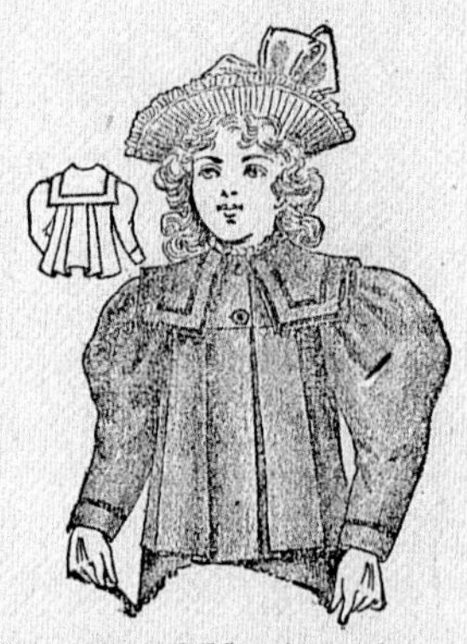

No. 302. Children's reefers in all-wool cloth, navy, red, bluette and green, 2 rows of black braid on sailor collar, Empire back and front, sizes 2 to 6 years, $1.50.

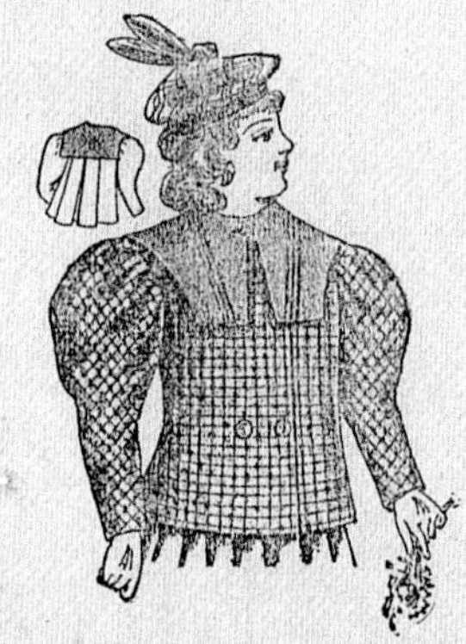

No. 303. Children's reefers of all-wool check boucle tweed, with braided plain cloth collars, colors red and bluette, sizes 2 to 6 years, $1.50.

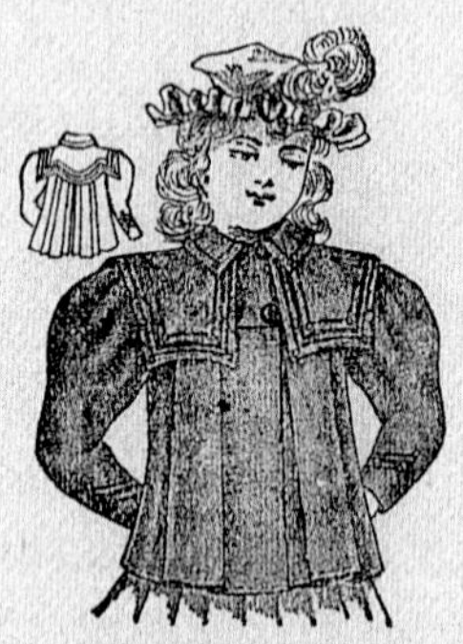

No. 304. Children's all-wool plain cloth reefers, colors navy, red and cadet, white mohair braid trimmed, roll collar, Empire front and back, sizes 2 to 6 years, $1.75.

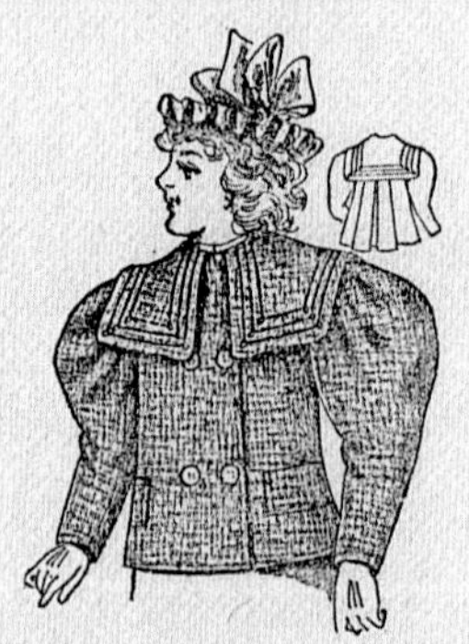

No. 305. Children's reefers of all-wool fancy tweed, brown soutaschè braid trimming, sizes 2 to 6 years, $2.00.

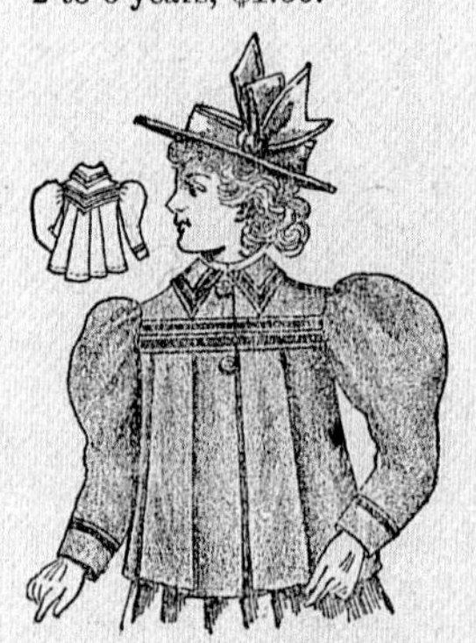

No. 306. Children's reefers of all-wool plain cloth, colors red and bluette, sizes 2 to 6 years, $2.25.

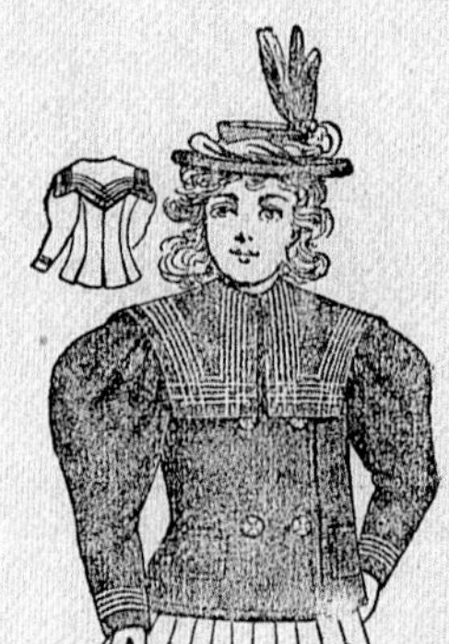

No. 307. Children's reefers of all-wool plain cloth, colors cardinal, green and bluette, pointed sailor collar, trimmed with white soutasche braid, pearl buttons, sizes 2 to 6 years, $2.50.

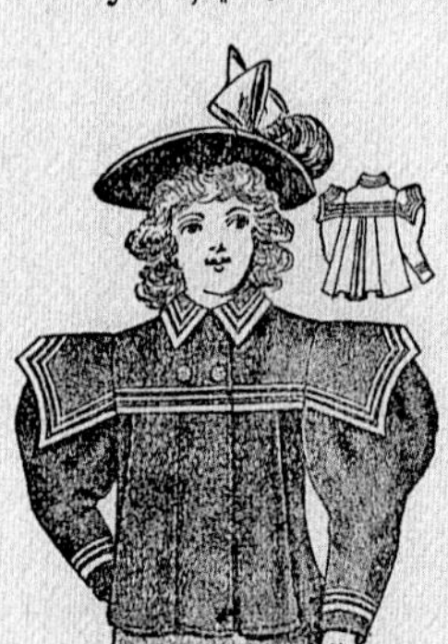

No. 308. Children's all-wool plain cloth reefers, colors navy, cardinal and light blue, white braid and pearl button trimming, sizes 2 to 6 years, $2.50.

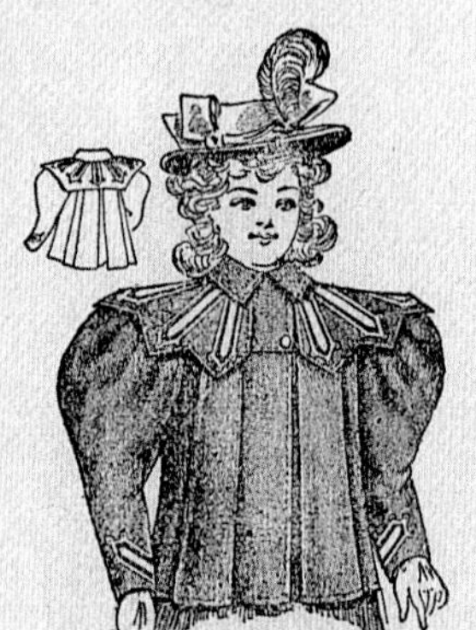

No. 309. Children's reefers of all-wool plain cloth, colors green, light blue and red, fancy pointed sailor collar, trimmed with white braid and pearl buttons, sizes 2 to 6 years, $3.00.

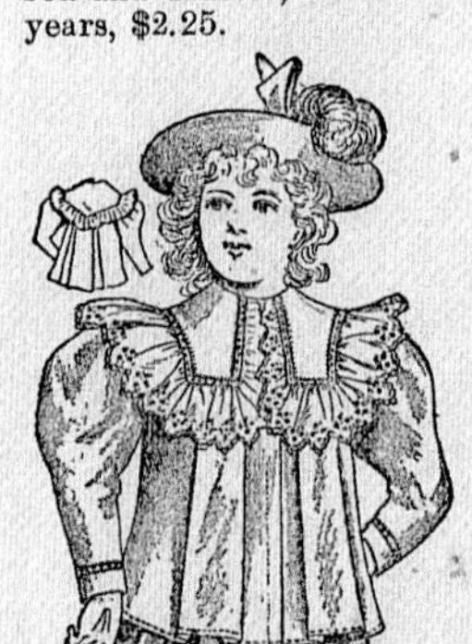

No. 310. Child's white pique wash reefer, deep collar, trimmed with Swiss embroidery edge, fancy braid on collar and cuffs, Empire style, sizes 1, 2, 3 and 4 years, $1.35.

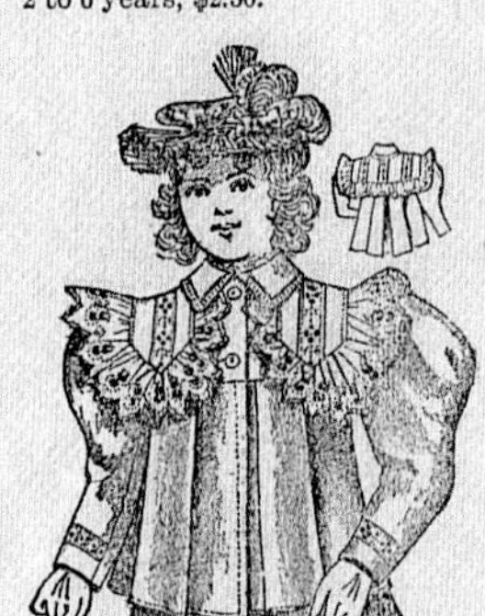

No. 311. Child's white pique reefer, roll collar, trimmed with fancy braid, deep sailor collar, with 3 rows of Swiss insertion and edged with embroidery, embroidery insertion on cuffs, Empire style, sizes 1, 2, 3 and 4 years, $1.75.

SIZES of all garments should be clearly stated, also size of boots, gloves, hats, etc.

Children's summer reefers. *Eaton's Spring and Summer Catalogue*, 1898.

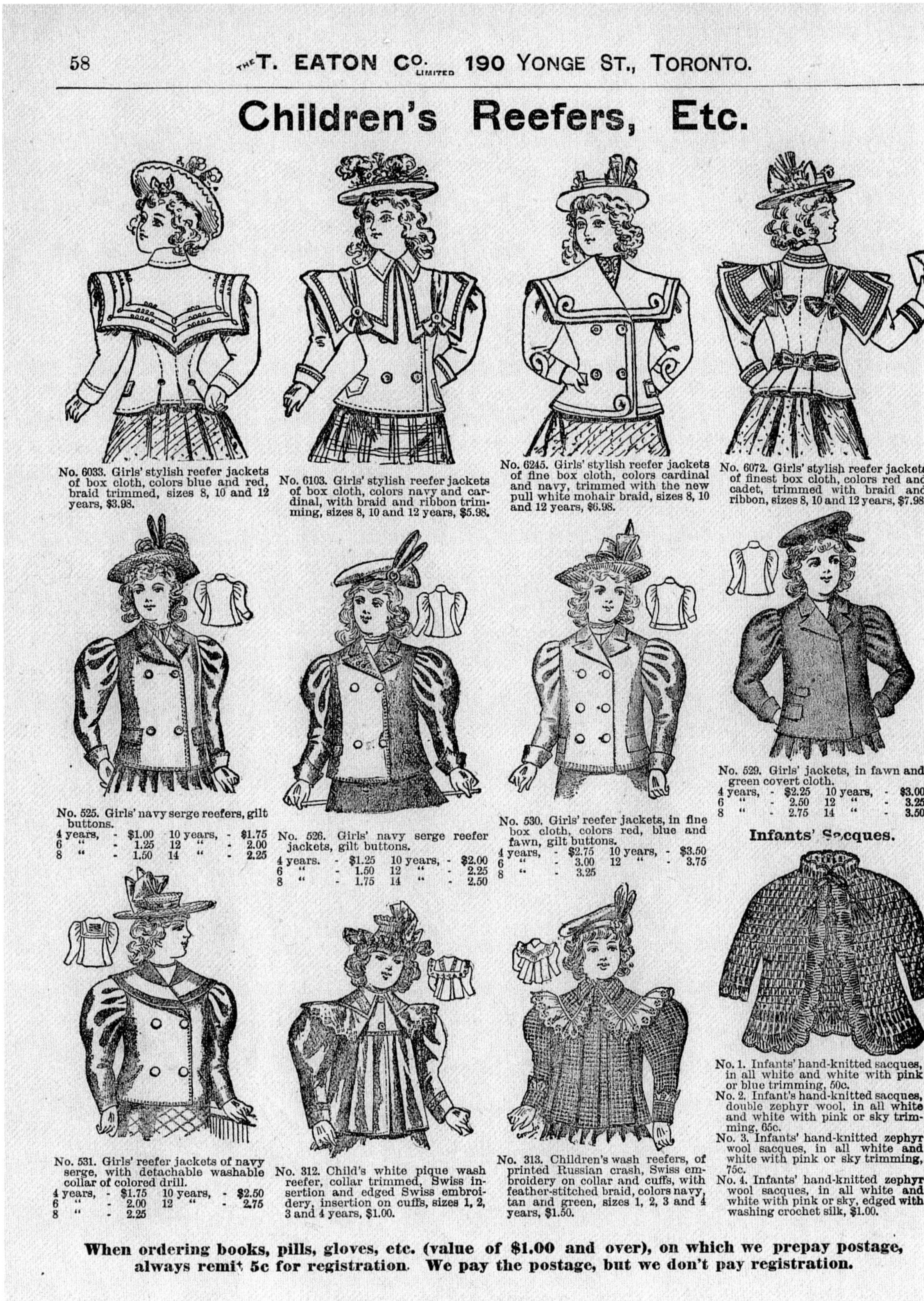

58 THE T. EATON Co. LIMITED 190 YONGE ST., TORONTO.

Children's Reefers, Etc.

No. 6033. Girls' stylish reefer jackets of box cloth, colors blue and red, braid trimmed, sizes 8, 10 and 12 years, $3.98.

No. 6103. Girls' stylish reefer jackets of box cloth, colors navy and cardinal, with braid and ribbon trimming, sizes 8, 10 and 12 years, $5.98.

No. 6245. Girls' stylish reefer jackets of fine box cloth, colors cardinal and navy, trimmed with the new pull white mohair braid, sizes 8, 10 and 12 years, $6.98.

No. 6072. Girls' stylish reefer jackets of finest box cloth, colors red and cadet, trimmed with braid and ribbon, sizes 8, 10 and 12 years, $7.98.

No. 525. Girls' navy serge reefers, gilt buttons.

4 years,	- $1.00	10 years,	- $1.75
6 "	- 1.25	12 "	- 2.00
8 "	- 1.50	14 "	- 2.25

No. 526. Girls' navy serge reefer jackets, gilt buttons.

4 years.	- $1.25	10 years,	- $2.00
6 "	- 1.50	12 "	- 2.25
8 "	- 1.75	14 "	- 2.50

No. 530. Girls' reefer jackets, in fine box cloth, colors red, blue and fawn, gilt buttons.

4 years,	- $2.75	10 years,	- $3.50
6 "	- 3.00	12 "	- 3.75
8 "	- 3.25		

No. 529. Girls' jackets, in fawn and green covert cloth.

4 years,	- $2.25	10 years,	- $3.00
6 "	- 2.50	12 "	- 3.25
8 "	- 2.75	14 "	- 3.50

Infants' Sacques.

No. 531. Girls' reefer jackets of navy serge, with detachable washable collar of colored drill.

4 years,	- $1.75	10 years,	- $2.50
6 "	- 2.00	12 "	- 2.75
8 "	- 2.25		

No. 312. Child's white pique wash reefer, collar trimmed, Swiss insertion and edged Swiss embroidery, insertion on cuffs, sizes 1, 2, 3 and 4 years, $1.00.

No. 313. Children's wash reefers, of printed Russian crash, Swiss embroidery on collar and cuffs, with feather-stitched braid, colors navy, tan and green, sizes 1, 2, 3 and 4 years, $1.50.

No. 1. Infants' hand-knitted sacques, in all white and white with pink or blue trimming, 50c.
No. 2. Infant's hand-knitted sacques, double zephyr wool, in all white and white with pink or sky trimming, 65c.
No. 3. Infants' hand-knitted zephyr wool sacques, in all white and white with pink or sky trimming, 75c.
No. 4. Infants' hand-knitted zephyr wool sacques, in all white and white with pink or sky, edged with washing crochet silk, $1.00.

When ordering books, pills, gloves, etc. (value of $1.00 and over), on which we prepay postage, always remit 5c for registration. We pay the postage, but we don't pay registration.

Hats and Bonnets

"In selecting a hat, especially when it is one that is to be developed in an artistic way, it is wisest to buy the largest felt hat untrimmed and bend it to suit the face, cutting the brim if it is needed."—Isabel A. Mallon, *Ladies' Home Journal,* October 1894

"A young baby going out-of-doors in the winter should have a worsted Shetland veil over its face. One can be purchased for from twenty-five to fifty cents. White is the best color. Veils can be injurious as soon as a child begins to use its eyes, as the effort to see through the meshes strains them."—Elizabeth Robinson Scovil, *Ladies' Home Journal,* October 1896

On the subject of millinery, magazine advice columnists doled out their share of dress reform guidance. In regard to the long-standing practice that girls' hats be held in place with tight inner banding, *Ladies' Home Journal* scribe Elizabeth Scovil directed mothers to remove the rubber insert and instead secure the hat with ribbon ties. She stepped further into their business with the comment, "You will make it impossible for a careless nurse to put the rubber band behind

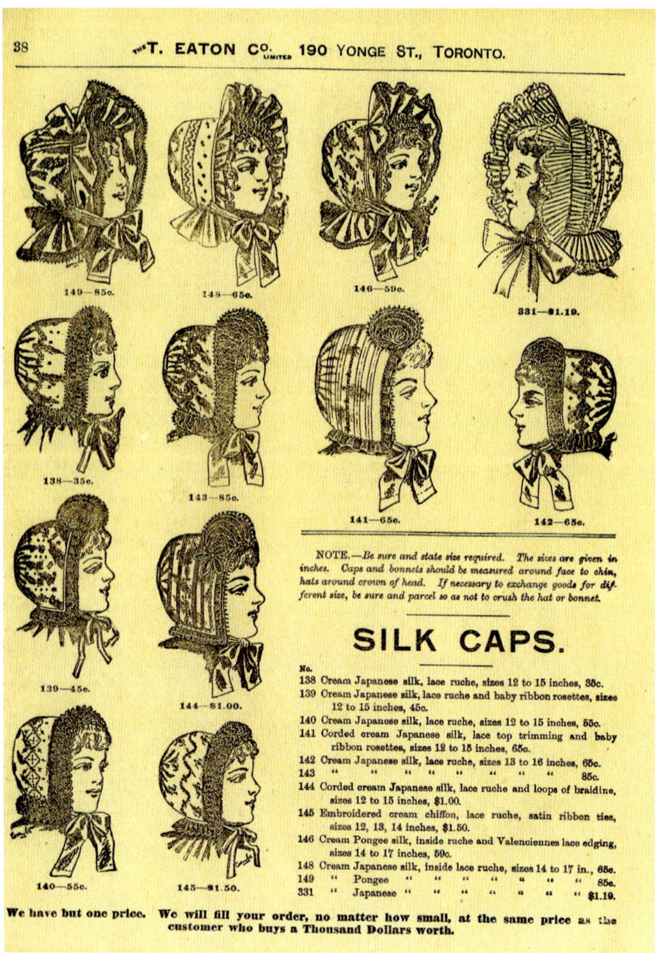

38 THE T. EATON CO. LIMITED 190 YONGE ST., TORONTO.

NOTE.—*Be sure and state size required. The sizes are given in inches. Caps and bonnets should be measured around face to chin, hats around crown of head. If necessary to exchange goods for different size, be sure and parcel so as not to crush the hat or bonnet.*

SILK CAPS.

No.
138 Cream Japanese silk, lace ruche, sizes 12 to 15 inches, 35c.
139 Cream Japanese silk, lace ruche and baby ribbon rosettes, sizes 12 to 15 inches, 45c.
140 Cream Japanese silk, lace ruche, sizes 12 to 15 inches, 55c.
141 Corded cream Japanese silk, lace top trimming and baby ribbon rosettes, sizes 12 to 15 inches, 65c.
142 Cream Japanese silk, lace ruche, sizes 13 to 16 inches, 65c.
143 " " " " " " " " 85c.
144 Corded cream Japanese silk, lace ruche and loops of braidine, sizes 12 to 15 inches, $1.00.
145 Embroidered cream chiffon, lace ruche, satin ribbon ties, sizes 12, 13, 14 inches, $1.50.
146 Cream Pongee silk, inside ruche and Valenciennes lace edging, sizes 14 to 17 inches, 59c.
148 Cream Japanese silk, inside lace ruche, sizes 14 to 17 in., 65c.
149 " Pongee " " " " " " " 85c.
331 " Japanese " " " " " " " $1.19.

We have but one price. We will fill your order, no matter how small, at the same price as the customer who buys a Thousand Dollars worth.

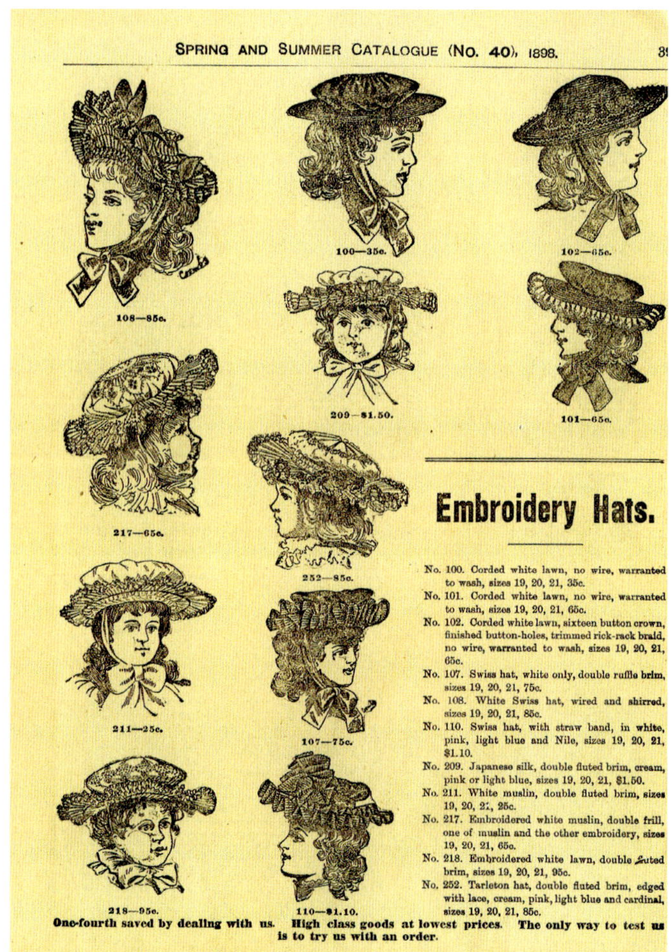

SPRING AND SUMMER CATALOGUE (NO. 40), 1898. 39

Embroidery Hats.

No. 100. Corded white lawn, no wire, warranted to wash, sizes 19, 20, 21, 35c.
No. 101. Corded white lawn, no wire, warranted to wash, sizes 19, 20, 21, 65c.
No. 102. Corded white lawn, sixteen button crown, finished button-holes, trimmed rick-rack braid, no wire, warranted to wash, sizes 19, 20, 21, 65c.
No. 107. Swiss hat, white only, double ruffle brim, sizes 19, 20, 21, 75c.
No. 108. White Swiss hat, wired and shirred, sizes 19, 20, 21, 85c.
No. 110. Swiss hat, with straw band, in white, pink, light blue and Nile, sizes 19, 20, 21, $1.10.
No. 209. Japanese silk, double fluted brim, cream, pink or light blue, sizes 19, 20, 21, $1.50.
No. 211. White muslin, double fluted brim, sizes 19, 20, 21, 25c.
No. 217. Embroidered white muslin, double frill, one of muslin and the other embroidery, sizes 19, 20, 21, 65c.
No. 218. Embroidered white lawn, double fluted brim, sizes 19, 20, 21, 95c.
No. 252. Tarleton hat, double fluted brim, edged with lace, cream, pink, light blue and cardinal, sizes 19, 20, 21, 85c.

One-fourth saved by dealing with us. High class goods at lowest prices. The only way to test us is to try us with an order.

Various styles and fabrications of misses' and children's hats and bonnets. *Eaton's Spring and Summer Catalogue,* 1898.

her ears and so cause them to lose their shape *Ladies' Home Journal*, October 1896)." Veils for children remained in vogue despite warnings that they may be injurious to young eyes.

As with dresses, hats selected for female children varied in style according to age groups. By mid-decade, girls twelve to fourteen years of age were wearing very small hats trimmed with large ribbon bows, while the high Normandy bonnets and very large hats trimmed with drooping plumes held with sparkling buckles were reserved for preschoolers. Babies' bonnets were equally large, arguably to provide shade in summer. Round turbans were chosen for older girls. The novel close-fitting Dutch cap, devoid of trimming, was advertised as keeping "the most sensitive parts of the head warm and comfortable, driving away many an attack of earache and toothache (*Ladies' Home Journal*, October 1896)."

Winter hats for outdoor play and skating parties were often hand-knit at home in a bonnet style with pompom decorations and plaited wool ties. Matching mittens kept little hands warm.

Church and other formal winter occasions called for more luxurious fabrics such as velvet or embroidered wool. These were fashioned into simple head-hugging bonnet styles that were either purchased or machine stitched at home. Contrast ribbon ties and silk linings or edgings added decorative interest.

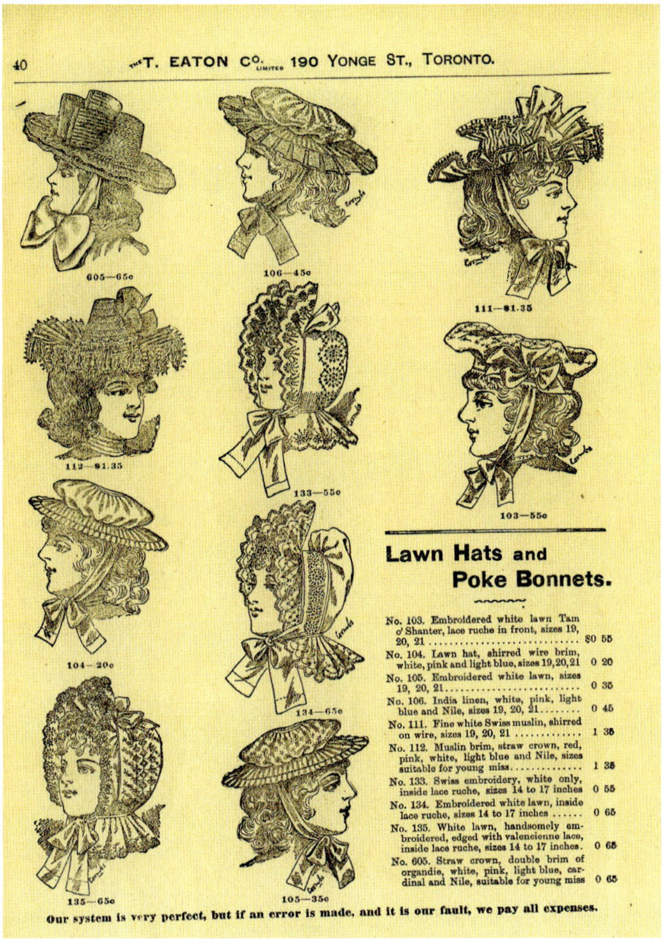
40 THE T. EATON CO. LIMITED 190 YONGE ST., TORONTO.

605—65c 106—45c 111—$1.35 112—$1.35 133—55c 103—55c 104—20c 134—65c 135—65c 105—35c

Lawn Hats and Poke Bonnets.

No. 103. Embroidered white lawn Tam o' Shanter, lace ruche in front, sizes 19, 20, 21	$0 55
No. 104. Lawn hat, shirred wire brim, white, pink and light blue, sizes 19, 20, 21	0 20
No. 105. Embroidered white lawn, sizes 19, 20, 21	0 35
No. 106. India linen, white, pink, light blue and Nile, sizes 19, 20, 21	0 45
No. 111. Fine white Swiss muslin, shirred on wire, sizes 19, 20, 21	1 35
No. 112. Muslin brim, straw crown, red, pink, white, light blue and Nile, sizes suitable for young miss	1 35
No. 133. Swiss embroidery, white only, inside lace ruche, sizes 14 to 17 inches	0 55
No. 134. Embroidered white lawn, inside lace ruche, sizes 14 to 17 inches	0 65
No. 135. White lawn, handsomely embroidered, edged with valencienne lace, inside lace ruche, sizes 14 to 17 inches	0 65
No. 605. Straw crown, double brim of organdie, white, pink, light blue, cardinal and Nile, suitable for young miss	0 65

Our system is very perfect, but if an error is made, and it is our fault, we pay all expenses.

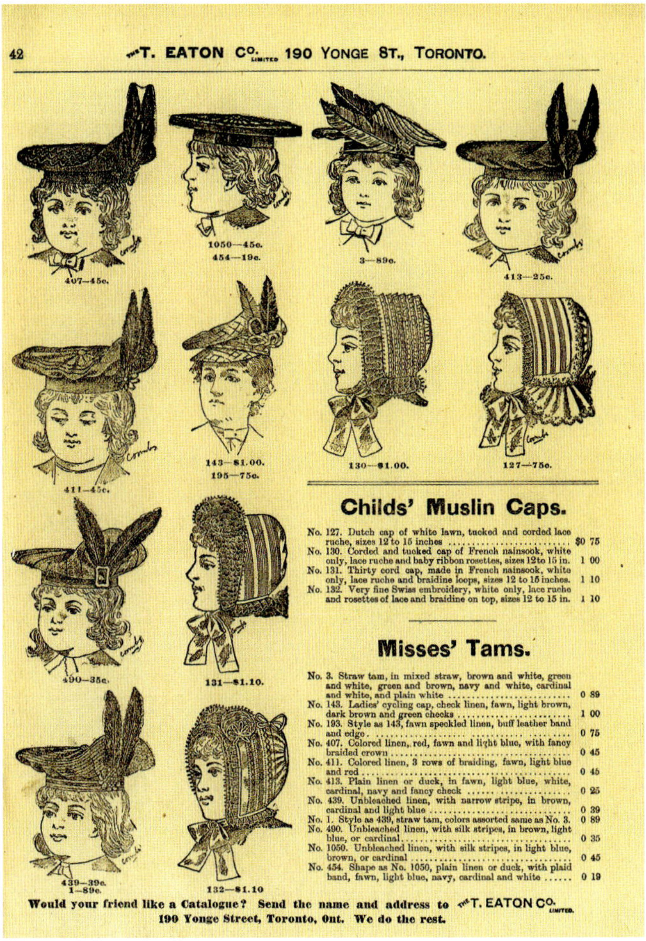
42 THE T. EATON CO. LIMITED 190 YONGE ST., TORONTO.

407—45c. 1050—45c. 454—19c. 3—89c. 413—25c. 411—45c. 143—$1.00. 193—75c. 130—$1.00. 127—75c. 490—35c. 131—$1.10. 439—39c. 1—89c. 132—$1.10

Childs' Muslin Caps.

No. 127. Dutch cap of white lawn, tucked and corded lace ruche, sizes 12 to 15 inches	$0 75
No. 130. Corded and tucked cap of French nainsook, white only, lace ruche and baby ribbon rosettes, sizes 12 to 15 in.	1 00
No. 131. Thirty cord cap, made in French nainsook, white only, lace ruche and braidine loops, sizes 12 to 15 inches.	1 10
No. 132. Very fine Swiss embroidery, white only, lace ruche and rosettes of lace and braidine on top, sizes 12 to 15 in.	1 10

Misses' Tams.

No. 3. Straw tam, in mixed straw, brown and white, green and white, green and brown, navy and white, cardinal and white, and plain white	0 89
No. 143. Ladies' cycling cap, check linen, fawn, light brown, dark brown and green checks	1 00
No. 193. Style as 143, fawn speckled linen, buff leather band and edge	0 75
No. 407. Colored linen, red, fawn and light blue, with fancy braided crown	0 45
No. 411. Colored linen, 3 rows of braiding, fawn, light blue and red	0 45
No. 413. Plain linen or duck, in fawn, light blue, white, cardinal, navy and fancy check	0 25
No. 439. Unbleached linen, with narrow stripe, in brown, cardinal and light blue	0 39
No. 1. Style as 439, straw tam, colors assorted same as No. 3.	0 89
No. 490. Unbleached linen, with silk stripes, in brown, light blue, or cardinal	0 35
No. 1050. Unbleached linen, with silk stripes, in light blue, brown, or cardinal	0 45
No. 454. Shape as No. 1050, plain linen or duck, with plaid band, fawn, light blue, navy, cardinal and white	0 19

Would your friend like a Catalogue? Send the name and address to THE T. EATON CO. LIMITED. 190 Yonge Street, Toronto, Ont. We do the rest.

Home and School

"The clothes necessary for a young girl's school outfit will depend entirely upon the class of school to which she may be going."—Emma M. Hooper, *Ladies' Home Journal,* October 1896

Many a woman's periodical carried patterns for children's everyday wear, serviceable garments that would stand up to harsh treatment and frequent wear. Aprons for girls who wanted to help around the home were simply made with consideration for altering for growth.

When making up school frocks, mothers were advised to create durable aprons without elaborate trimmings. Often the same garment was made up for two or more children. To distinguish ownership, identifying initials would be sewn on the interior of the garment. By the second decade of the twentieth century, seamstresses could purchase strips of initials printed on linen tape for this purpose, saving time and effort.

Sporting Attire

With dress reform came a focus on comfort as well as health. As children participated in sporting and leisure activities, a disdain for woolen materials, popular in the Victorian age, was met with an acceptance of cooler fabrics such as linen for warm weather activities.

For bicycling, special consideration was given to leggings for girls. These were close fitting and made of leather, canvas, corduroy, or plain cloth. In 1898, these cost from between sixty-five cents a pair and two dollars and forty cents a pair.

Although simplicity and comfort were factored into the design of play clothes, so too were style features. Overalls for girls came into fashion at the same time as those for boys, toward the end of the nineteenth century. A small notation in the September 1898 *Ladies' Home Journal* revealed these were made of blue or brown denim and cut almost to the throat in front and equally high in the back. What is most interesting is that they were open to the hip and cut wide enough to accommodate the insertion of skirts.

Undergarments

"If they are properly attended to and sewed securely in place, then tapes are better than buttons for the underwear of little people, but this is something that each mother must decide for herself."—Isabel A. Mallon, *Ladies' Home Journal,* October 1894

Undergarments of wool or cotton were selected for children according to the weather and chosen activity. These included cotton drawers, cotton or flannel petticoats, wool stockings and vests, as well as corset-like waists fitted with garters for the suspension of stockings.

Seasonal accommodations to children's garments were made through the layering or lessoning of undergarments. As always, fashion considerations came first. In the April 1898 issue of *Ladies' Home Journal* columnist Emma Hooper observed, "Baby girls of three years wear white cambric dresses through the winter, with amply warm flannels and very heavy outdoor coats." In summer, a simple cotton dress was preferred with a removable matching guimpe, "so that on very warm days, the little frock may become a low necked one."

By the 1890s, when a fashion for all-white dressing came into vogue, easily made up colored slips in an inexpensive dimity (twenty-five cents a yard) were worn by very young children under frilly white lingerie dresses.

Woven undergarments for children could be purchased at department stores or mail order services, often with incentives such as that offered by the Northwestern Knitting Company, which promised a free miniature doll's undershirt "to every mother stating for how many children she buys underwear (*Ladies' Home Journal*, April 1898)."

Formal Wear

"Many a child has been unhappy because she has been forced to wear a gown, a hat or a coat that is shapeless and ugly. . . . Many of us have known a girl to sulk for hours because she hated her frock, and, though this may seem like a little unhappiness to older people, it means much to those who are young and supersensitive. To love color and to wear a dingy brown when it would have been just as easy to have gotten a red that would have delighted the eyes and sent a glow to the heart seems like nothing, but it is a great deal."—Isabel A. Mallon, *Ladies' Home Journal*, October 1894

Throughout history, fashion designers have drawn inspiration from a number of sources. In 1894, for example, Paris was setting the trend for five- to ten-year-old "little women" to adopt a style for formal wear known as the Charles the Second pelisse, based on that worn by the seventeenth-century British king when he was a boy. The garment was comprised of a coat cut from the shoulders in box pleats reaching beyond the gown to below the ankles. A deep, self-fabric square collar added a regal air to the special occasion garment, as did the cuffed and deeply puffed sleeves. Typically, a self-fabric belt, three-inches in width, was placed under the arms and fastened with a steel buckle. *Ladies' Home Journal* columnist Isabel Mallon suggested the coat be made of gray cashmere trimmed

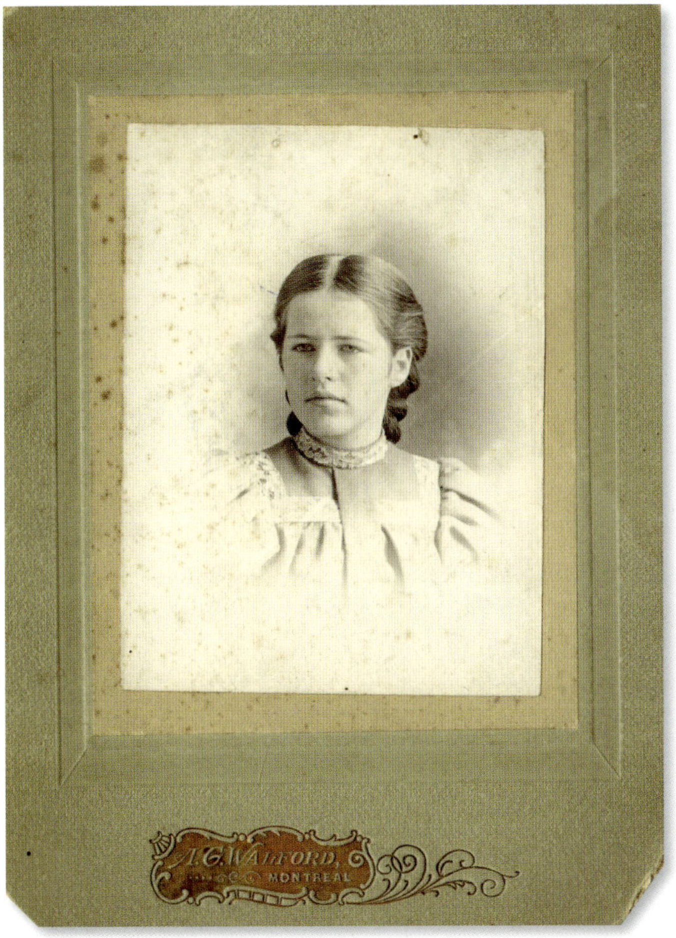

April 1898: Young Mildred Forbes' lace-trimmed bodice is cut in the prevailing style for women and girls of the late 1890s, with large gathers in the sleeve cap and above the bust. A shallow, stand-up collar presides over a lace-banded yoke. Cabinet card by A. G. Walford, Montreal.

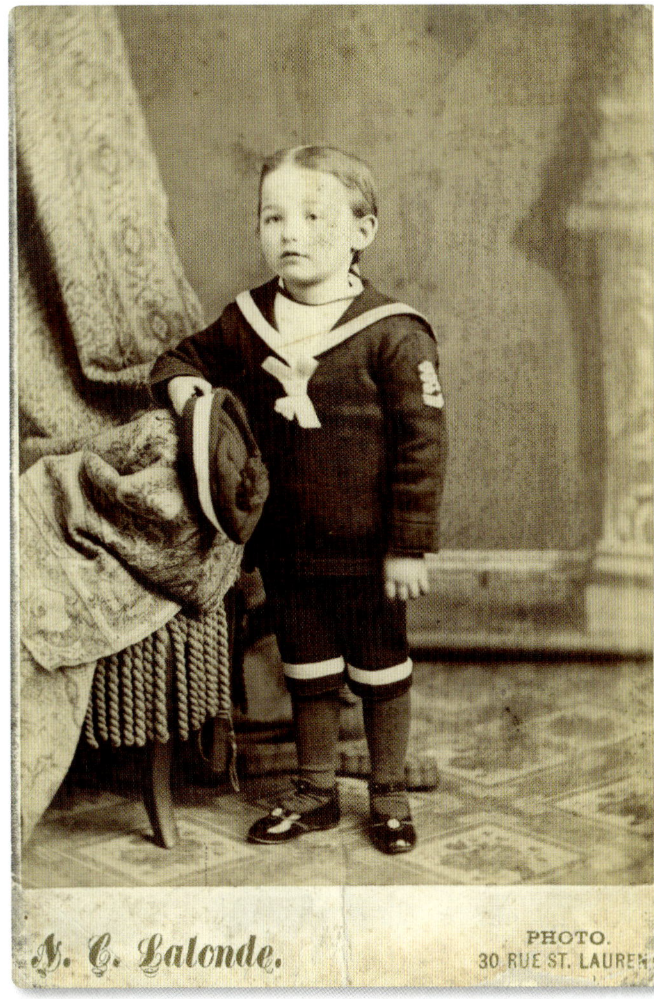

Johnnie Croll, in a nautical suit with matching tam, wears decorated, gender-neutral patent leather ankle straps over his dark stockings. Lalonde Photo Studio, Montreal, Quebec.

at the cuffs with white lace, "unless it is designed for a bridesmaid, in which case white corded silk trimmed with coffee colored lace and a hat of 'dead white' with coffee colored plumes, would be the better choice" (April 1894).

Some four years later, a less complicated design for children's formal occasion wear was sanctioned in the April 1898 issue of *Ladies' Home Journal*. "Frocks of China silk or taffeta, if simply made, are permissible," wrote Emma M. Hooper. "Lace and ribbons are the trimmings used, and the little dresses are worn to weddings, home entertainments, etc."

In keeping with styles for women in the Gay Nineties, children's formal garments featured bishop sleeves, triple- and quadruple-width box-pleated skirts, coachman's cape collars, self-fabric bridal collars, double and triple-layer collars, large, white mother-of-pearl buttons, and wide flouncings on skirts and pinafores.

Season by season, subtle changes in style and ornamentation were reported on in the fashion journals with specific recommendations for girls of different ages. In a column entitled "The Little Girls' Gowns," Isabel Mallon recommended ankle-length yoked dresses of brown scarlet or blue serge with small trimmings of fur or velvet for girls aged six to ten. Mallon sites an example of a scarlet serge gown, its high collar and cuffed full sleeves trimmed with black astrakhan. "In the early autumn, if her underwear were chosen properly, a small girl could wear this frock without an outer wrap, but a little later the wise mother would make, to wear with it, a long coat of the same material trimmed with black fur, and she would, at the same time, remove the black fur from the gown and put black braid in its place (*Ladies' Home Journal*, October 1894)."

Mallon describes a typical gown for a girl of fourteen as a full-skirted olive green wool sateen, plain across the

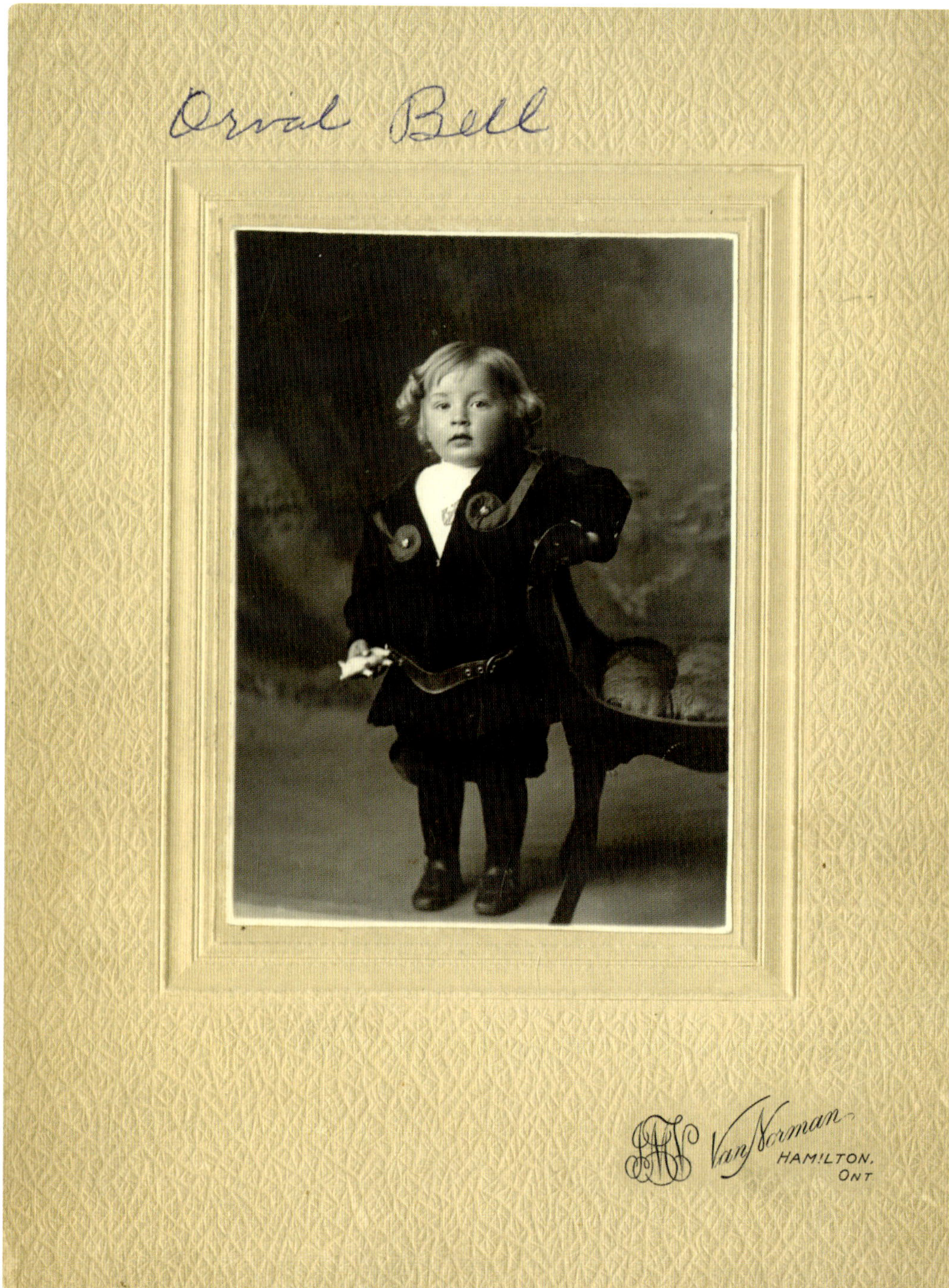

Orval Bell appears overwhelmed in his dark velvet bloomer costume with low-slung belt. The ribbon appliqués, which terminate in frontal rosettes, add interest to what would otherwise be a nondescript jacket.

front and lain in coarse gathers in the back. A high-collared round bodice with full sleeves is arranged in front in folds with revers to provide a vest effect. A three-inch-wide olive ribbon bands the waist to hang long and straight in back. Black stockings, shoes, and a black cloth coat complete the ensemble. "In the very cold weather a small black muff will be carried and black undressed kid gloves will be worn."

Evening dress for boys was given equal consideration. Especially popular toward the end of the nineteenth century were the Eton suit and the tuxedo suit; the former was comprised of a high buttoned vest, long trousers, and a short jacket; the latter was designed with a rolling collar, short trousers, and a low-cut waistcoat, the collar and lining of which was to be fashioned of silk.

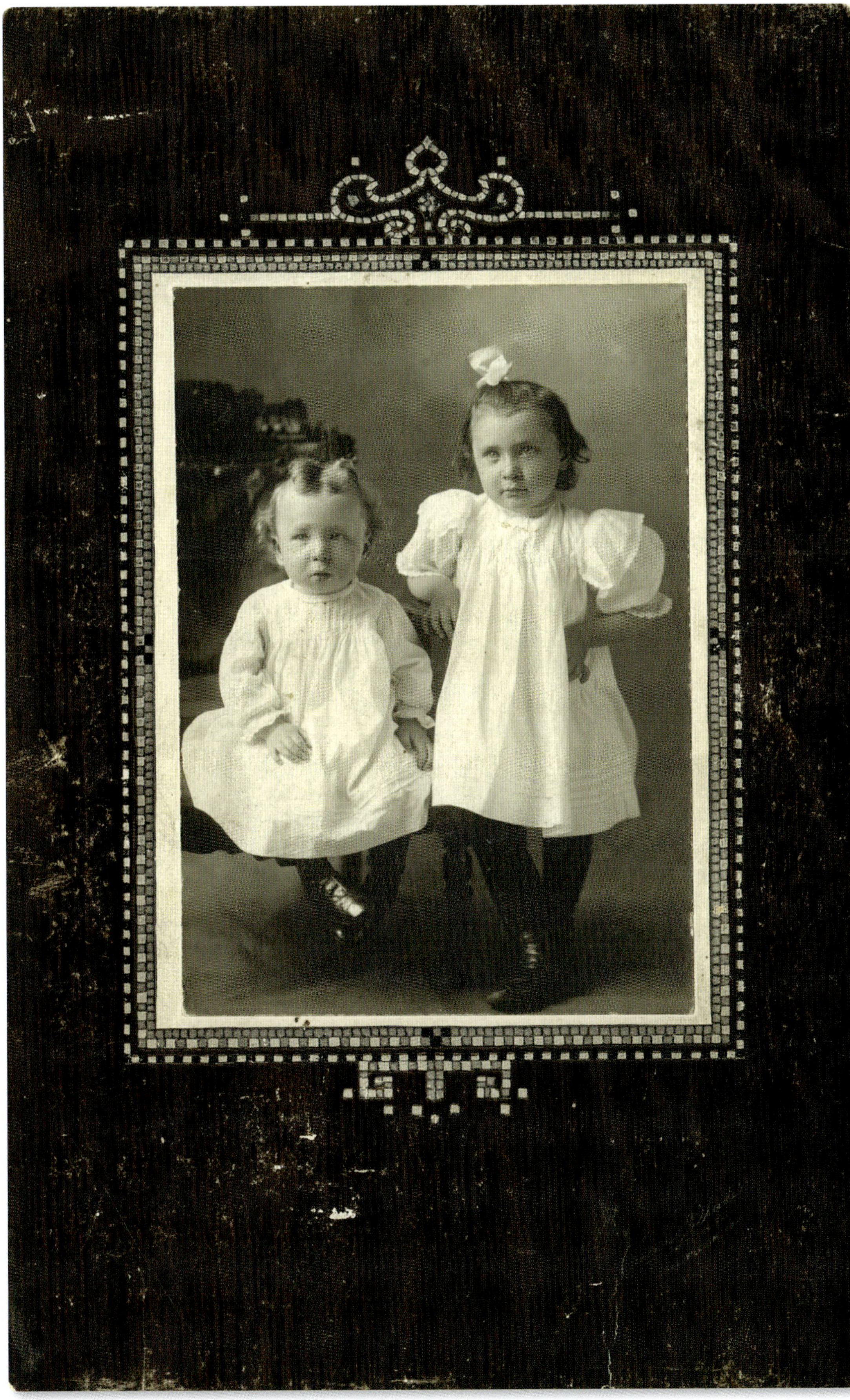

A pair of sassy tots in white cotton gowns, dark stockings, and leather shoes.

Shoes

"The wrinkled shapelessness of a baby's shoe, creased into numberless wrinkles by the restless little foot, is the only thing in footwear that is sweeter and dearer for being worn."—Robert F. Burdette, *Ladies' Home Journal*, April 1898

"Everything that a child wears should be firmly fastened, for nothing will make her so unhappy as to find that she is coming undone. Allow her shoes to be a little large, giving the foot a chance to grow."—Isabel A. Mallon, *Ladies' Home Journal*, October 1894

In an October 1894 issue of *Ladies' Home Journal*, Isabel A. Mallon advised mothers to select laced footwear for their daughters over those that button, because "the lacings will permit the boot to be easy in fit or not, as is most comfortable." Questions regarding the proper use of rubber boots for children were also addressed in the popular periodical. Then, as now, rubber boots were clumsy when worn over shoes, and mothers were advised that lamb's wool insoles could be worn inside the boots in place of shoes. Care was to be taken, however, that children should not wear their rubber boots in the house or while sitting in school. "The moisture from the perspiration cannot escape through the rubber and the feet become damp," argued *Ladies' Home Journal* columnist Elizabeth Robinson Scovil in October 1894.

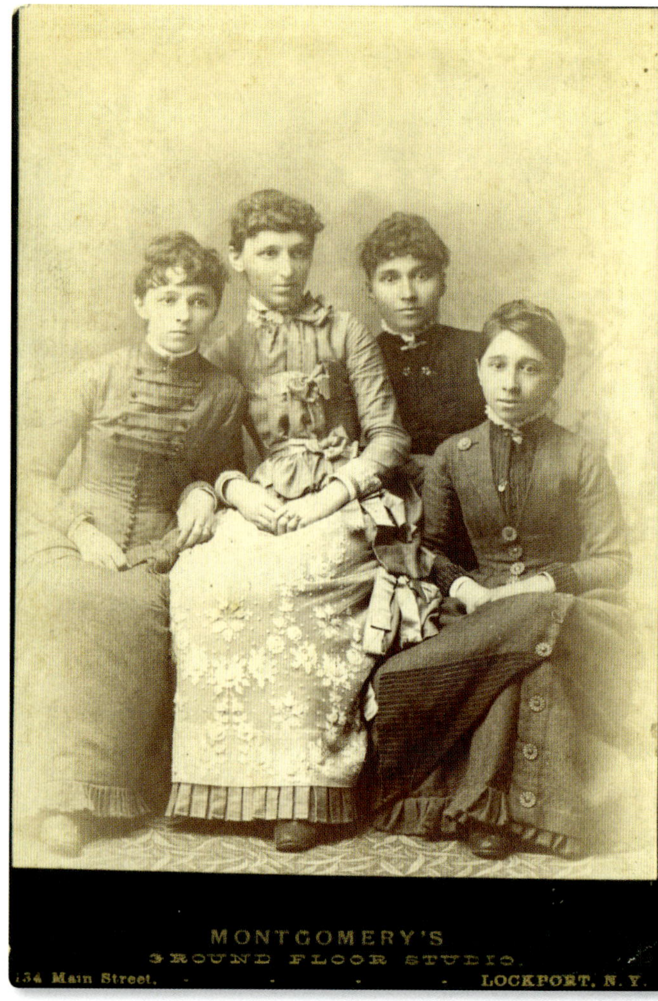

Cabinet card portrait of the Wendel sisters Agnes, Mary, Margaret, and Ella in 1890s daywear. While the dresses are different, the style elements of each are the same. Box and knife-pleated petticoat hems sweep the floor, keeping their dresses clean. The bodices are tightly corseted. Three of the girls wear bar brooches at the neckline. Montgomery's Photo Studio, Lockport, New York.

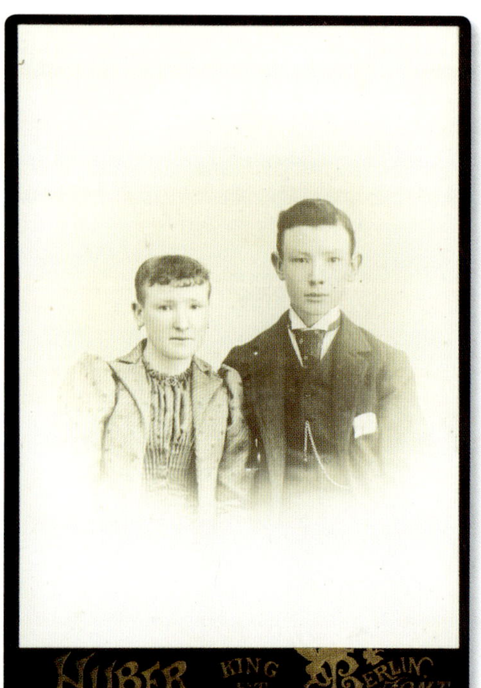

C.1890: A teen couple dressed as adults in their Sunday best. The boy wears a white shirt under a Milton collar with a vested suit with sloping shoulders and notched collar. A pocket watch and silk tie—patterned to match the girl's suit—formalize the look. She wears a jacket with leg-o-mutton sleeves over a dress of the same fabric which is dotted in an Easter egg motif. Cabinet card photograph by H. A. Huber, King St. Berlin, Ontario.

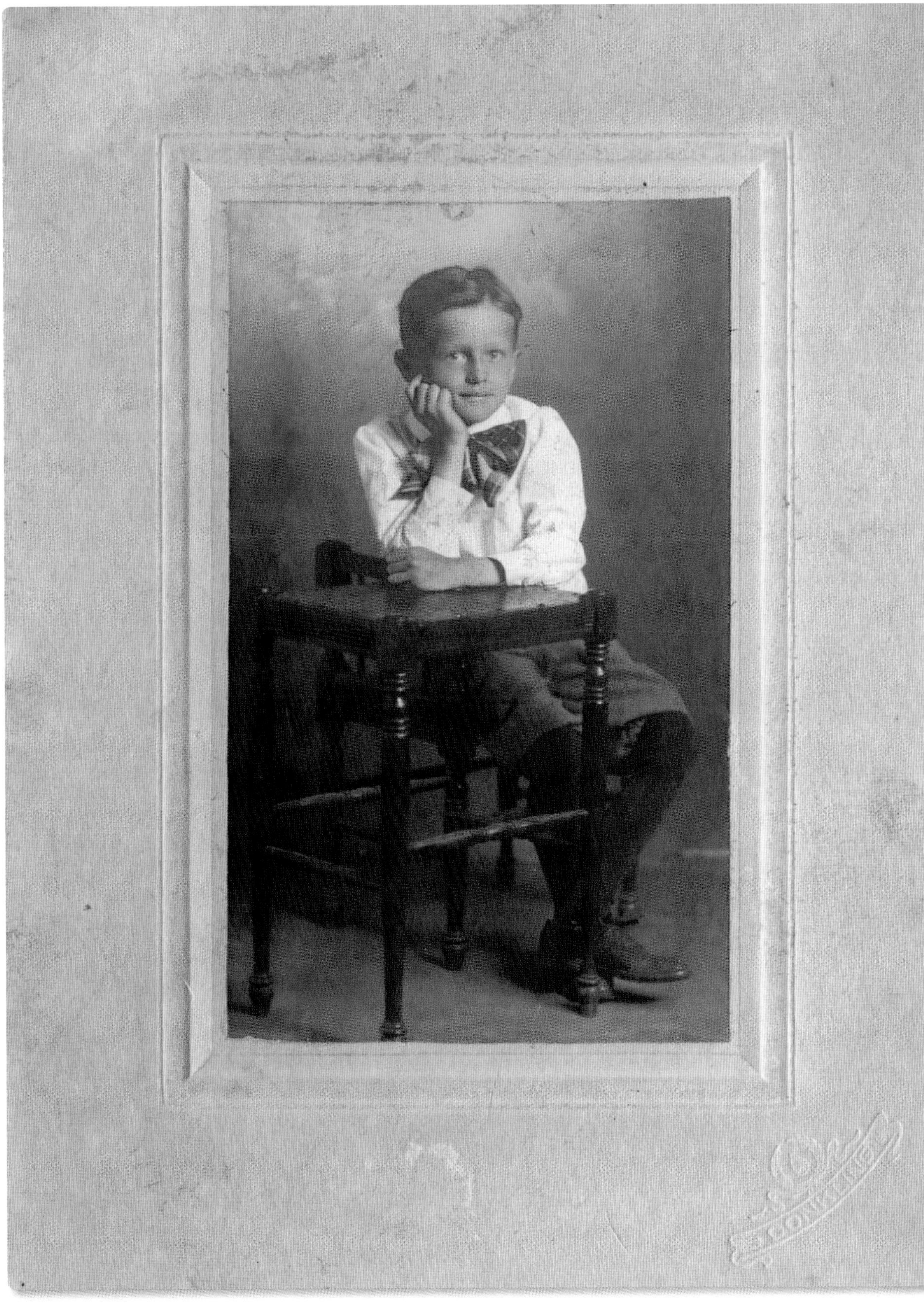

A school boy in knee pants and long stockings appears nonchalant despite the floppy tartan bow that adorns his neck.

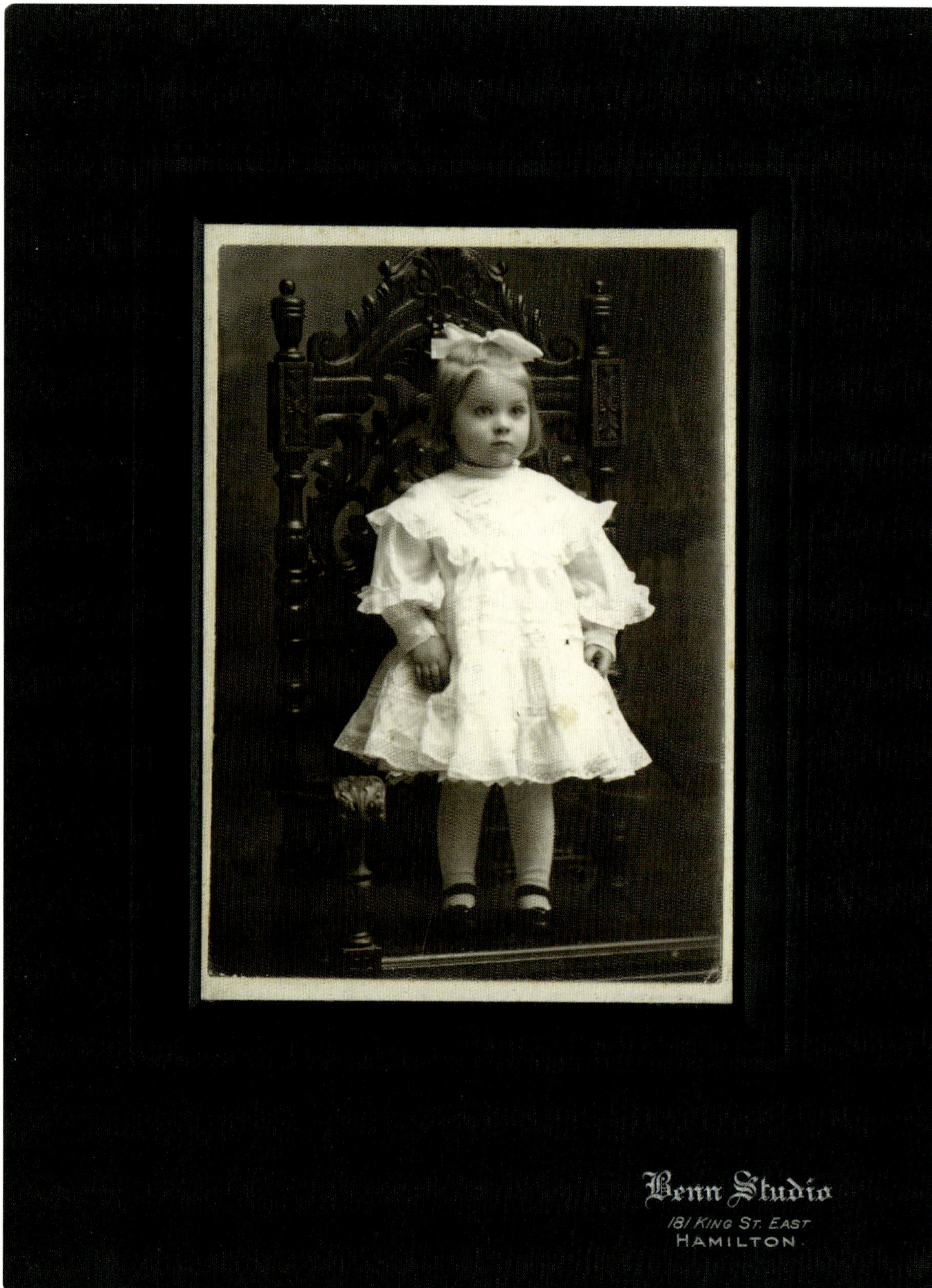

An intricately carved ecclesiastical chair forms the perfect backdrop for a young girl's photographic debut. The fullness of the crisp white dress is likely supported by several petticoats. Cabinet card by Benn Studio, Hamilton, Ontario.

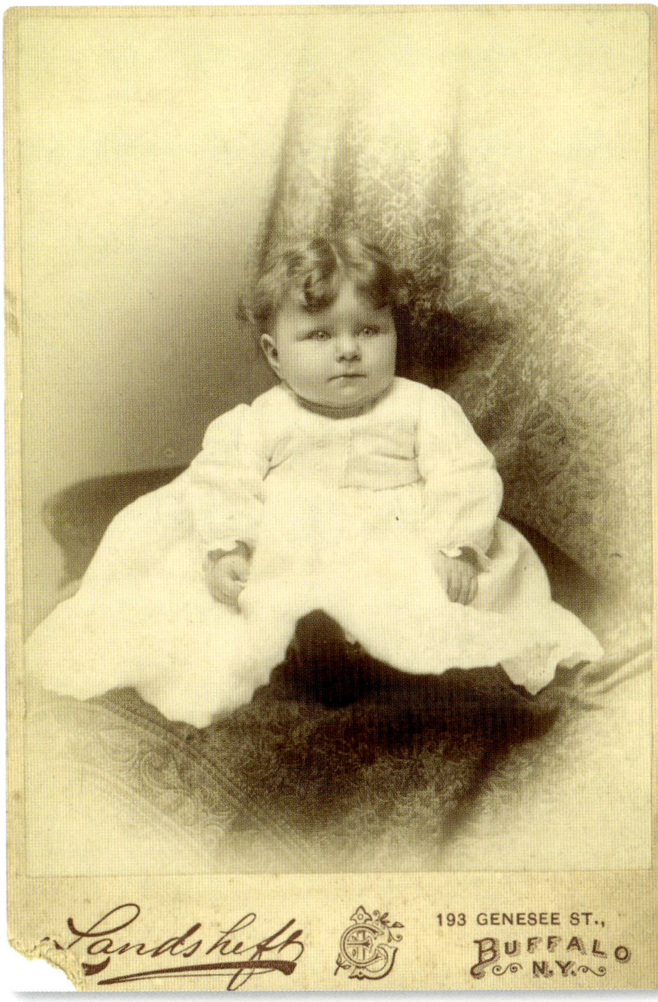

Victorian cabinet image of a healthy infant in a gender-neutral white long-sleeved gown. Fashionable curls cascade from a center part.

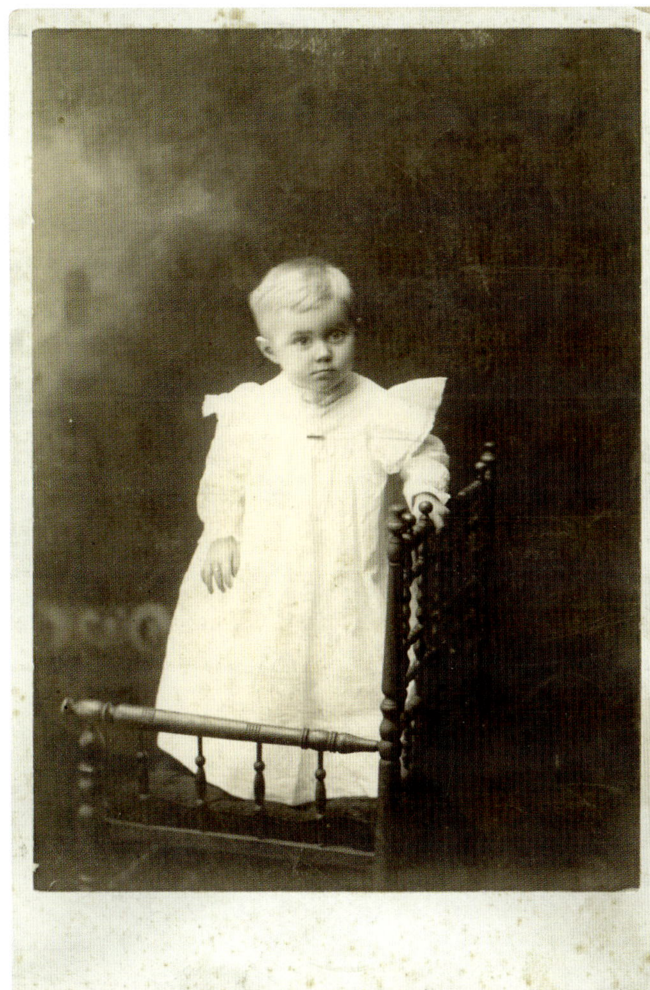

Cabinet card image of a young boy standing on a chair to show off his long white gown with trendy butterfly sleeves.

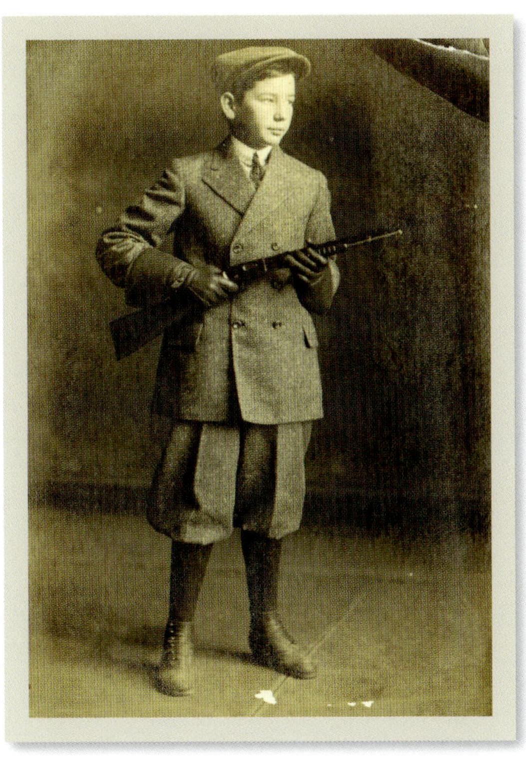

Dressed for the hunt in a newsboy cap and smart wool suit with creased knickers. The button-down collar is secured behind a narrow tie. High button boots and leather gauntlet gloves complete the outfit.

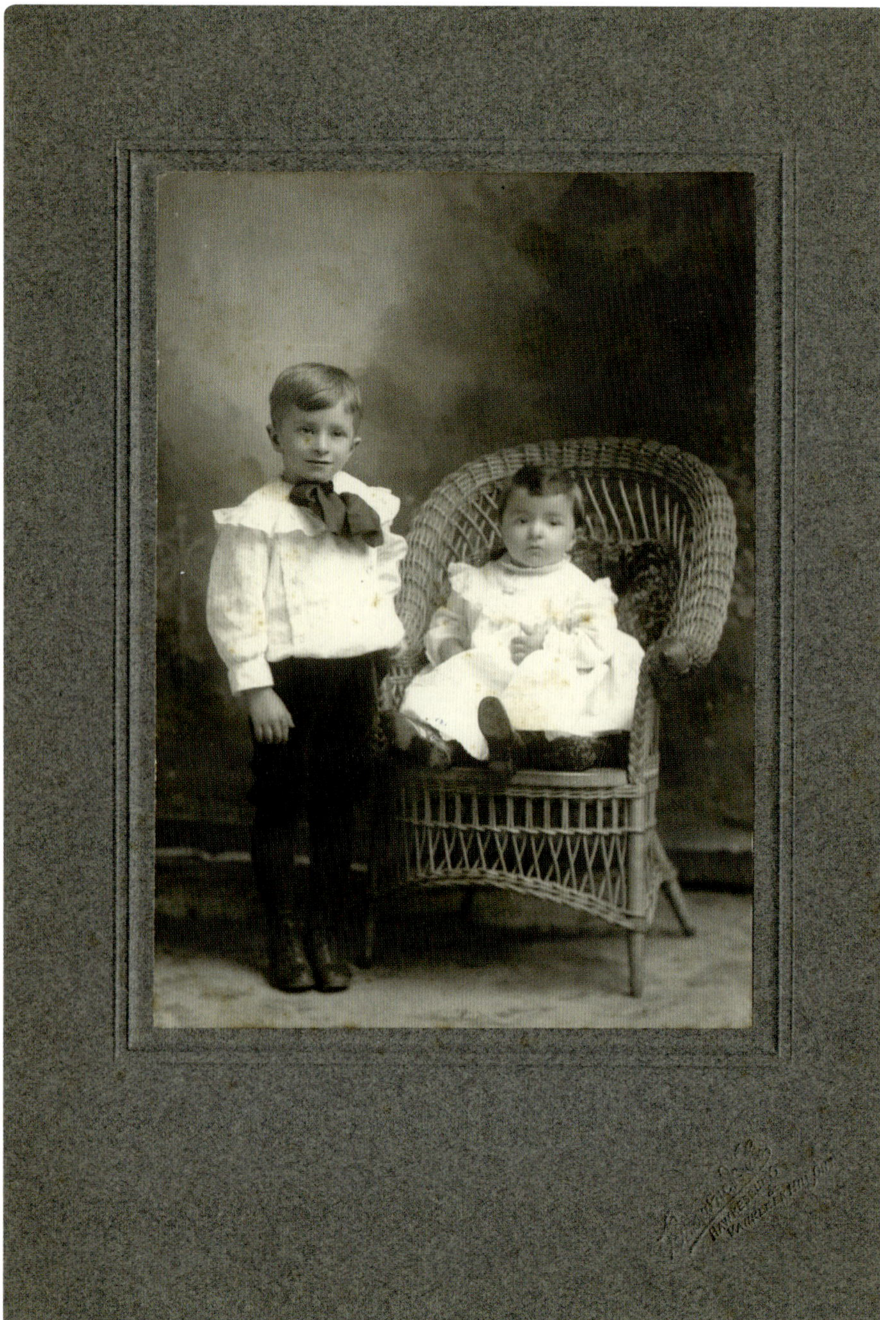

Garth Irvine, dressed á la Little Lord Fontleroy in velvet knickers and a white double breasted blouse with ruffled yoke, stands beside his infant brother Norman, who is attired in a long-sleeved, lace-trimmed dress. Garth wears ankle-high leather boots over dark woolen stockings. Cabinet card photographed in Vankleek Hill, Ontario.

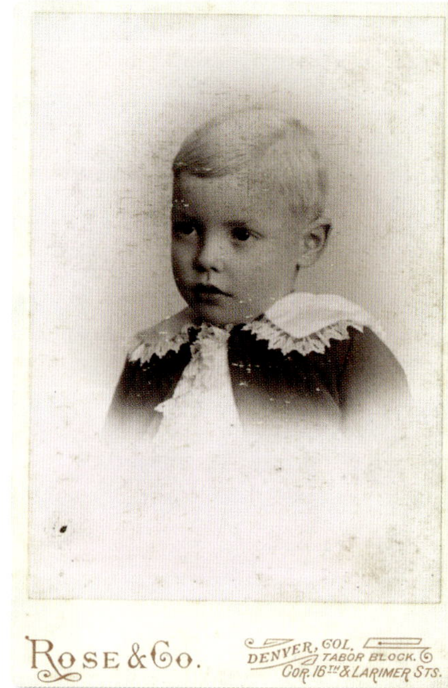

This tot's cutaway jacket shows off a contrast blouse with exquisite lace-trimmed jabot and collar. Cabinet card by Rose & Co., Denver, Colorado.

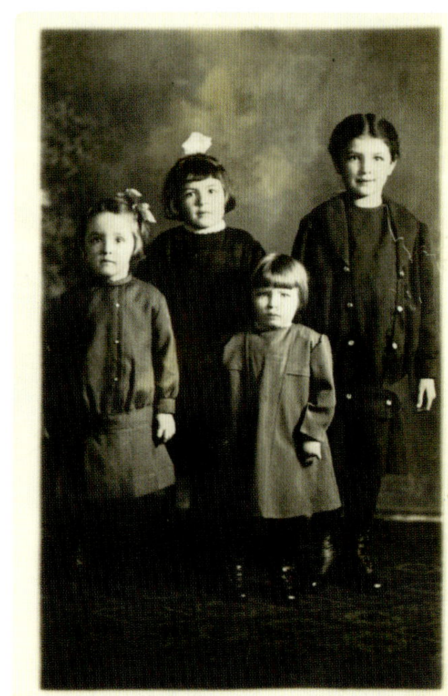

An 1890s postcard image of four female siblings. Note the severity of the drop waist dresses on the far left and far right.

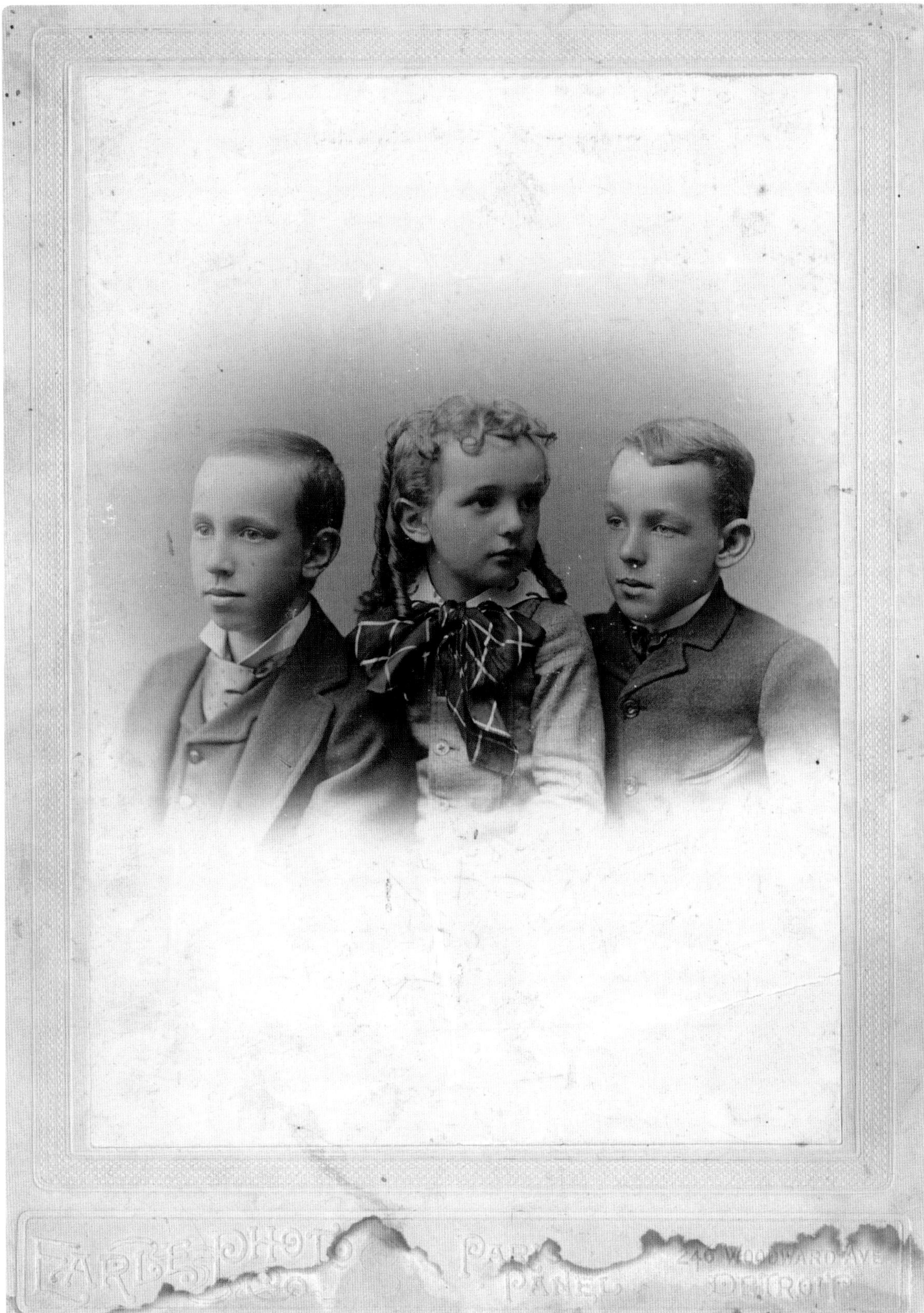

1890s studio portrait of fashionably buttoned-up siblings. The fashion details of each costume draw attention to the neck: the first boy's open collar and knotted tie, the girl's giant bow, the second boy's short lapels and apparent ascot.

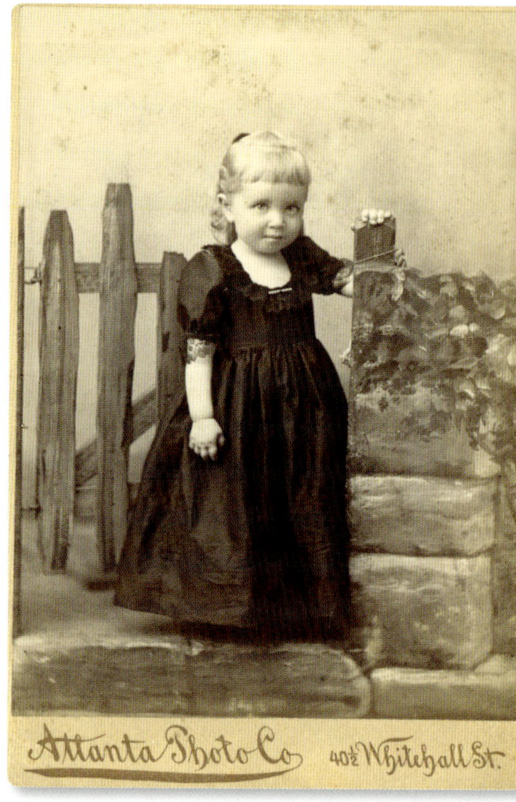

July 15, 1891: This well-groomed tot (aged thirty-eight months) poses in a short-sleeved, richly toned gown with lace-trimmed collar and short puffed sleeves. Cabinet card image by Atlanta Photo Co.

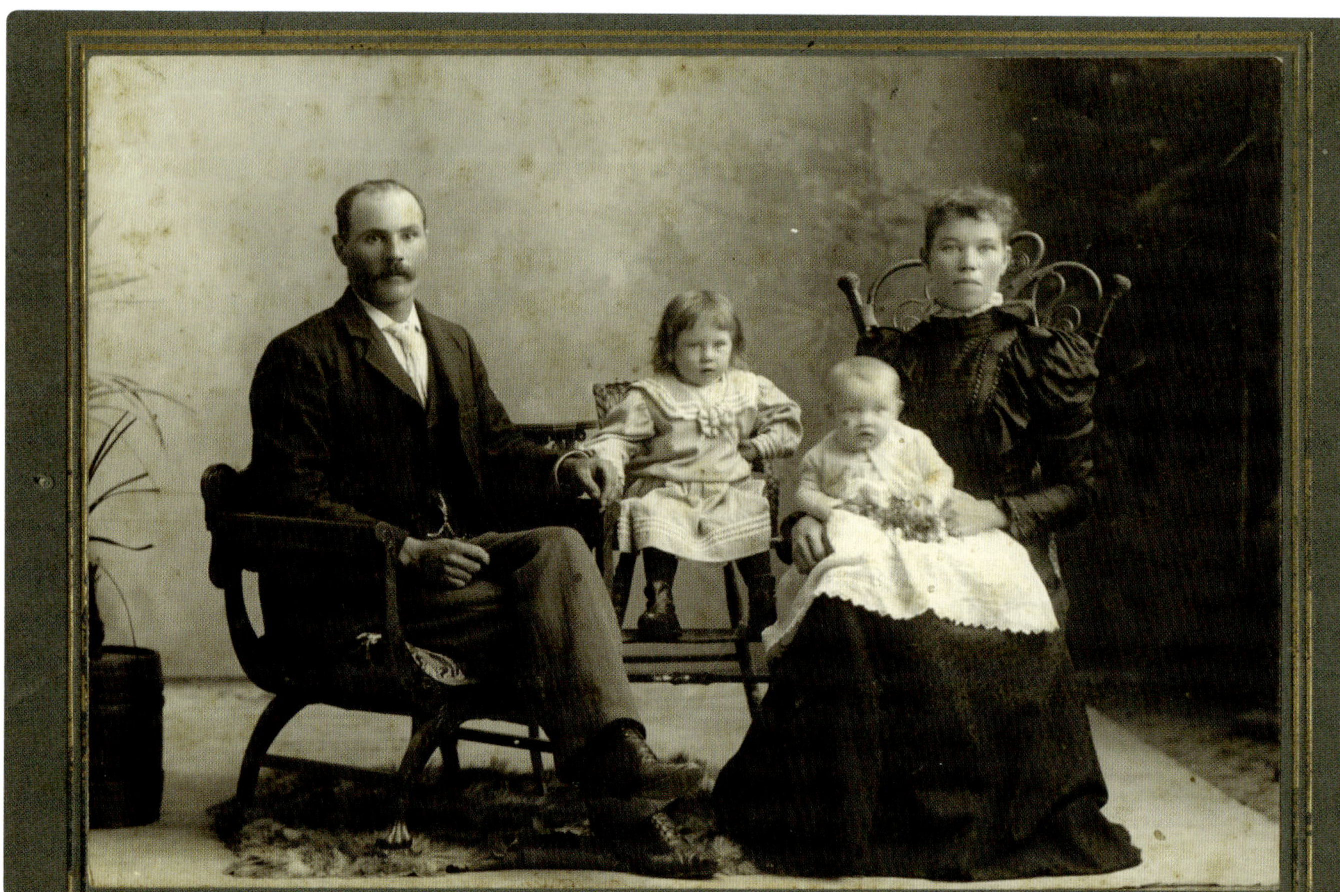

1890s family portrait in dress typical of the era.

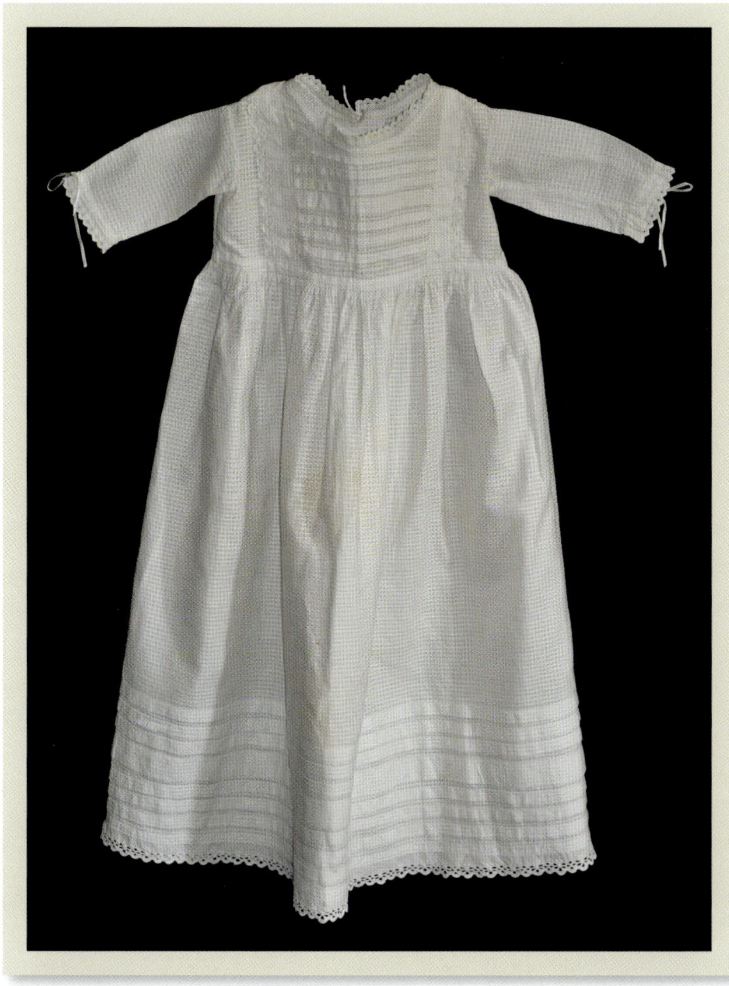

Young child's cotton gown with three-quarter sleeve and lace edging.

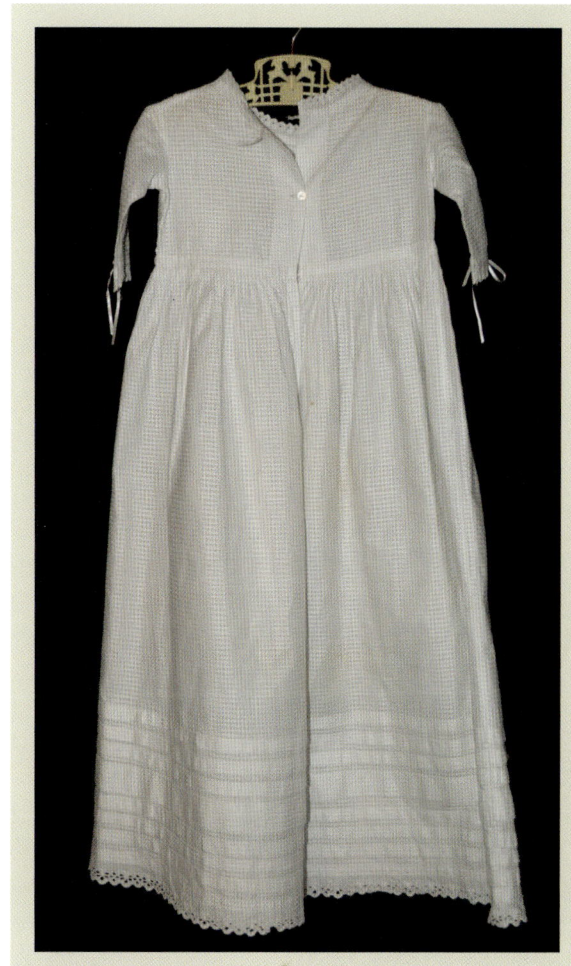

Back view.

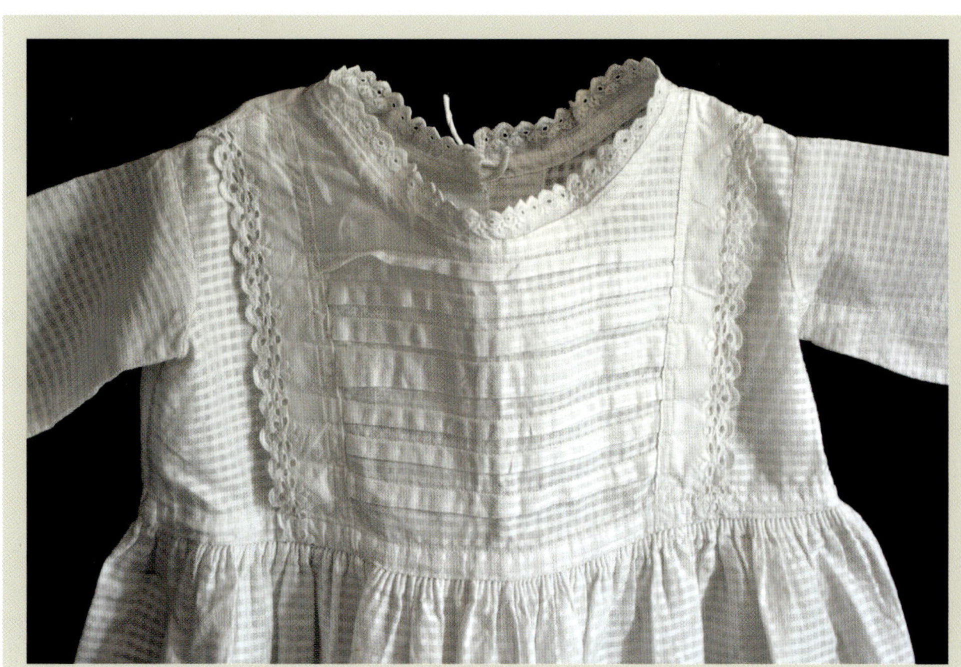

Detail: bodice.

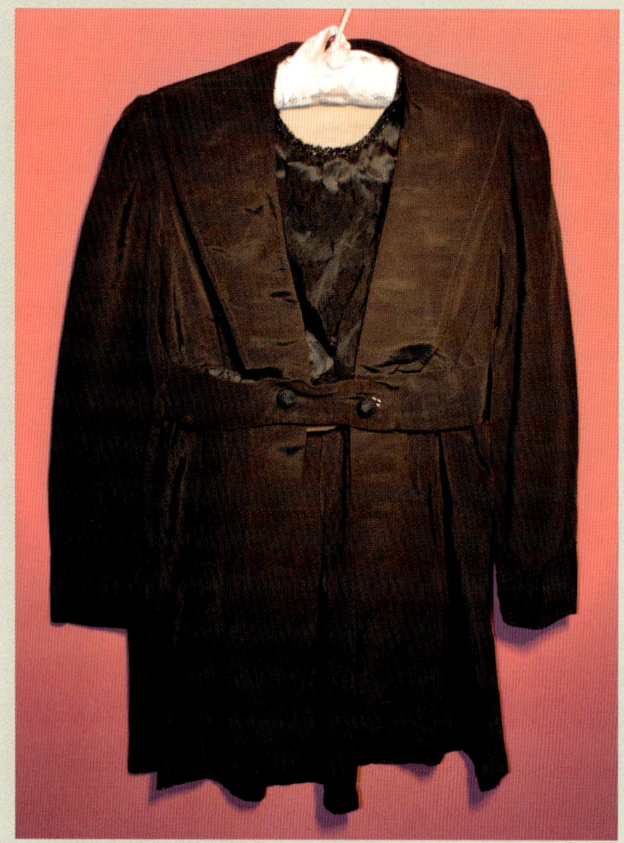

Black taffeta jacket with pouched bodice. Fabric covered buttons, roll collar, and black silk inset vestee trimmed with jet beads.

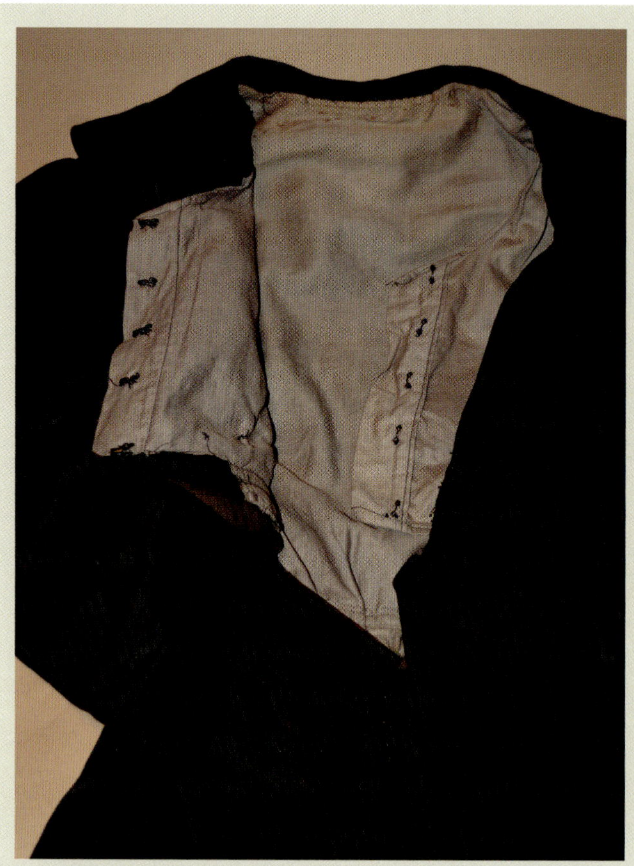

Cotton lined interior. Note the lack of boning.

Bead-trimmed vestee.

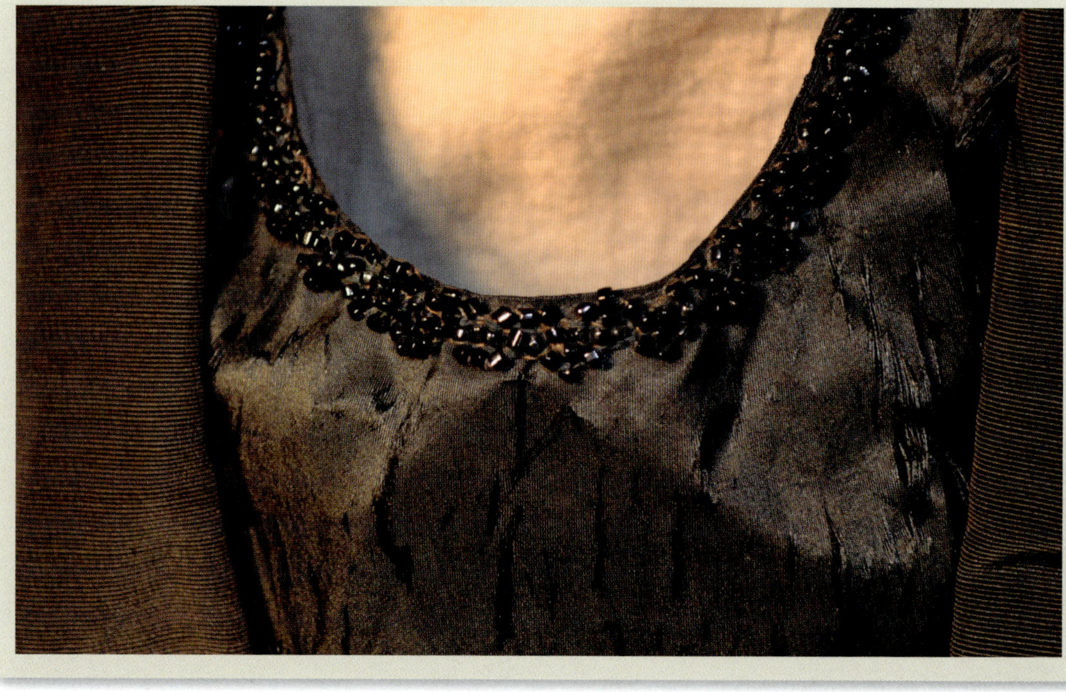

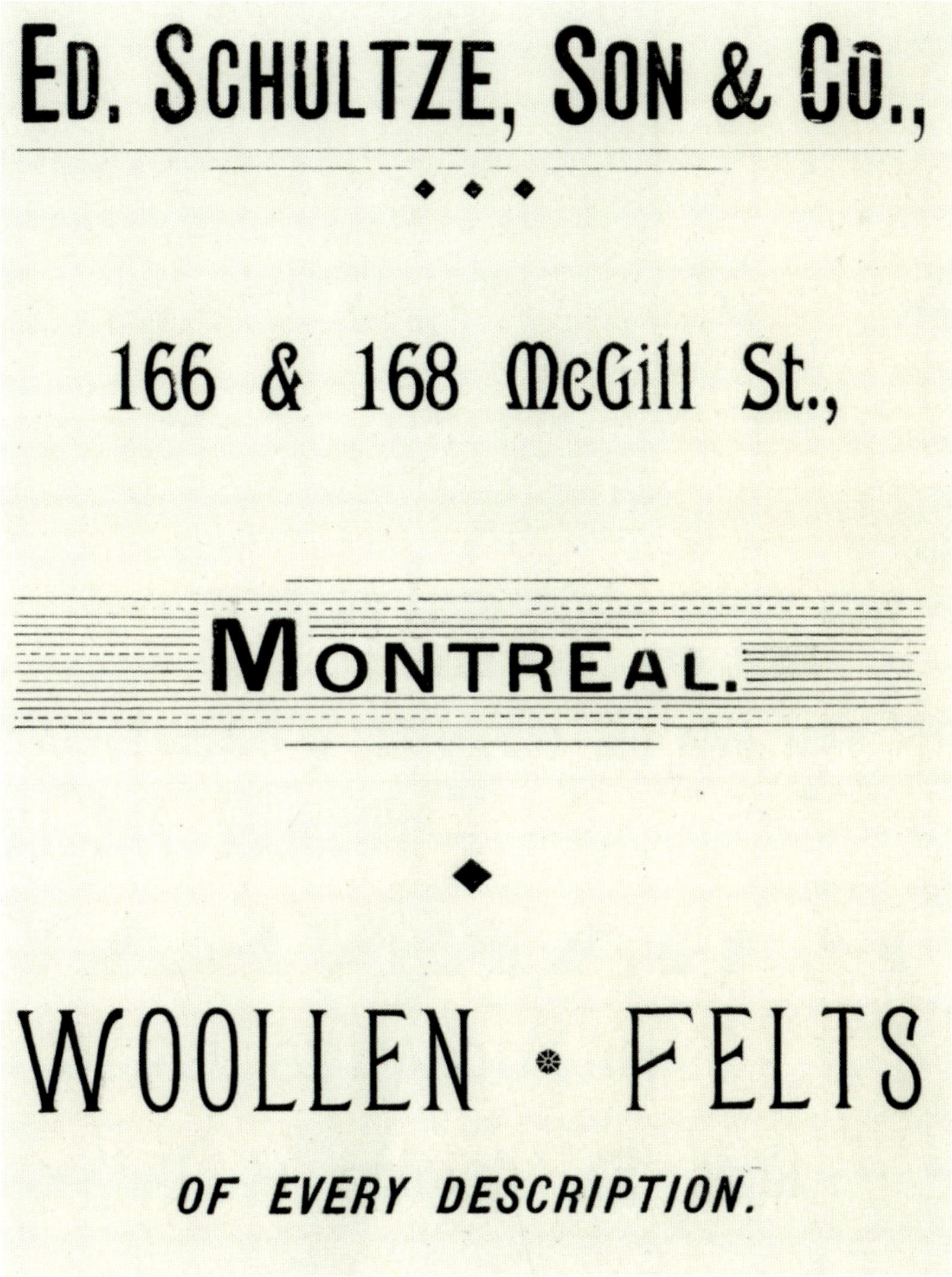

Advertisement for a downtown Montreal textile retailer specializing in woolens and felt. *Canada and Her Commerce*, 1894.

CHAPTER FIVE

Ease and Elegance
1900–1910

"Maternal vanity and linen-drapers' profits demand fashions for children . . . the result of which is generally gratifying to the eye, ruinous to the parental purse, and injudicious from the point of view of health."—What's What, *1902*

"Bands of briar-stitch make a strong and pretty trimming for children's aprons and dresses."—Elizabeth Robinson Scovil, *Ladies' Home Journal*, February 1900

Cultural Influences

Each new century comes with its own sense of newness and excitement. When that change on the calendar coincides, even roughly, with the passing of one monarch and the coronation of another, a mood of expectancy is created. Following as it did on the heels of the second industrial revolution, at a time when synergistic technological advancements allowed for an increasingly prosperous middle class, the Edwardian era promised a life of ease and elegance that was reflected in the costume of the day as well as the slang term "in the swim."

While the Edwardian era owes its name to King Edward VII, who ascended the British throne following the death of Queen Victoria in 1901, the Edwardian aesthetic derives from the sense of lightness that characterized the tone of the era—a welcome contrast to the heaviness of Victorian sensibility, costume, and décor. Edward himself embraced a lavish lifestyle, which contributed to the era's optimism.

Throughout the Belle Epoque, sartorial celebrities like Poiret and Lucile created art-inspired couture for the elite that was broadly imitated, creating, where dress was concerned, less of a divide between the social elite and the common man.

Extensive coverage of the Boxer Rebellion and the Russo-Japanese War early in the decade fostered an interest in all things Oriental, a phenomenon that designers exploited in their construction of gowns and walking suits for women. Designs for children borrowed from the Western interpretation of Far East costume concepts as well.

Designers and fashionistas embraced pastel colors and flimsy fabrics such as silk, which tends to reflect light. Textile merchants developed a number of fabrics from this resource including net, tulle, lace, and *mousseline-de-soie*, to name but a few. Other delicate cotton fabrics such as batiste, georgette, voile—more durable than silk—were particularly suited to the construction of children's clothing.

The number of new sporting pursuits available to adults and children at the turn of the century contributed to the development of less restrictive clothing, with functionality a prime concern when it came to children's play clothes. Dress reform efforts and anti-corset initiatives initiated in the mid-Victorian period were only now beginning to see results, but parents were left with conflicting advice from notable doctors who offered advice on how best to dress children from a health standpoint.

Most agreed that children's corsets or stays were injurious to health. One famous surgeon who specialized in hip joint disorders railed against waistbands, advising that petticoats be hung from the shoulders with braces.

On the other hand, specialists in spinal disorders urged parents to ensure that their sons' and daughters' spinal health be supported through the wearing of padded waistbands. In 1902, *What's What* concluded, "Bare feet and woolly gaiters, boots, shoes, hoods and hats, they are all right and all wrong, according to somebody." The guide suggested parents select light, warm clothes, few in number, that could be easily enlarged and that "do not pull or press upon the body in any manner."

The book provided an example of what a typical seven-year-old girl would ordinarily wear under her dress in winter: a combination or vest, a chemise, stays, drawers, a flannel petticoat, a cotton petticoat with or without an attached bodice, stockings, and suspenders. *What's What* (1902) suggested the following dress reform improvements: a thick woolen vest, woolen knickerbockers with a detachable lining, a sleeveless flannel bodice, stockings gartered at the knee, a short pilot jacket for walking and running, or a woolen Spencer jacket. All of the above were to be worn under dresses, shirt and skirt sets, or smock frocks, with substitutions of thinner material in summer. Typically, socks replaced woolen stockings from May until October.

Style Retrospective

"Among the newest colors are foliage-green and emerald shades of green, blue in the corn-flower shadings, geranium and poppy reds, dahlia, plum, and aubergine. Shaded mousseline is used for entire frocks as well as for scarfs and trimmings."—*New Idea Woman's Magazine*, October 1903.

Early into the century, fashion dictators declared velvet—no longer popular for indoor wear— to be the most popular fabric for little boys' and girls' outerwear. A coat depicted in *The Delineator* in November 1902 shows an attractive, gender-neutral number in black, trimmed with bands of matching taffeta, "the buttons being of dull black enamel." The double-breasted knee-length coat boasts "drooping" sleeves decorated with turn-back cuffs. A rolling collar provides glamour and warmth at the neck.

A second coat, deemed suitable for a young child of either gender, presents a similar silhouette, this time with a cape collar and bishop's sleeves with optional turn-back cuffs. Kersey, moiré silk, corduroy, melton cloth, beaver felt, and taffeta are suggested for fabrication, with limerick lace for trim, and rose-pink taffeta for lining. Such a garment would be a sentient delight to eyes, ears, and fingers.

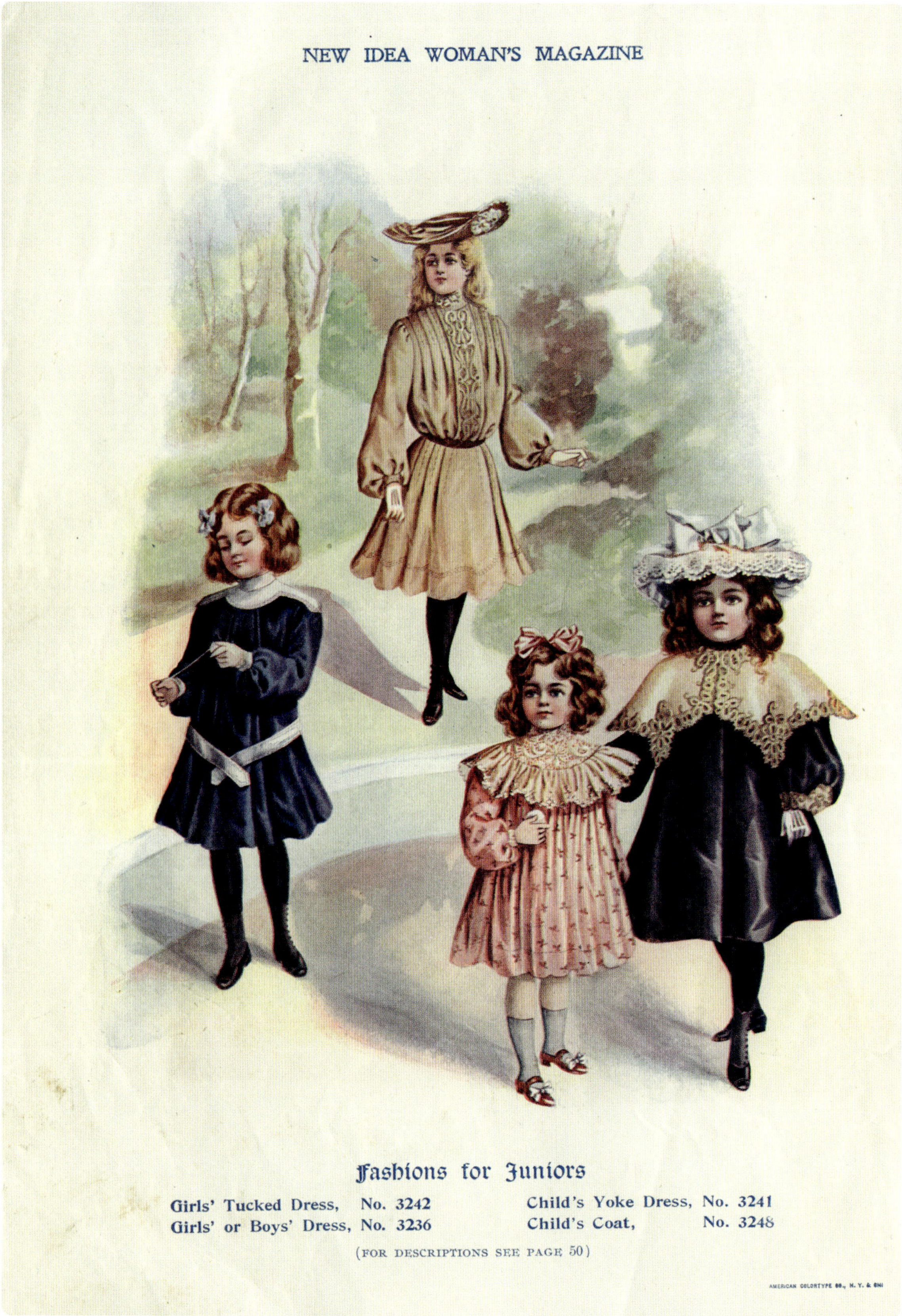
NEW IDEA WOMAN'S MAGAZINE
Fashions for Juniors
Girls' Tucked Dress, No. 3242
Girls' or Boys' Dress, No. 3236
Child's Yoke Dress, No. 3241
Child's Coat, No. 3248
(FOR DESCRIPTIONS SEE PAGE 50)

Fashion plate of three fall dresses and a coat styled for girls and boys from the pages of *New Idea Woman's Magazine*, October 1903.

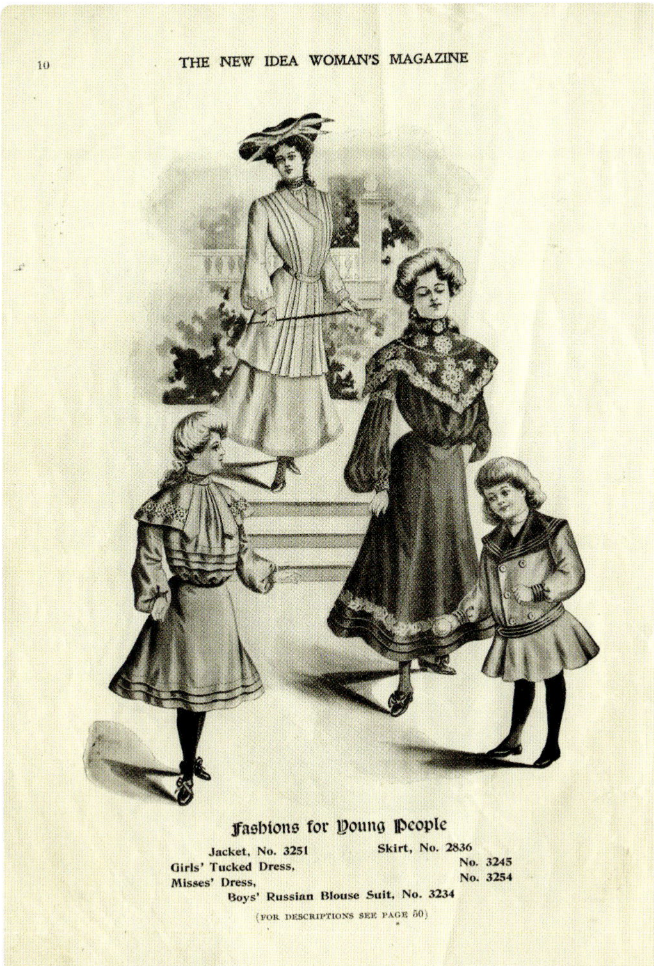

Fashion plate of "Fashions for Young People" including a boy's Russian blouse suit. *New Idea Woman's Magazine*, October 1903.

Equally lavish are the winter outerwear patterns outlined for older girls or misses. A mother or dressmaker making up these patterns would be required to purchase plenty of fabric—velvet, Sicilian, or beautifully patterned snowflake cloth—to create the multi-gored long skirt and peplum jacket described. Further yardages would be required for lining, as well as *peau-de-soie* for facings. Additionally, the trimmings selected range from fur to lace to Russian braid, specially chosen for the then up-to-date arrowhead trim.

Further into the decade, as silk gained popularity, it was widely used for frills, flounces, and insertions on children's clothing. For Edwardians, lightness in color was as important as lightness in weight when considering textiles for children's clothing. Pale blues, pinks, and lavenders along with soft browns and bright whites made the grade. White was also used to temper stronger blues and browns, while soft creams were paired with red, purple, or black, particularly in winter when wools and flannels prevailed.

As the heavy fabrics and layering practices of the Victorian era fell by the wayside, striped cottons and linens along with eyelets lent a fresh appearance to summer dressing. Visual interest was created through tucking, belting, ruffling, pleating, or lace insertion.

Heavy lace figured prominently in the trimming of children's costume early in the twentieth century, whether it was used to adorn a collar and cuffs, delineate a cape or dress band, or add flair to a millinery marvel. Ribbons found favor in the form of sashes on children's dresses designed for afternoon wear. These were tied fashionably at the left side.

Styles for girls and teen girls featured high-necked pouter pigeon bodices with bishop sleeves and flared skirts, hem length marking the only age distinction. A tailored look was also emerging with crisp lines delineated with fabric tucks and top stitching. *New Idea Magazine,* October 1903, recommended fabrics of canvas or zibeline for everyday fall ensembles and challis or *peau-de-soie* for dressier garments.

A watered down version of the S-curve and mono-bosom silhouette, immortalized in the romantic drawings of Dana Gibson, was represented in children's wear as well. By 1901, *The Delineator* was showing low-belted dresses for girls with fullness built into the front to mimic the pigeon-breasted aesthetic worn by their mothers. Box pleats created fullness at the waist with most frocks closing at the center back.

A good deal of fabric was required to complete the prevailing style, as many a skirt boasted a full three layers of lace-trimmed ruffles at the hem, as well as elbow-length self-fabric sleeves fitted over full bishop sleeves.

Early Edwardian frocks are easily recognizable by their high-waisted flowing appearance and top-heavy silhouette, a look further enhanced by the draping of sashes, or fur and feather boas, or by pinning the bodice with soft textile floral sprays.

Bolero suit styles worn over pouter pigeon blouses made the scene for younger girls, while misses enjoyed the new trumpet or tulip skirt styles. These were cut in three sections with circular hem flounces and dart-fitted hips. For these, *The Delineator* suggested textile selections of Lansdowne, albatross, cashmere, and Henrietta.

Girls' coats were similarly fashioned to resemble the prevailing styles for women, nicely imitating the newly popular tailored coats and walking suits. Angular collars, contrast cuffs, and bold buttons took their cue from styles for men. With women's hat buttons sometimes matching coat buttons, thanks to designers like Lucille, how could large, flashy buttons not find their way onto children's wear?

When it came to older boys, suit styles closely imitated those designed for men, and many a youth pedalled his bicycle while clad in a tweed or shepherd's-plaid knicker

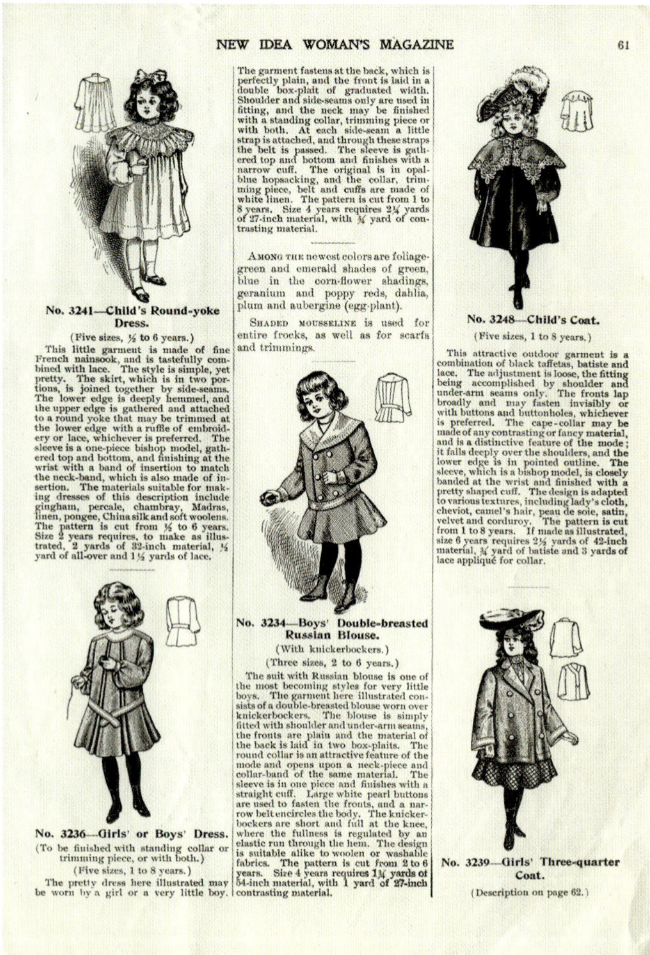

NEW IDEA WOMAN'S MAGAZINE 61

No. 3241—Child's Round-yoke Dress.

(Five sizes, ½ to 6 years.)

This little garment is made of fine French nainsook, and is tastefully combined with lace. The style is simple, yet pretty. The skirt, which is in two portions, is joined together by side-seams. The lower edge is deeply hemmed, and the upper edge is gathered and attached to a round yoke that may be trimmed at the lower edge with a ruffle of embroidery or lace, whichever is preferred. The sleeve is a one-piece bishop model, gathered top and bottom, and finishing at the wrist with a band of insertion to match the neck-band, which is also made of insertion. The materials suitable for making dresses of this description include gingham, percale, chambray, Madras, linen, pongee, China silk and soft woolens. The pattern is cut from ½ to 6 years. Size 2 years requires, to make as illustrated, 2 yards of 32-inch material, ½ yard of all-over and 1½ yards of lace.

No. 3236—Girls' or Boys' Dress.

(To be finished with standing collar or trimming piece, or with both.)

(Five sizes, 1 to 8 years.)

The pretty dress here illustrated may be worn by a girl or a very little boy. The garment fastens at the back, which is perfectly plain, and the front is laid in a double box-plait of graduated width. Shoulder and side-seams only are used in fitting, and the neck may be finished with a standing collar, trimming piece or with both. At each side-seam a little strap is attached, and through these straps the belt is passed. The sleeve is gathered top and bottom and finishes with a narrow cuff. The original is in opal-blue hopsacking, and the collar, trimming piece, belt and cuffs are made of white linen. The pattern is cut from 1 to 8 years. Size 4 years requires 2¼ yards of 27-inch material, with ¾ yard of contrasting material.

Among the newest colors are foliage-green and emerald shades of green, blue in the corn-flower shadings, geranium and poppy reds, dahlia, plum and aubergine (egg-plant).

Shaded mousseline is used for entire frocks, as well as for scarfs and trimmings.

No. 3234—Boys' Double-breasted Russian Blouse.

(With knickerbockers.)

(Three sizes, 2 to 6 years.)

The suit with Russian blouse is one of the most becoming styles for very little boys. The garment here illustrated consists of a double-breasted blouse worn over knickerbockers. The blouse is simply fitted with shoulder and under-arm seams, the fronts are plain and the material of the back is laid in two box-plaits. The round collar is an attractive feature of the mode and opens upon a neck-piece and collar-band of the same material. The sleeve is in one piece and finishes with a straight cuff. Large white pearl buttons are used to fasten the fronts, and a narrow belt encircles the body. The knickerbockers are short and full at the knee, where the fullness is regulated by an elastic run through the hem. The design is suitable alike to woolen or washable fabrics. The pattern is cut from 2 to 6 years. Size 4 years requires 1¾ yards of 54-inch material, with 1 yard of 27-inch contrasting material.

No. 3248—Child's Coat.

(Five sizes, 1 to 8 years.)

This attractive outdoor garment is a combination of black taffetas, batiste and lace. The adjustment is loose, the fitting being accomplished by shoulder and under-arm seams only. The fronts lap broadly and may fasten invisibly or with buttons and buttonholes, whichever is preferred. The cape-collar may be made of any contrasting or fancy material, and is a distinctive feature of the mode; it falls deeply over the shoulders, and the lower edge is in pointed outline. The sleeve, which is a bishop model, is closely banded at the wrist and finished with a pretty shaped cuff. The design is adapted to various textures, including lady's cloth, cheviot, camel's hair, peau de soie, satin, velvet and corduroy. The pattern is cut from 1 to 8 years. If made as illustrated, size 6 years requires 2½ yards of 42-inch material, ¾ yard of batiste and 3 yards of lace appliqué for collar.

No. 3239—Girls' Three-quarter Coat.

(Description on page 62.)

A variety of children's fashions popular in 1903. *New Idea Woman's Magazine*, October 1903.

suit, the pants carefully strapped and buckled at the knee. The popular sack suit was well named as the jackets and coats lacked waist definition.

Mothers still found favor with Fontleroy suits for younger boys, particularly when paired with colorful blouses and shirtwaists. Cotton and linen sailor suits, the new smaller-collared vestee suits, and Man of War outfits also tempted buyers.

Undergarments took on a new, less weighty appearance as well. Saying goodbye to the five or six rustling taffeta petticoats, which were *de rigueur* in the Victorian age, Edwardian girls relied on narrow silk, chiffon, fine lace, or handkerchief linen underskirts. Despite dress reform efforts, infants and children approached the new century still attired in cotton or cambric waists, although lacings were not employed for girls under the age of seven. Garters were supplied separately in sets of four to be sewn onto waists where appropriate.

Hats and Bonnets

Early in the decade, straw boaters capped boys' and girls' summer ensembles, but the hats designed for boys were primarily of natural straw with black ribbon bands, while boaters for girls were fashioned with smaller crowns and garnished with ribbons, plumes, and other vertical trims. These hats were occasionally dyed to match a particular ensemble. Left plain, they became the uniform of North American school girls *à la* Anne of Green Gables.

By 1906, fashion scribes had much to say about the variety of children's hat styles and fabrications available to retail shoppers. Copywriters used terms such as "Japanese ties" to evoke a sense of the fashionable Orient.

The May 1906 cover of *The Delineator* features a sketch of two young girls dressed in white summer frocks with exaggerated puffy sleeves, self-fabric bands creating a ruffle effect just above the elbow. Wide-brimmed cartwheel hats complete the ensembles, although one of the girls, hat in hand, wears an oversized yellow bow in her hair.

The heads of babies and young children were tied up warm and tight under flared, tucked, ruched, and shirred hoods, or bonnets, revere caps, and ear-hugging turbans. Winter bonnets of Zephyr wool and silken floss competed for attention with bear cloth bonnets, crocheted angora caps, and velveteen poke bonnets. While most winter bonnets came in a natural cream color only, purveyors of the velveteen variety offered a choice of cardinal, myrtle, brown, or navy faced with white, if desired.

Hats and bonnets for little girls were suited to the season, with woolen tam o' shanters preferred in winter, and straw or fabric bonnets approved for summer. Bonnets mimicked those worn by adult women and continued to be fashioned on wire frames until about 1910. These were tied with pastel silk or satin sashes and showed off lace trims and/or clusters of cloth flowers.

Older girls might be seen in wide-brimmed straws to balance the flounced hems of their longer skirts. Accoutrements such as ribbon belts and sleeve bands, walking stick parasols, and lace collars added to the romantic aesthetic of girls who were not quite but soon to be women.

Seasonal style changes kept milliners busy, not only serving custom clients, but supplying the latest chapeaux to high-end retailers as well. Department stores, such as Eaton's, made sure to inform their mail order customers that they did not keep a stock of seasonal headwear beyond a certain date. Additionally, when ordering children's headwear from a catalog, mothers were reminded to first measure their child's head size.

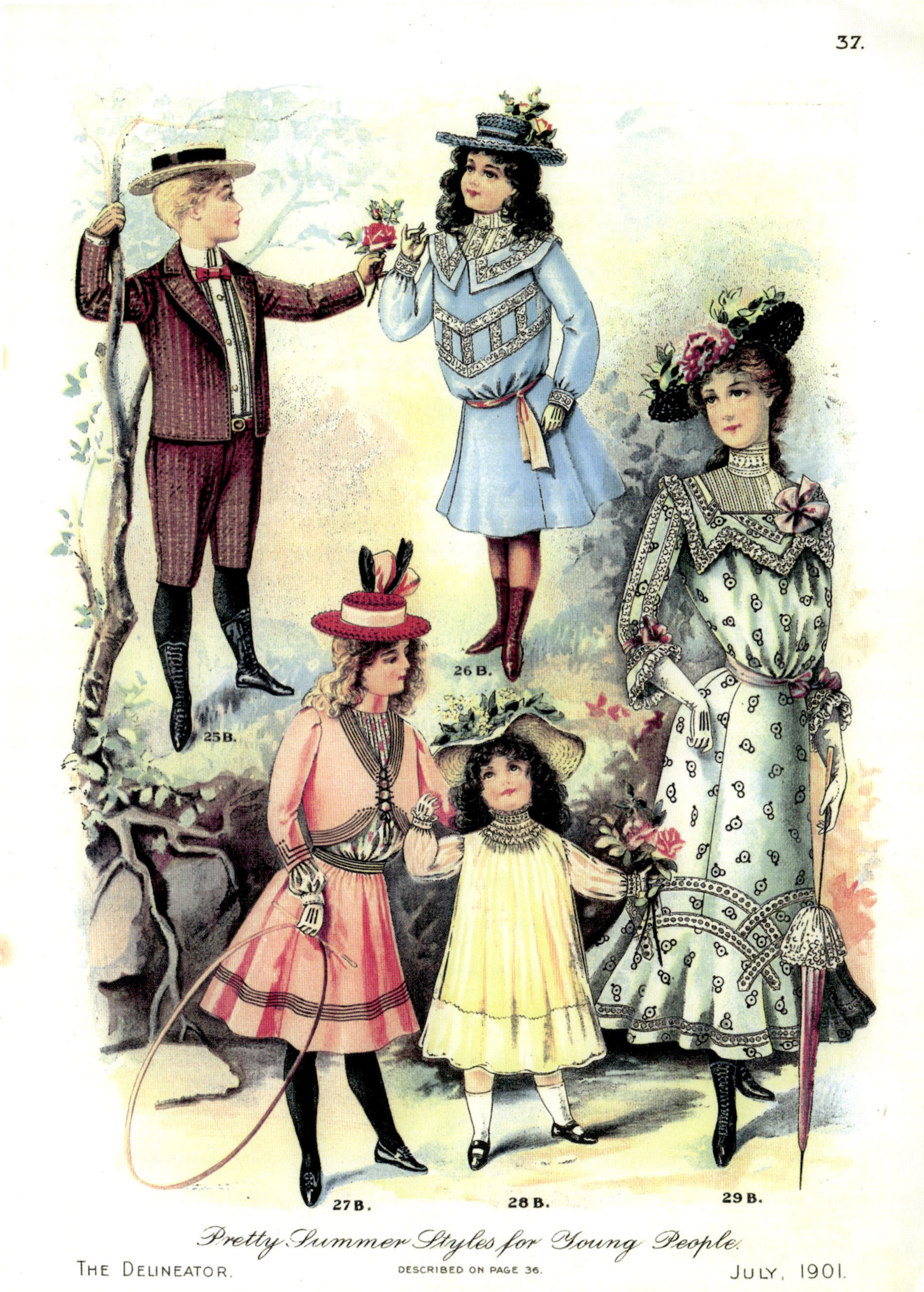

Children's and misses summer fashions. *The Delineator*, July 1901.

Children's Ulsters and Automobile Coats.

Schedule of Sizes for Children's Ulsters

Length,	27 inches;	30 inches;	33 inches;	36 inches;	39 inches.
Age,	4 years;	6 years;	8 years;	10 years;	12 years.

When ordering Children's Ulsters state age and length downward from bottom of collar band (back).
When ordering Children's Automobile Coats state age.

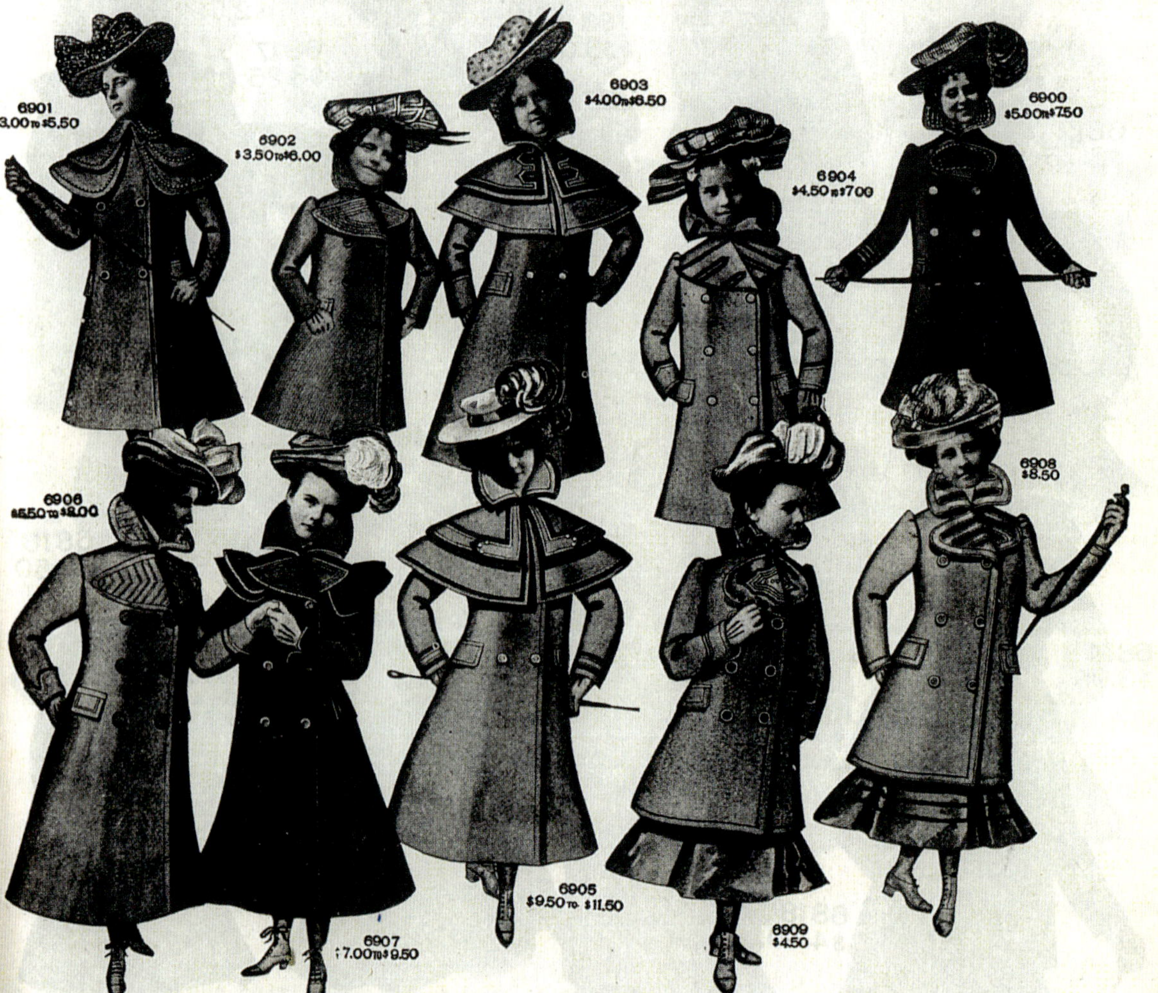

No. 6901. ENGLISH CHEVIOT SERGE ULSTER, colors navy, royal, fawn, brown and green, trimmed with fancy braid, 27-inch, **3.00**; 30-inch, **3.50**; 33-inch, **4.00**; 36-inch, **4.50**; 39 inch, **5.00**; 42-inch, **5.50.**

No. 6902. HEAVY FRIEZE ULSTER, colors Oxford, navy, green, brown, fawn, red, royal and blue mixture, finished with rows of stitching, 27-inch, **3.50**; 30-inch, **4.00**; 33-inch, **4.50**; 36-inch, **5.00**; 39-inch, **5.50**; 42-inch, **6.00.**

No. 6903. HEAVY FRIEZE ULSTER, colors fawn, brown, navy, red and royal, braid trimmed, 27-inch, **4.00**; 30-inch, **4.50**; 33-inch, **5.00**; 36-inch, **5.50**; 39-inch, **6.00**; 42-inch, **6.50.**

No. 6904. BEAVER CLOTH ULSTER, colors fawn, brown, navy, royal, red and green, trimmed with folds of satin, 27-inch, **4.50**; 30-inch, **5.00**; 33-inch, **5.50**; 36-inch, **6.00**; 39-inch, **6.50**; 42-inch, **7.00.**

No. 6900. ENGLISH BEAVER CLOTH ULSTER, colors fawn, brown, navy, royal, green and red, is trimmed with velvet, fancy braid and small buttons, 27-inch, **5.00**; 30-inch, **5.50**; 33-inch, **6.00**; 36-inch, **6.50**; 39-inch, **7.00**; 42-inch, **7.50.**

No. 6906. HEAVY ALL-WOOL FRIEZE ULSTER, colors blue mixture, fawn, brown, grey, green and navy, trimmed with velvet pipings and pearl buttons, 27-inch, **5.50**; 30-inch, **6.00**; 33-inch, **6.50**; 36-inch, **7.00**; 39-inch, **7.50**; 42-inch, **8.00.**

No. 6907. STYLISH ALL-WOOL KERSEY CLOTH ULSTER, navy only, finished with straps of self, and pearl buttons, 27-inch, **7.00**; 30-inch, **7.50**; 33-inch, **8.00**; 36-inch, **8.50**; 39-inch, **9.00**; 42-inch, **9.50.**

No. 6905. FINE ALL-WOOL KERSEY CLOTH ULSTER, colors fawn, brown, castor, royal and navy, trimmed with folds of satin, and pearl buttons, 27 inch, **9.50**; 30-inch, **10.00**; 33-inch, **10.50**; 36-inch, **11.00**; 39-inch, **11.50**; 42-inch, **12.00.**

No. 6909. CHILD'S AUTOMOBILE COAT, made of heavy all-wool frieze, colors blue, fawn, brown, green, navy and Oxford, trimmings of velvet and braid, 8, 10 and 12 years, **4.50.**

No. 6908. CHILD'S AUTOMOBILE COAT, made of fine all-wool kersey cloth, colors light fawn, dark fawn and red, lined throughout with serge silk, has velvet trimmings and pearl buttons, 8, 10 and 12 years, **8.50.**

Children's winter ulsters and automobile coats. *Eaton's Fall and Winter Catalogue*, 1901–1902.

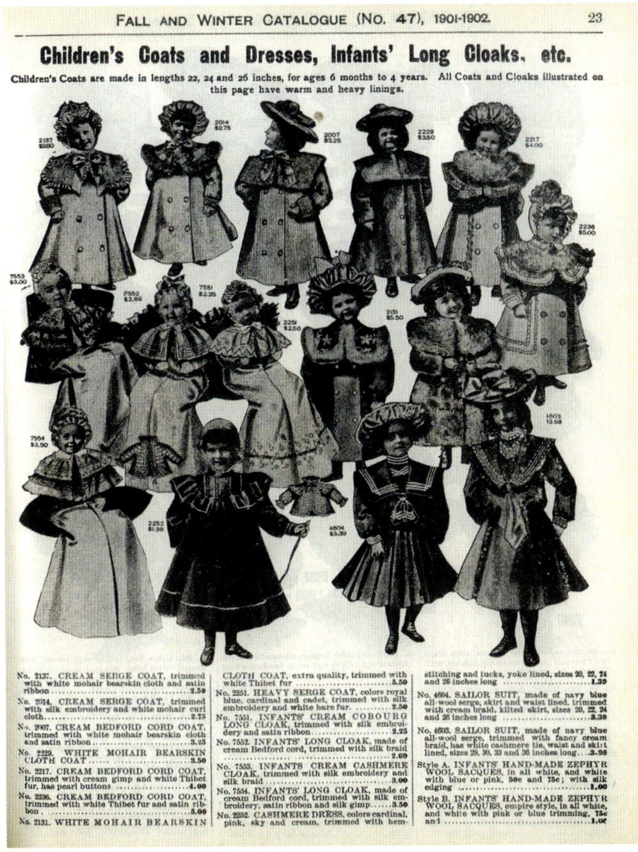
FALL AND WINTER CATALOGUE (NO. 47), 1901-1902.
23
Children's Coats and Dresses, Infants' Long Cloaks, etc.
Children's Coats are made in lengths 22, 24 and 26 inches, for ages 6 months to 4 years. All Coats and Cloaks illustrated on this page have warm and heavy linings.

Children's winter coats and dresses, infants' cloaks. *Eaton's Fall and Winter Catalogue*, 1901–1902.

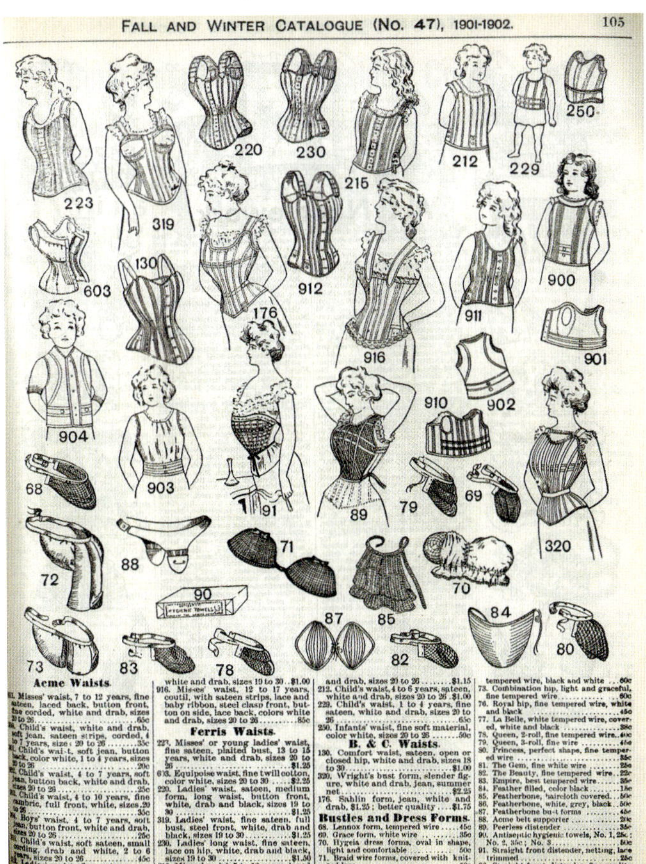
FALL AND WINTER CATALOGUE (NO. 47), 1901-1902.
105
Acme Waists.
Ferris Waists.
B. & C. Waists.
Bustles and Dress Forms.

Children's and misses' waists and bustles. *Eaton's Fall and Winter Catalogue*, 1901–1902.

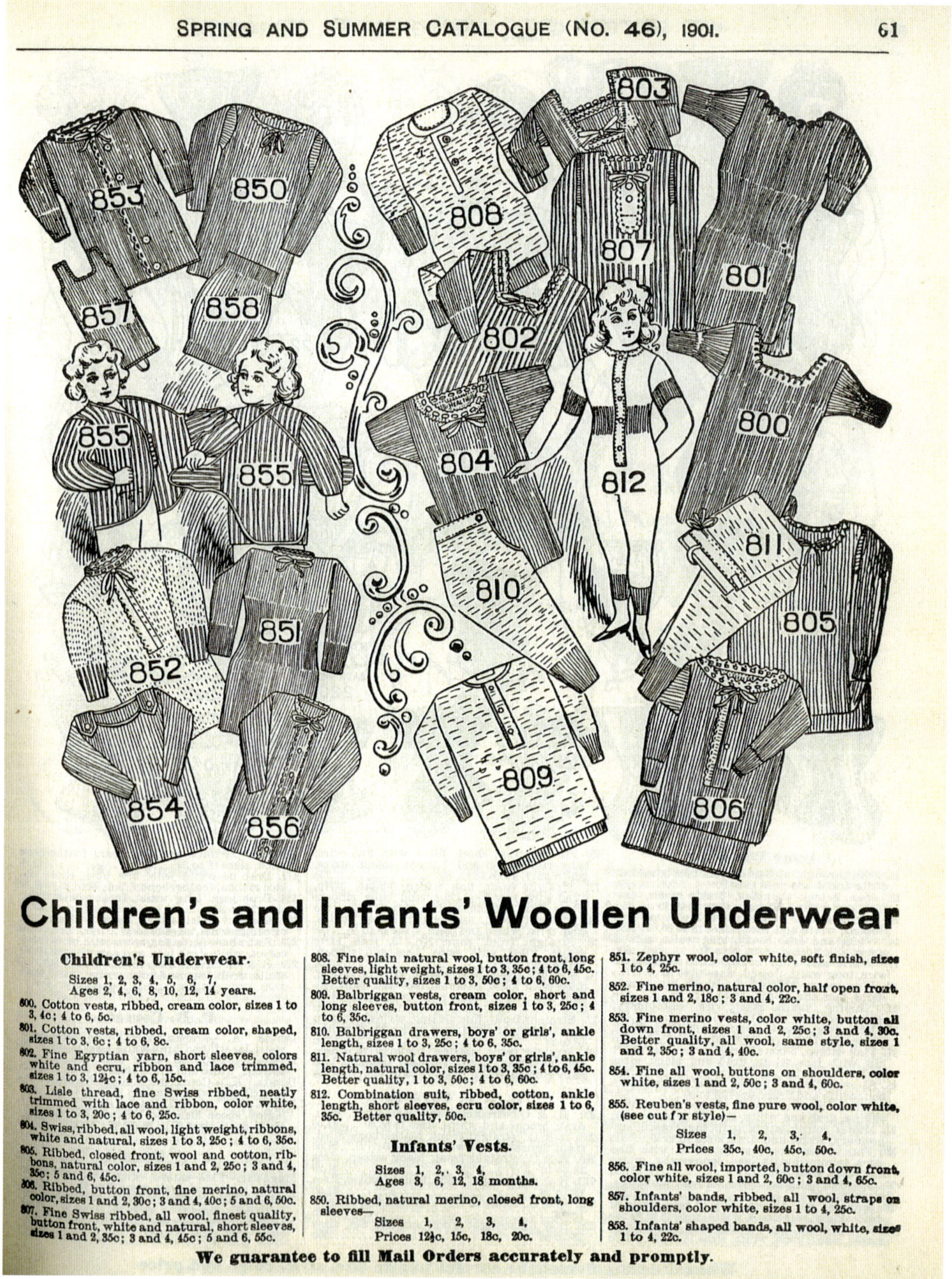

SPRING AND SUMMER CATALOGUE (NO. 46), 1901. 61

Children's and Infants' Woollen Underwear

Children's Underwear.

Sizes 1, 2, 3, 4, 5, 6, 7,
Ages 2, 4, 6, 8, 10, 12, 14 years.

800. Cotton vests, ribbed, cream color, sizes 1 to 3, 4c; 4 to 6, 5c.
801. Cotton vests, ribbed, cream color, shaped, sizes 1 to 3, 6c; 4 to 6, 8c.
802. Fine Egyptian yarn, short sleeves, colors white and ecru, ribbon and lace trimmed, sizes 1 to 3, 12½c; 4 to 6, 15c.
803. Lisle thread, fine Swiss ribbed, neatly trimmed with lace and ribbon, color white, sizes 1 to 3, 20c; 4 to 6, 25c.
804. Swiss, ribbed, all wool, light weight, ribbons, white and natural, sizes 1 to 3, 25c; 4 to 6, 35c.
805. Ribbed, closed front, wool and cotton, ribbons, natural color, sizes 1 and 2, 25c; 3 and 4, 35c; 5 and 6, 45c.
806. Ribbed, button front, fine merino, natural color, sizes 1 and 2, 30c; 3 and 4, 40c; 5 and 6, 50c.
807. Fine Swiss ribbed, all wool, finest quality, button front, white and natural, short sleeves, sizes 1 and 2, 35c; 3 and 4, 45c; 5 and 6, 55c.
808. Fine plain natural wool, button front, long sleeves, light weight, sizes 1 to 3, 35c; 4 to 6, 45c. Better quality, sizes 1 to 3, 50c; 4 to 6, 60c.
809. Balbriggan vests, cream color, short and long sleeves, button front, sizes 1 to 3, 25c; 4 to 6, 35c.
810. Balbriggan drawers, boys' or girls', ankle length, sizes 1 to 3, 25c; 4 to 6, 35c.
811. Natural wool drawers, boys' or girls', ankle length, natural color, sizes 1 to 3, 35c; 4 to 6, 45c. Better quality, 1 to 3, 50c; 4 to 6, 60c.
812. Combination suit, ribbed, cotton, ankle length, short sleeves, ecru color, sizes 1 to 6, 35c. Better quality, 50c.

Infants' Vests.

Sizes 1, 2, 3, 4,
Ages 3, 6, 12, 18 months.

850. Ribbed, natural merino, closed front, long sleeves—

Sizes	1,	2,	3,	4,
Prices	12½c,	15c,	18c,	20c.

851. Zephyr wool, color white, soft finish, sizes 1 to 4, 25c.
852. Fine merino, natural color, half open front, sizes 1 and 2, 18c; 3 and 4, 22c.
853. Fine merino vests, color white, button all down front, sizes 1 and 2, 25c; 3 and 4, 30c. Better quality, all wool, same style, sizes 1 and 2, 35c; 3 and 4, 40c.
854. Fine all wool, buttons on shoulders, color white, sizes 1 and 2, 50c; 3 and 4, 60c.
855. Reuben's vests, fine pure wool, color white, (see cut f)r style)—

Sizes	1,	2,	3,	4,
Prices	35c,	40c,	45c,	50c.

856. Fine all wool, imported, button down front, color white, sizes 1 and 2, 60c; 3 and 4, 65c.
857. Infants' bands, ribbed, all wool, straps on shoulders, color white, sizes 1 to 4, 25c.
858. Infants' shaped bands, all wool, white, sizes 1 to 4, 22c.

We guarantee to fill Mail Orders accurately and promptly.

Children's and infants' winter underwear. *Eaton's Fall and Winter Catalogue*, 1901–1902.

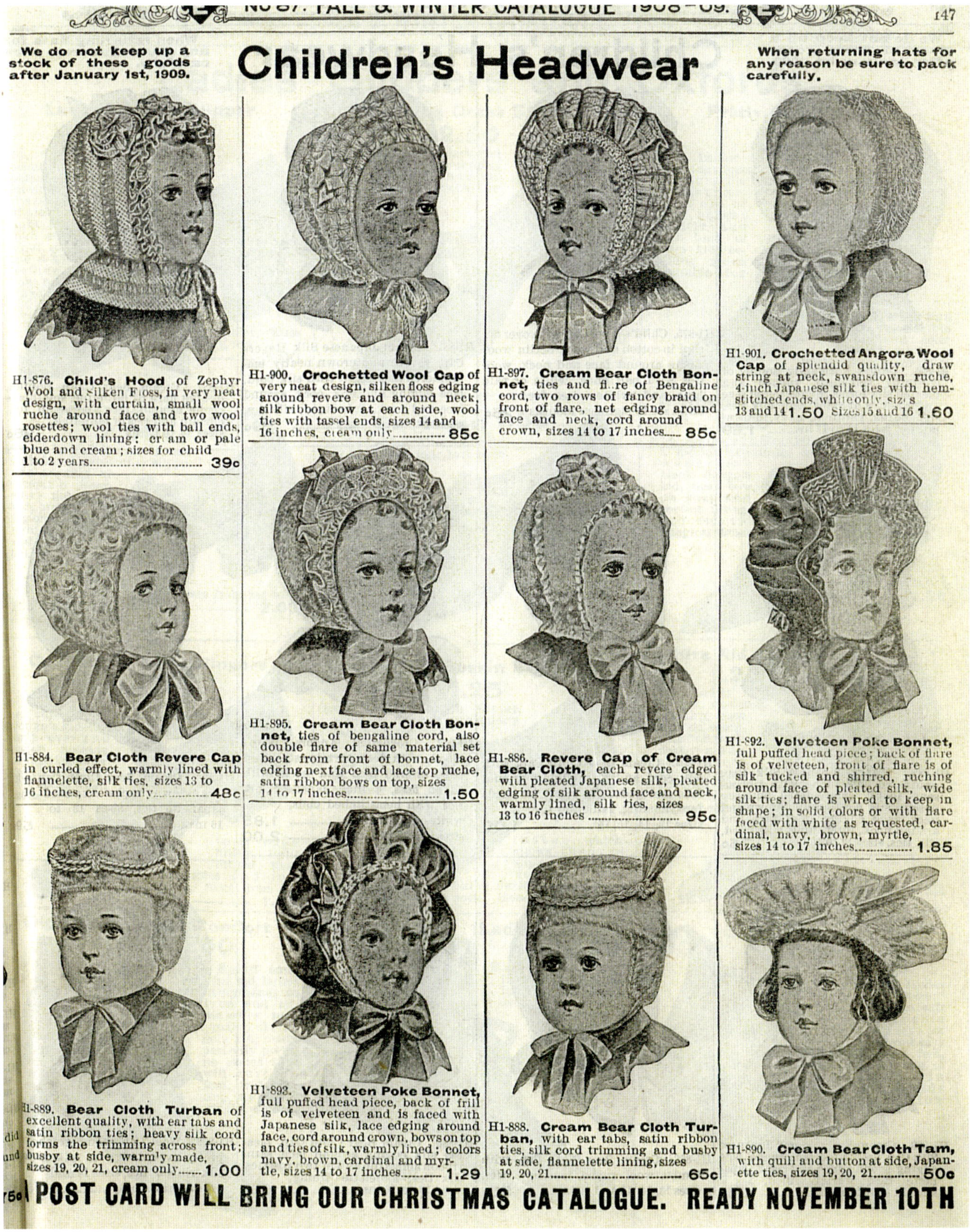

No. 87. FALL & WINTER CATALOGUE 1908–09. 147

We do not keep up a stock of these goods after January 1st, 1909.

Children's Headwear

When returning hats for any reason be sure to pack carefully.

H1-876. **Child's Hood** of Zephyr Wool and Silken Floss, in very neat design, with curtain, small wool ruche around face and two wool rosettes; wool ties with ball ends, eiderdown lining; cream and pale blue and cream; sizes for child 1 to 2 years........ 39c

H1-900. **Crochetted Wool Cap** of very neat design, silken floss edging around revere and around neck, silk ribbon bow at each side, wool ties with tassel ends, sizes 14 and 16 inches, cream only........ 85c

H1-897. **Cream Bear Cloth Bonnet,** ties and flare of Bengaline cord, two rows of fancy braid on front of flare, net edging around face and neck, cord around crown, sizes 14 to 17 inches..... 85c

H1-901. **Crochetted Angora Wool Cap** of splendid quality, draw string at neck, swansdown ruche, 4-inch Japanese silk ties with hem-stitched ends, white only, sizes 13 and 14 1.50 Sizes 15 and 16 1.60

H1-884. **Bear Cloth Revere Cap** in curled effect, warmly lined with flannelette, silk ties, sizes 13 to 16 inches, cream only........ 48c

H1-895. **Cream Bear Cloth Bonnet,** ties of bengaline cord, also double flare of same material set back from front of bonnet, lace edging next face and lace top ruche, satin ribbon bows on top, sizes 14 to 17 inches........ 1.50

H1-886. **Revere Cap of Cream Bear Cloth,** each revere edged with pleated Japanese silk, pleated edging of silk around face and neck, warmly lined, silk ties, sizes 13 to 16 inches........ 95c

H1-892. **Velveteen Poke Bonnet,** full puffed head piece; back of flare is of velveteen, front of flare is of silk tucked and shirred, ruching around face of pleated silk, wide silk ties; flare is wired to keep in shape; in solid colors or with flare faced with white as requested, cardinal, navy, brown, myrtle, sizes 14 to 17 inches........ 1.85

H1-889. **Bear Cloth Turban** of excellent quality, with ear tabs and satin ribbon ties; heavy silk cord forms the trimming across front; busby at side, warmly made, sizes 19, 20, 21, cream only...... 1.00

H1-893. **Velveteen Poke Bonnet,** full puffed head piece, back of frill is of velveteen and is faced with Japanese silk, lace edging around face, cord around crown, bows on top and ties of silk, warmly lined; colors navy, brown, cardinal and myrtle, sizes 14 to 17 inches........ 1.29

H1-888. **Cream Bear Cloth Turban,** with ear tabs, satin ribbon ties, silk cord trimming and busby at side, flannelette lining, sizes 19, 20, 21........ 65c

H1-890. **Cream Bear Cloth Tam,** with quill and button at side, Japanette ties, sizes 19, 20, 21........ 50c

A POST CARD WILL BRING OUR CHRISTMAS CATALOGUE. READY NOVEMBER 10TH

Hoods, bonnets, and caps for tiny youngsters. *Eaton's Fall and Winter Catalogue*, 1908–1909.

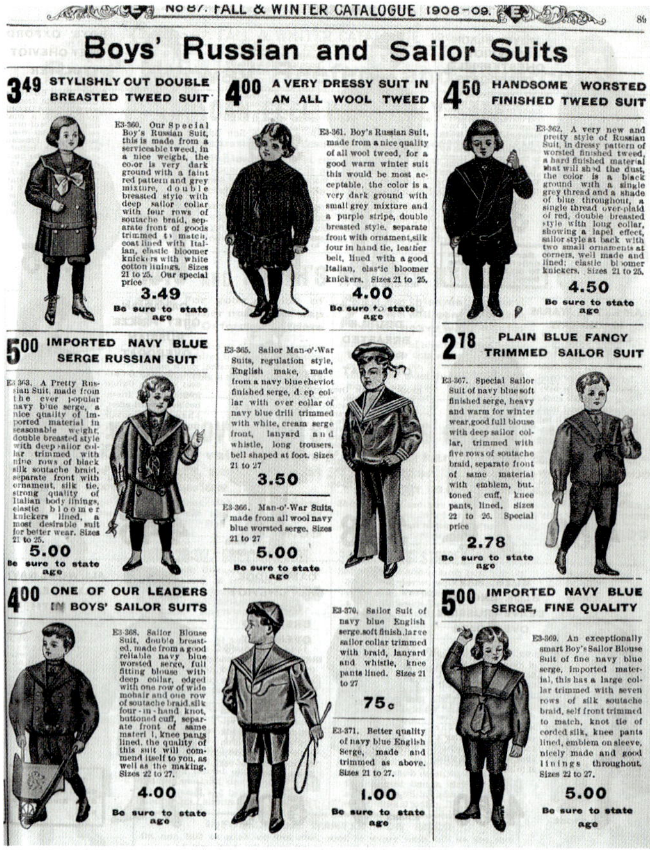

Boys' Russian and sailor suits. *Eaton's Fall and Winter Catalogue*, 1908–1909.

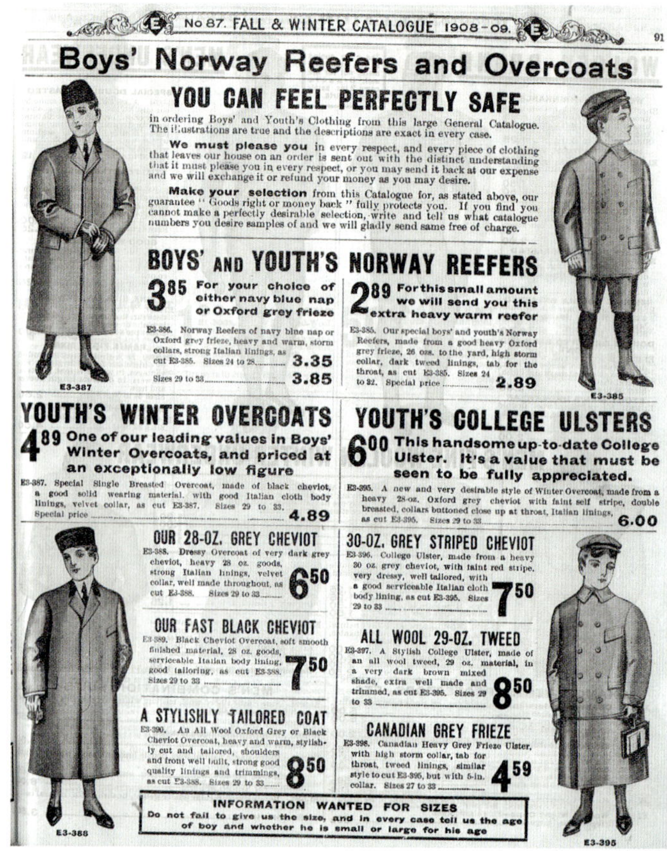

Jackets and overcoats for little gentlemen. *Eaton's Fall and Winter Catalogue*, 1908–1909.

Shoes and Boots

Shoes took on a more conservative appearance as the new century dawned, and the extremely pointed toe fell out of fashion. Despite style innovations, footwear for children at the turn of the century was well constructed, primarily of leather. The notion was widely held that a high leather shoe would support the ankles. It was argued that for active children this meant fewer falls, leading to fewer broken bones and doctor bills.

During the first decade of the twentieth century, little girls' dress shoes were similar in color (white or ivory) and workmanship to those of the late nineteenth century, but they took on a simpler aesthetic, rising to just below the ankle and fastening with a single button. Typically, they boasted elongated, squared-off toes, although in 1902 a trend for pointy-toed shoes emerged. The shoes sat on shallow, stacked heels and were decorated with satin, grosgrain, or self-fabric bows in the case of linen or canvas pairs.

Unadorned black leather Mary Janes were sanctioned for school or playtime, but high-button boots with wool uppers were also widely seen, particularly on boys.

Infants' Wear

> "Smocking is a pretty ornamentation for the yoke of a child's dress, particularly when the material is fine linen, soft silk or cashmere."—Elizabeth Robinson Scovil, *Ladies' Home Journal*, February 1900

The overall silhouette of infants' wear did not change with the dawning of the new century, but subtle changes in trim and fabrication, in keeping with dress reform influences and a trend to lightness in dress, were tracked and advocated in various fashion journals.

Furs and the Small Child

"Many of the children's coats this winter have a band of fur put on to imitate a yoke, even when the part above it is not filled in with silk."—Elizabeth Robinson Scovil, *Ladies' Home Journal*, February 1900

Fur served both a decorative and a practical purpose in late Victorian children's fashion. Yard goods stores carried a

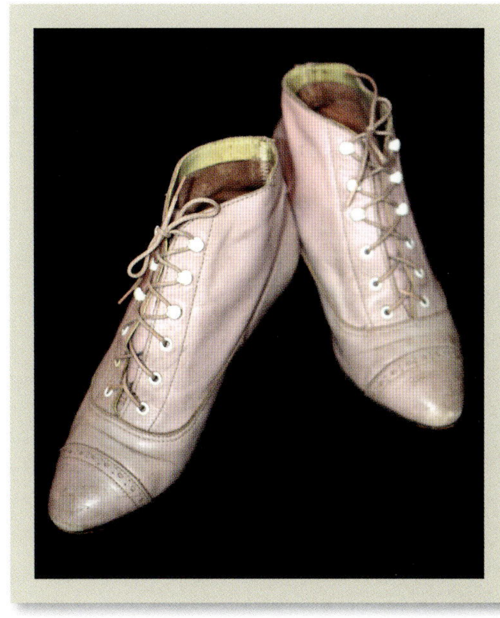

Misses lace-up pink leather boots with slight heel.

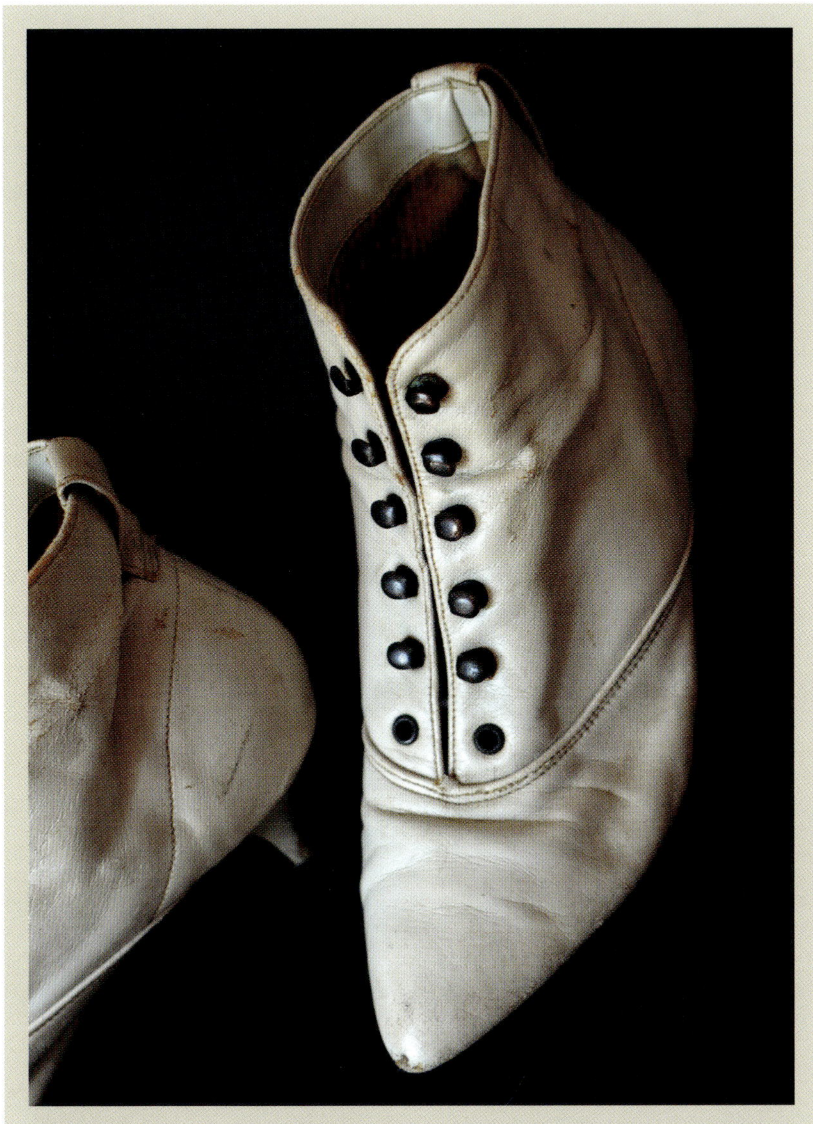

Similar high-top lace-up boots in white.

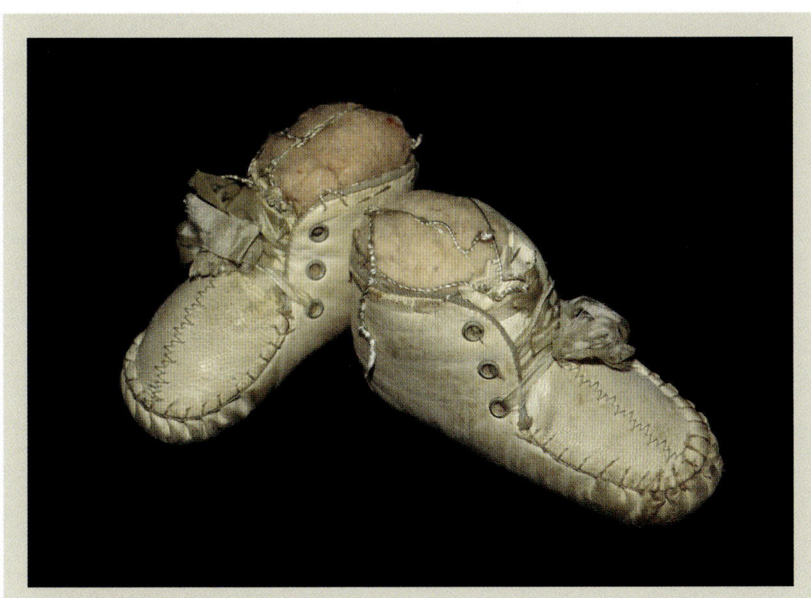

Infant's hand-stitched kid leather bootie with silk ribbon ties.

variety of common and exotic furs suitable for dressmaking. Fashion journals described the prevailing styles and offered suggestions for garment construction and fabric selection.

Under the heading "Coat for a Girl of Four," the February 1900 *Ladies' Home Journal* outlined instructions for a coat of blue silk and brown ladies' cloth cut with a wide cape outlined in brown fur. Otter and beaver are suggested. The contrast of texture and color of this simply styled garment is typical of turn-of-the-century children's patterning and reflects a move from heavier layered clothing to a lighter, streamlined aesthetic.

During this period, fur was favored in narrow bands of trimming to add contrast or give the impression of a more layered and detailed construction. This artifice was also applied to baby blankets and carriage covers. One pattern for a flannel-lined eiderdown baby carriage blanket suggested the application of a band of fur—black astrakhan on a jewel-toned red, gray astrakhan on cadet blue, white thibet on bright blue, or beaver fur on cream or dark green—to "simulate a flap turning over at the top" (*Ladies Home Journal*, February 1900).

> "White holds first rank this summer, as it did last, for children, young girls, and young women."—Emma M. Hooper, *Ladies' Home Journal,* May 1901

Paris fashion dictates of the early 1900s were widely reported in European and North American womens' magazines, with the new line described as expanded and inflated; ruffles adorn shoulders, skirts fall away from the body, and corsages are laid in plaits. Fancy buttons appear and shades of heliotrope, or *noisette*, nut-brown, and *sanglier*, dominate for fall and winter. Zibeline cloth is favored, as are chemisettes of lace and satin.

Ladies' Home Journal columnist Emma H. Hooper advised in May 1901 that a "pretty summer costume for a young girl would be a thin white gown trimmed with beading through which black velvet ribbon is run; a black velvet belt, with a sash of soft white ribbon tied on the left side, with large natural-looking pink roses run through it. The sash would slip under the belt at the side, be knotted twice at the lower edge, and have long ends cut rounded reaching to the very edge of the skirt." As confounding as this might seem to a contemporary reader, such a description would be enough for many a reader to create the garment described.

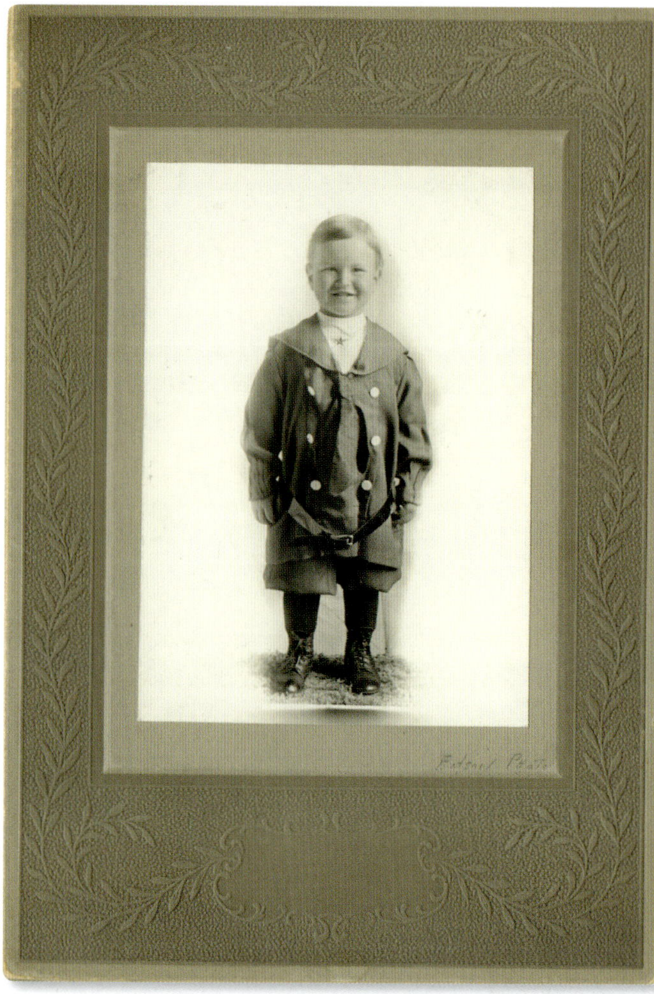

C. 1908: Three-year-old Rupert John Champion in a stylish Russian suit with giant contrast buttons and low, buckled belt.

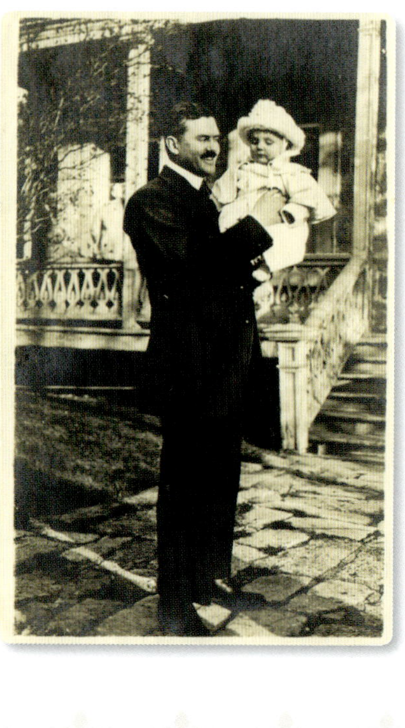

This young child's coat retains vestiges of Victorian styling, as does the bonnet.

This sweet Edwardian miss took care to dress for her portrait. In addition to the Dolly Dingle bow that tops her long, sleek sausage curls, she has decorated her freshly starched blouse with a heart pendant, ladies pocket watch, and cameo brooch.

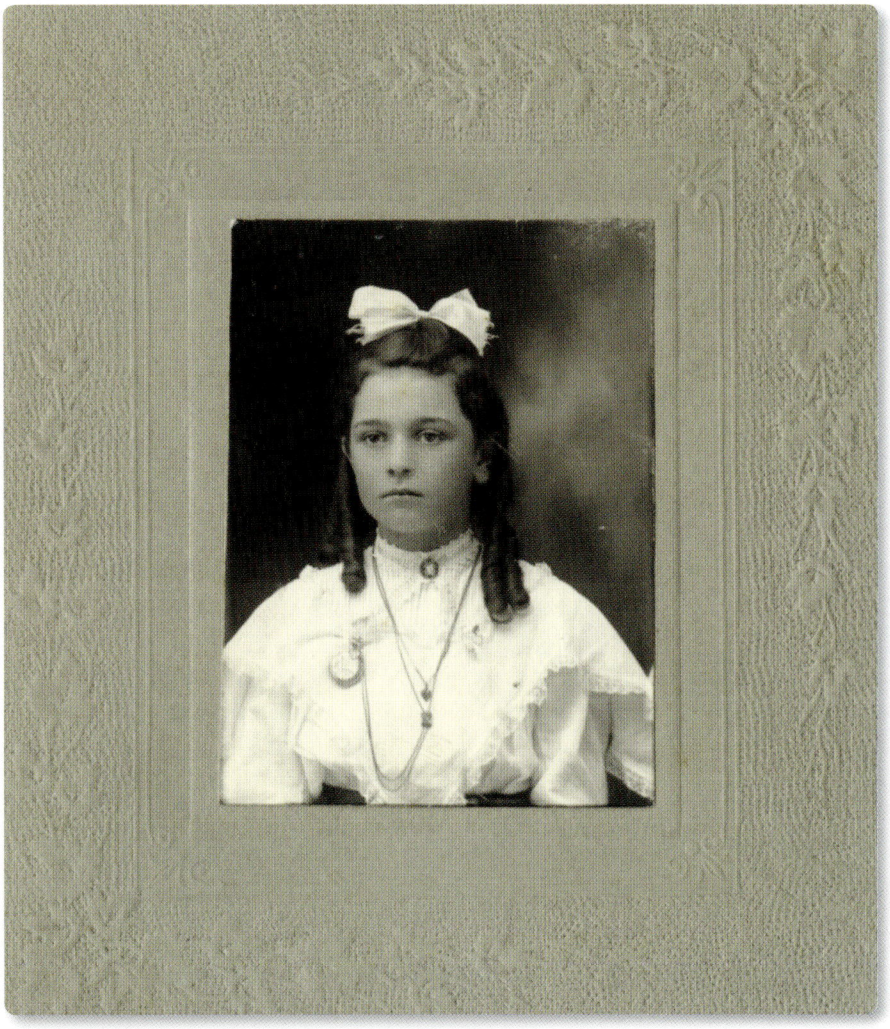

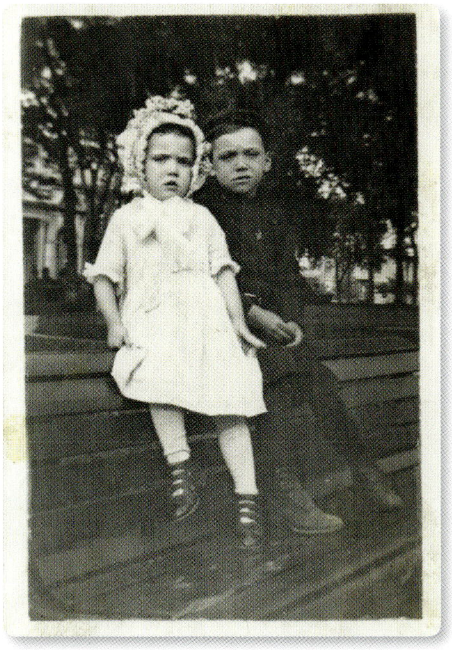

A young miss in Edwardian dress with three-quarter sleeves, her frilly bonnet similar to those shown in the 1908–1909 Eaton's catalog for approximately one dollar.

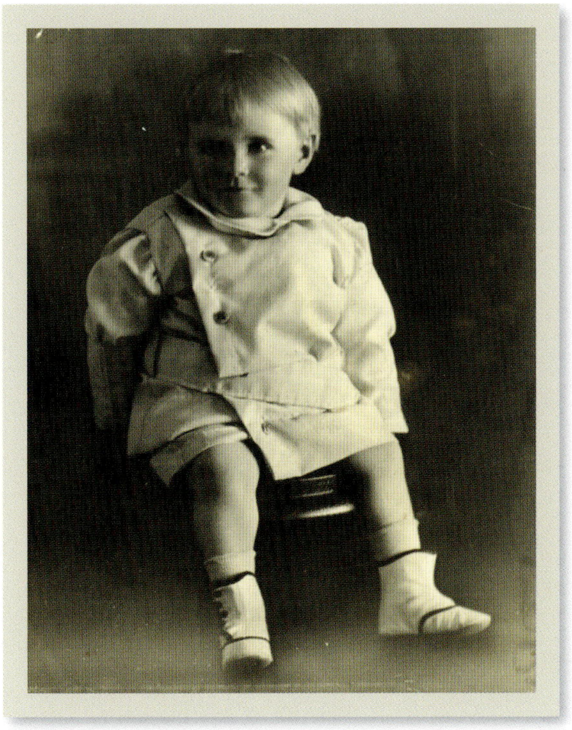

A handsome tyke in a light-colored boxy suit with wide buckled belt. Note the fashionable two-tone shoes.

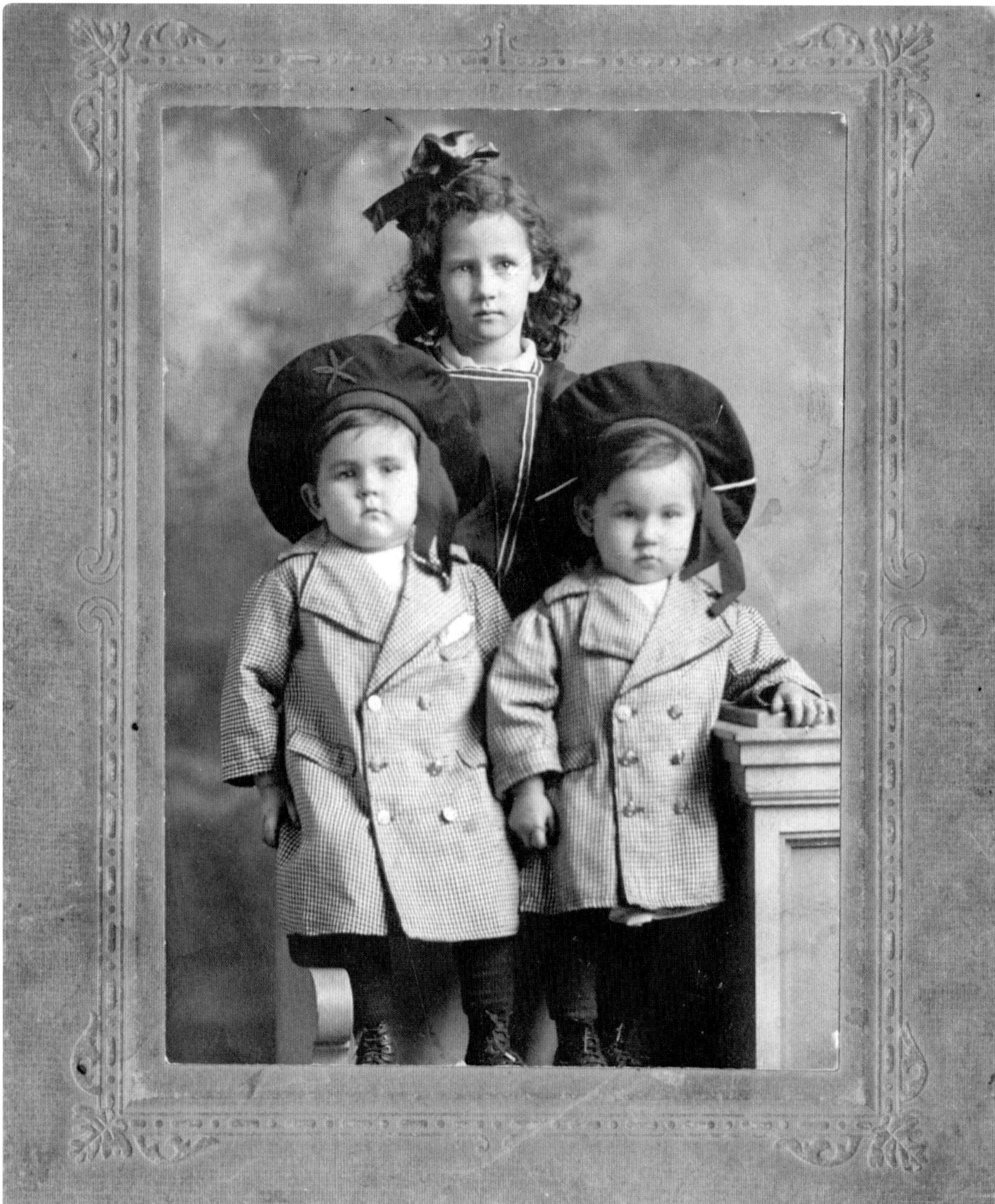

Cabinet card image of three fashionably dressed children c. 1902. The pair in front are dressed alike in double-breasted coats and giant tams with trailing ribbons.

The Hunter family c.1905: Jason and George wear matching nautical jackets over woolen britches with black stockings and leather boots. Their older brother, Jim, pictured in the front row, far right, is dressed in knee-length britches and a close-fitting suit jacket with narrow lapels. Blanche and Jane (second and third, top row) are dressed in skirt and blouse ensembles similar to styles for adult women, but with shorter skirts. They have all come from the funeral of the children's mother, Alice Jewett Hunter. Even the dog looks somber.

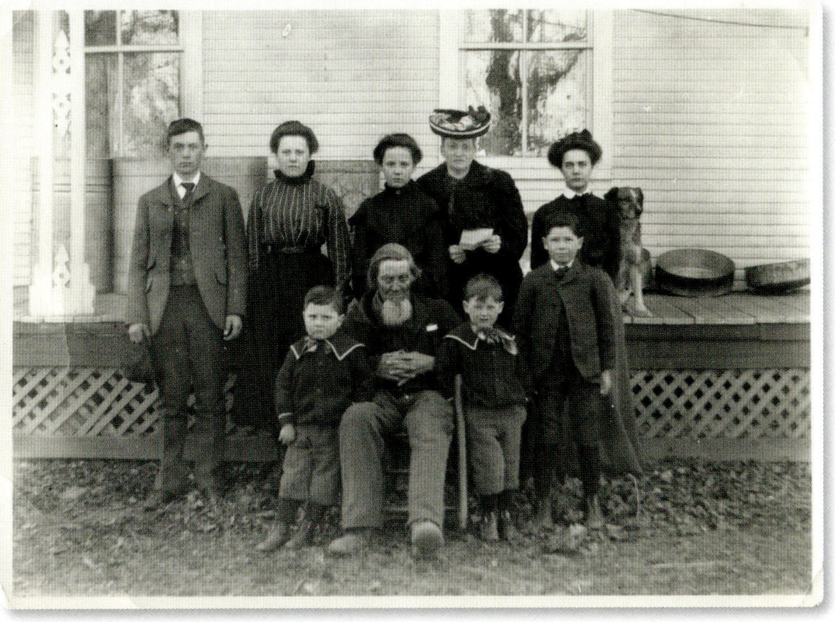

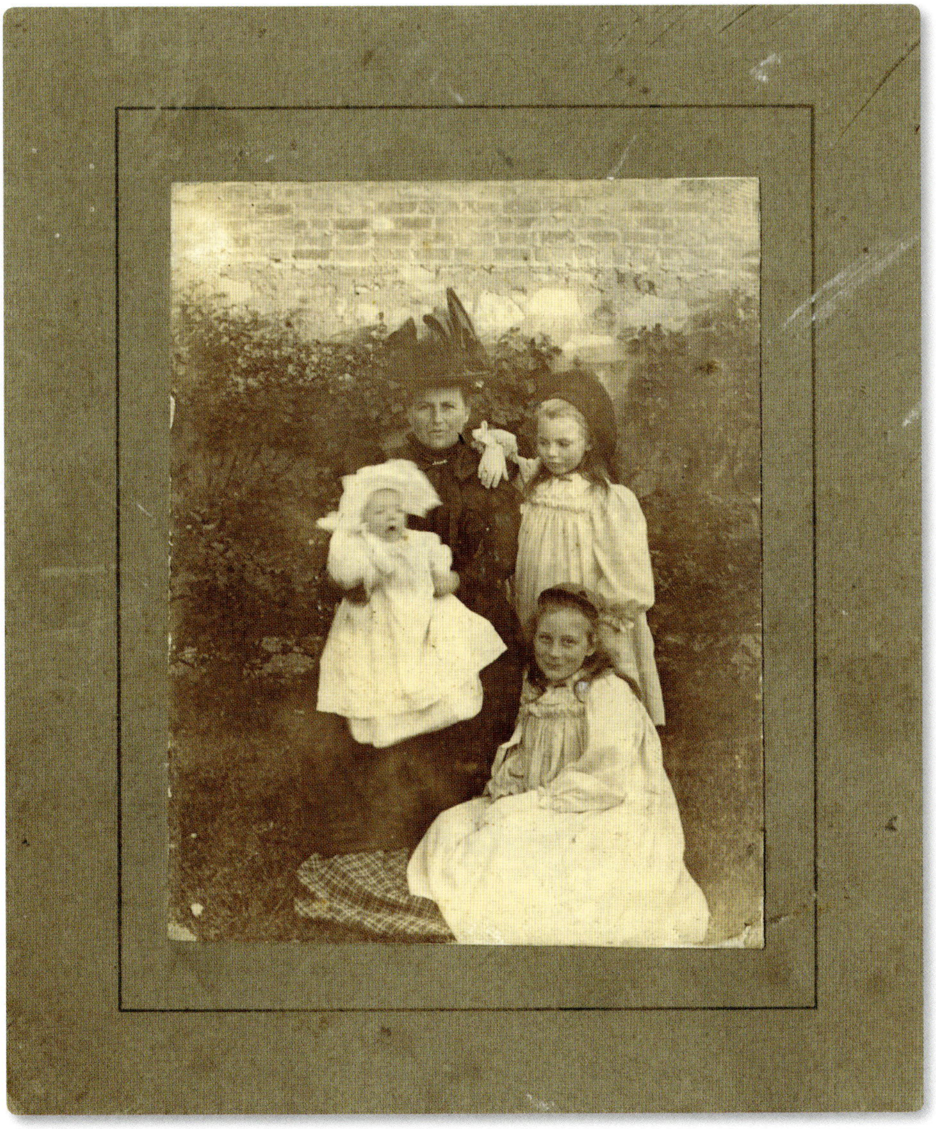

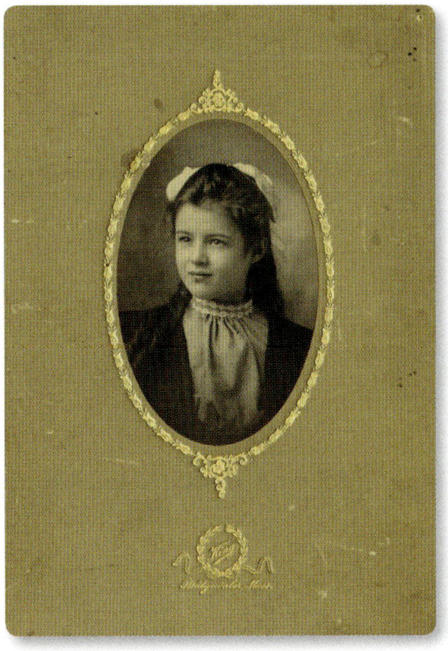

The wings of a giant butterfly bow can be seen atop the head of this pretty young girl dressed in a dark jacket with deep V-neck over a pigeon-breasted blouse. The blouse is gathered at the neck into a stand-up collar trimmed with double rows of lace braid.

Edwardian fashion, Scottish style: Addie and Gertie, in yoked, blousey dresses that look like modern-day nightgowns, wear their long hair drawn back under chic hats specially designed for children, one a large tam, the other a helmet style. Baby brother Seaton tops his white gown with a wired flare bonnet. The cabinet card photograph was sent to Maggie Philip from her cousins in Scotland.

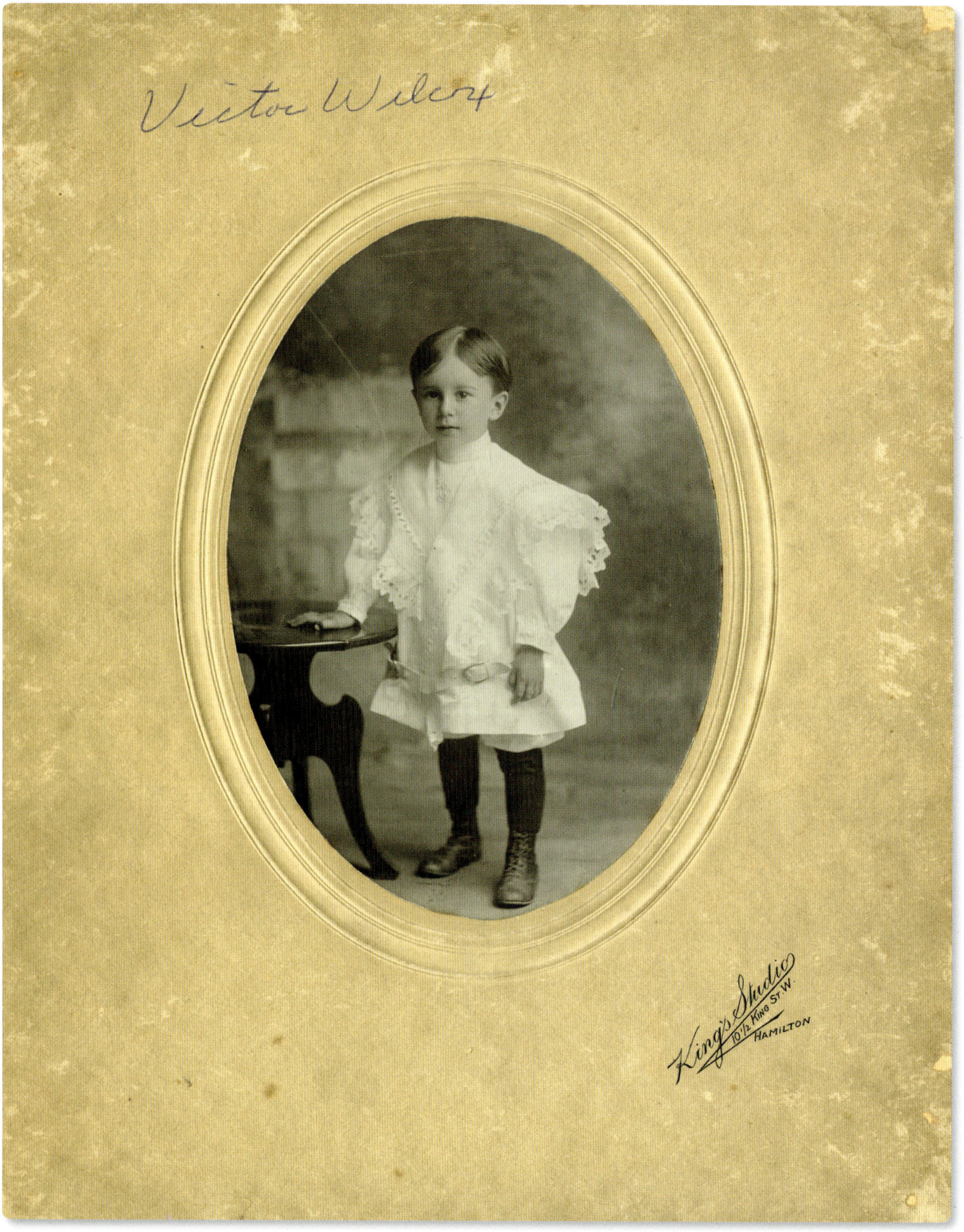

Victor Wilcox's crisp, white bloomer-knickers suit is low belted in the Russian style and features a lavish lace-trimmed collar that extends extravagantly beyond the shoulders.

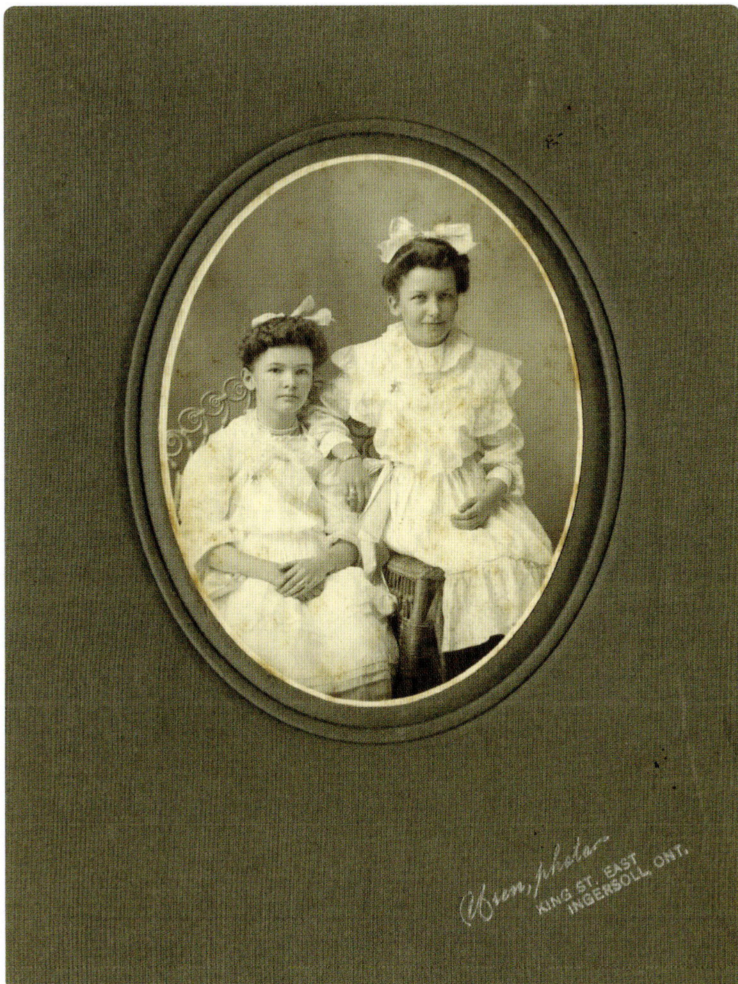

A pair of Edwardian sisters with grown-up Gibson girl hairdos and ruffle-trimmed dresses.

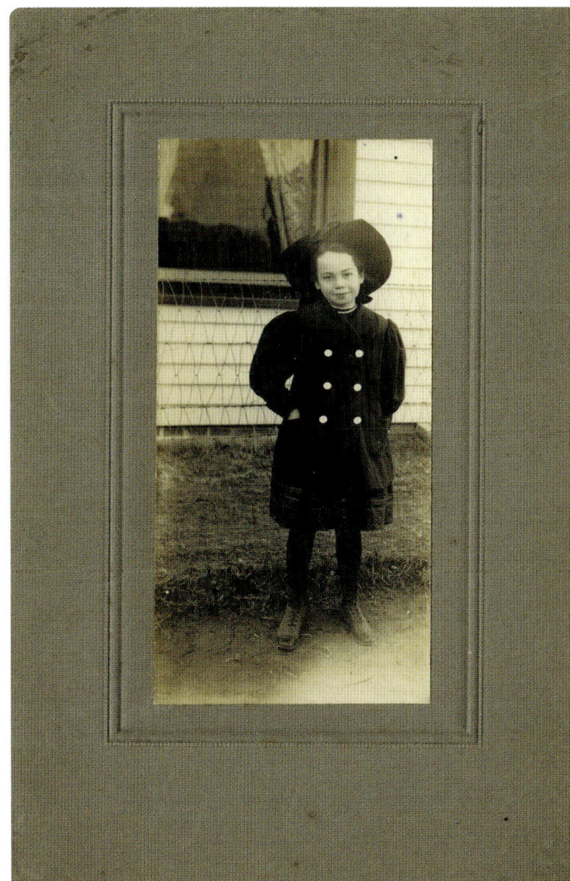

Erma Newton c.1902 in a double-breasted automobile coat and giant tam.

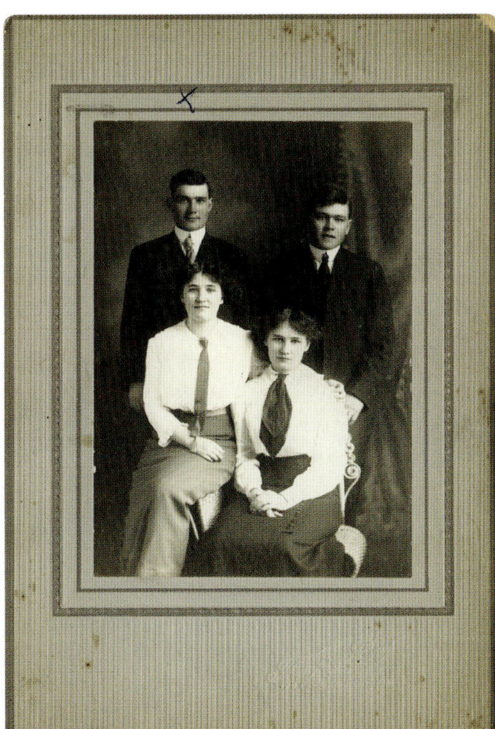

These teen girls are fashionably dressed in white cotton shirtwaists, accessorized with silk ties and bar pins. The girl on the left poses to ensure that the silk tassels of her tie can be seen draped across her hand.

Pearl Earl's box-pleated skirt and square-cut jacket with sailor collar are in keeping with the fashion aesthetic of the Edwardian era. Functional, giant white buttons add to the decorative simplicity of this outfit. Postcard image.

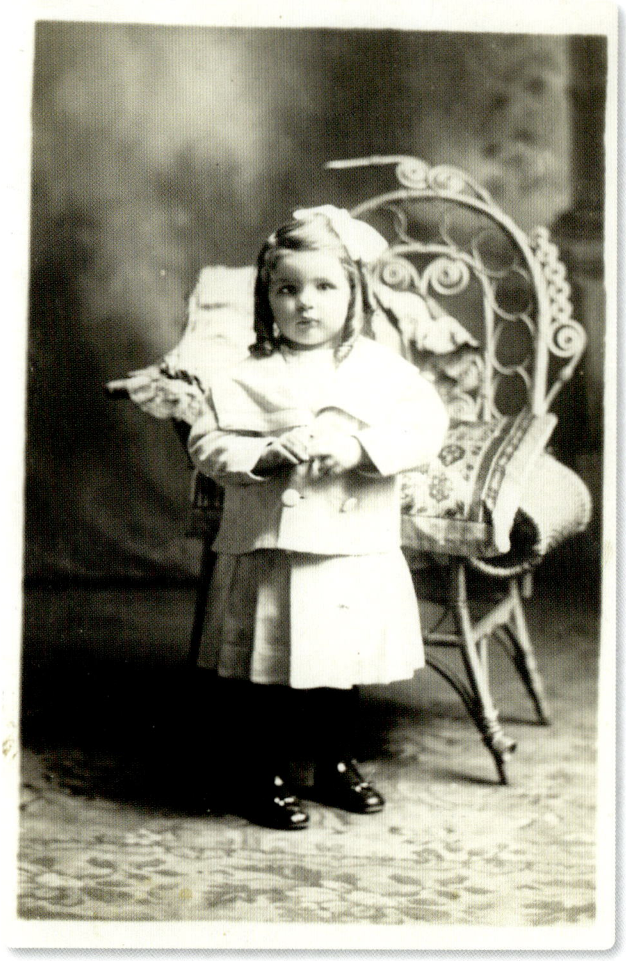

This pre-schooler's blousey white bloomer suit contrasts nicely with his fancy socks.

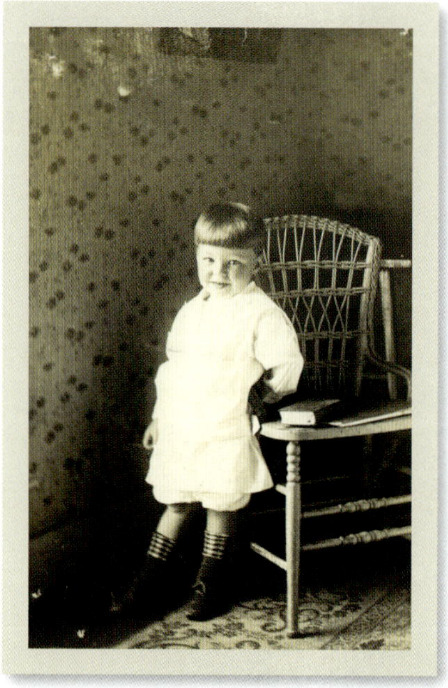

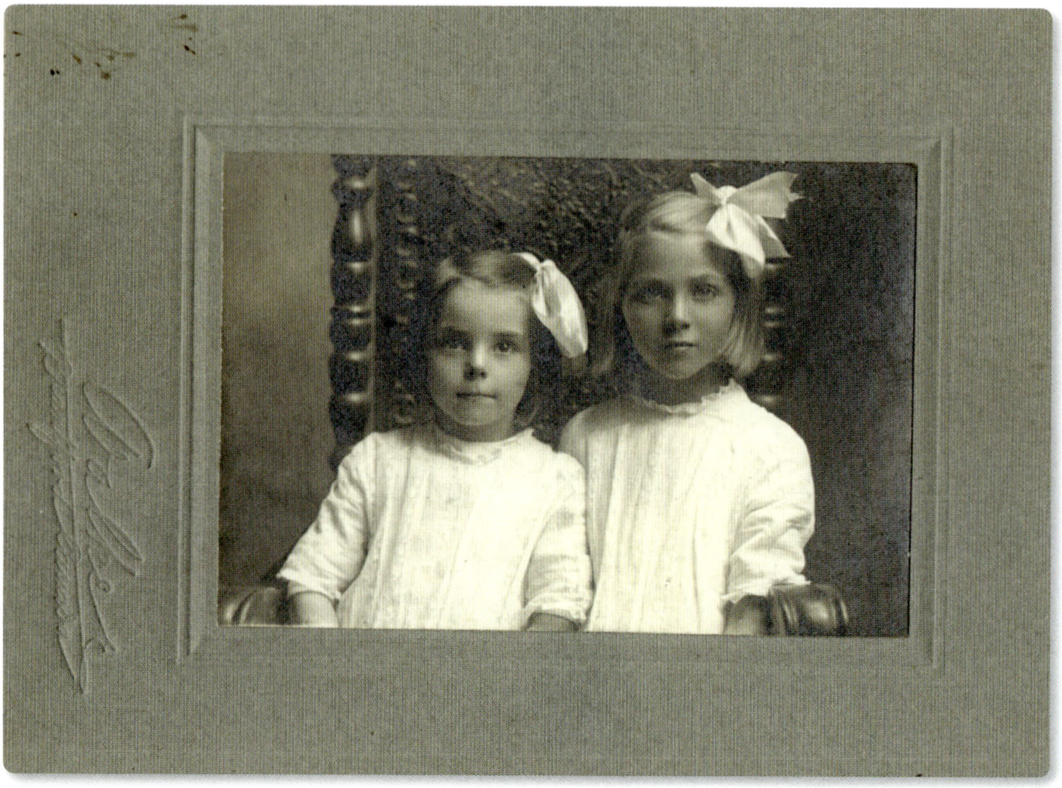

A lovely Edwardian image featuring sisters in white cotton dresses, their locks set with Dolly Dingle bows.

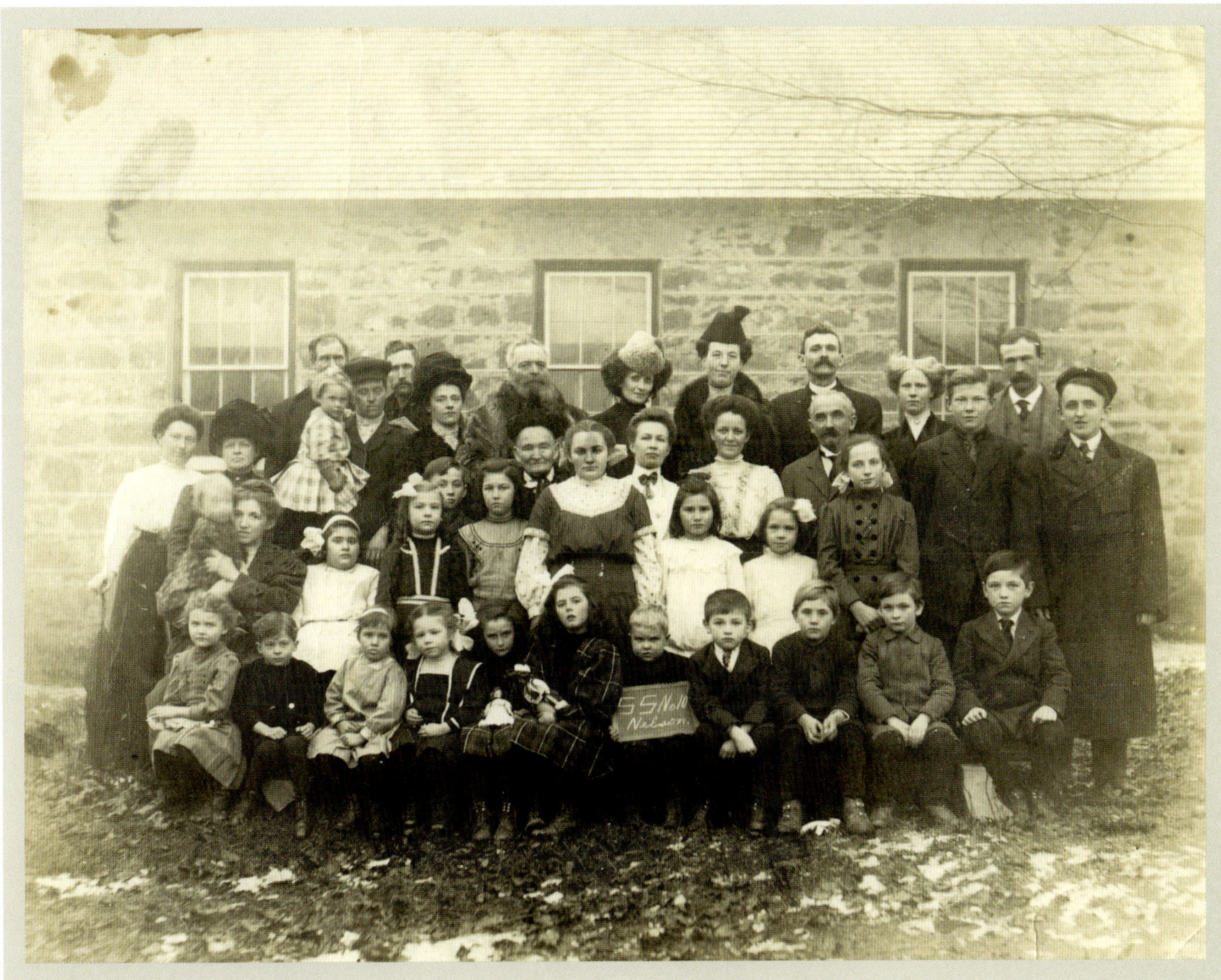

Several examples of late Victorian fashion can be seen in this early twentieth-century photo in which little Burdge Gunby holds the sign identifying the Nelson School in rural Ontario. Furs, early Edwardian hairstyles, shirt waists, tartans, and a walking stick umbrella reveal this group's interest in fashion.

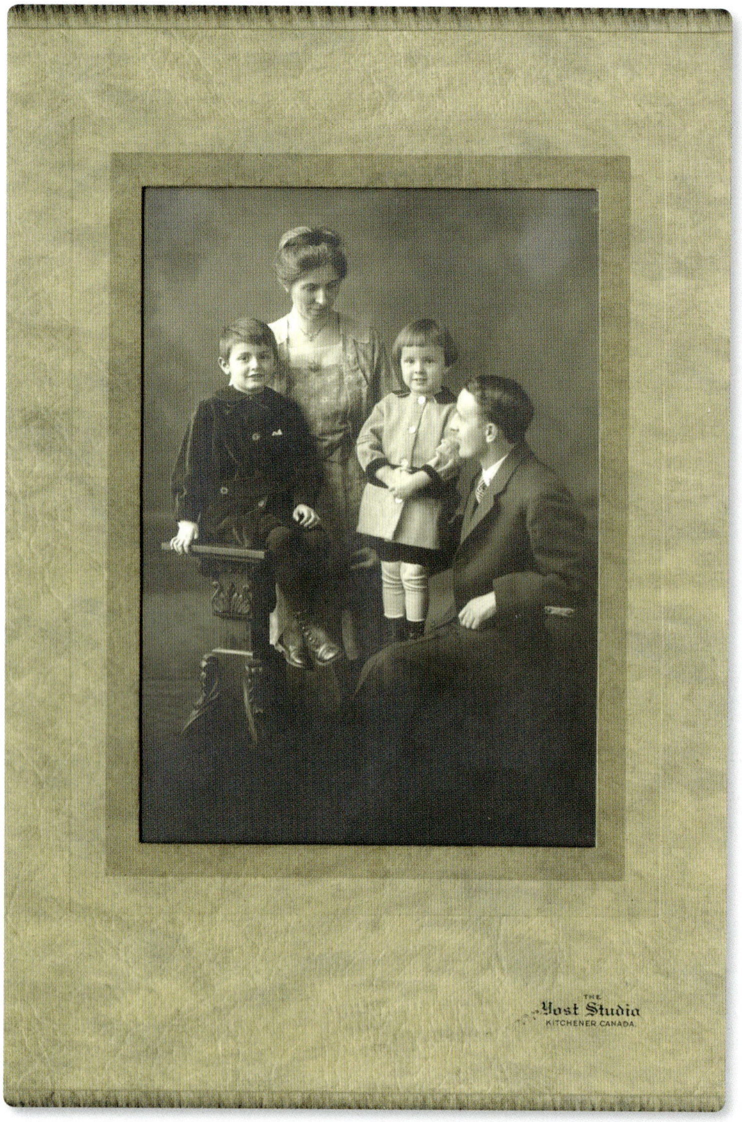

This family portrait is beautifully posed, placing the focus on the children. Both ensembles feature Peter Pan collars, large buttons, and full cuffed sleeves.

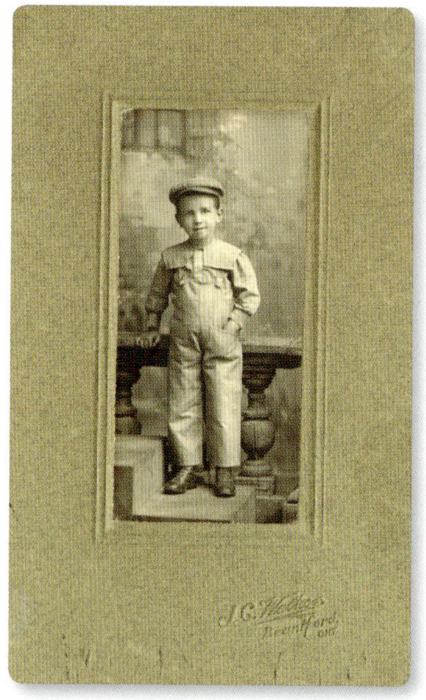

A young boy in snappy sailor blouse and crisp overalls poses in what appears to be a woolen newsboy cap. It would be interesting to know the color of his ensemble.

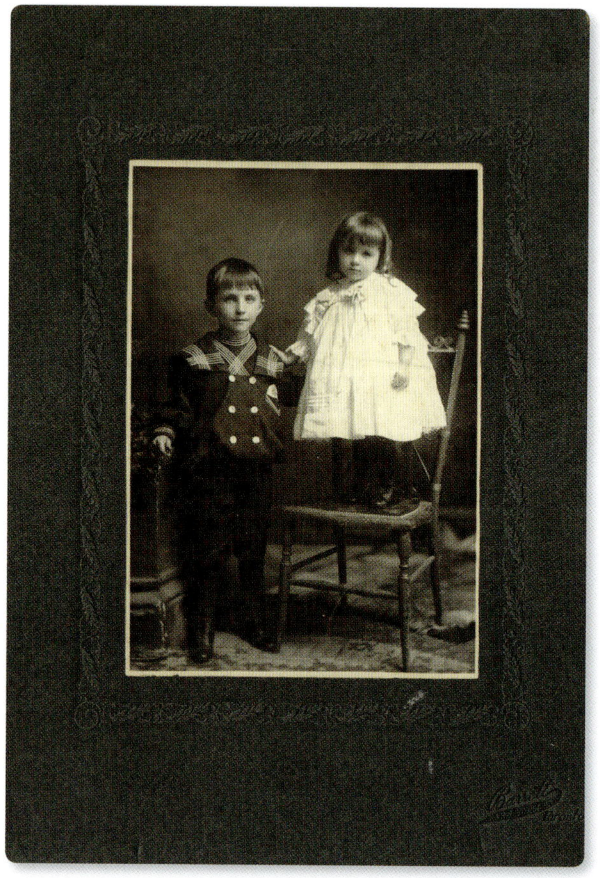

Cabinet card image of a boy smartly attired in a dark-colored sailor suit and woolen stockings. The boy poses with a young girl in yoked puffy sleeved dress.

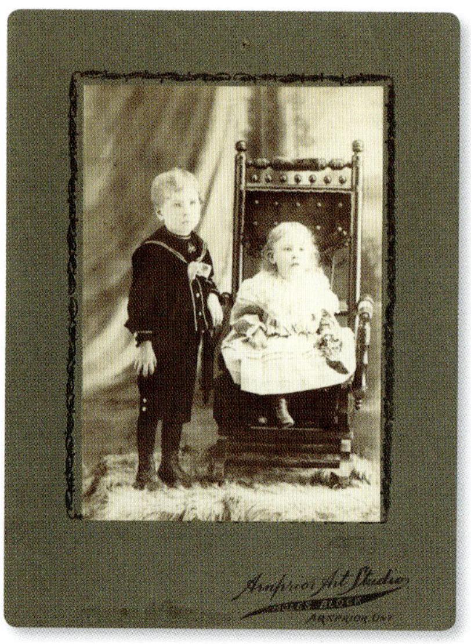

Buttons, a bow, and applied contrast braid decorate this youngster's long-sleeved sailor suit. The boy's female companion wears a long-sleeved dress with lacy bertha.

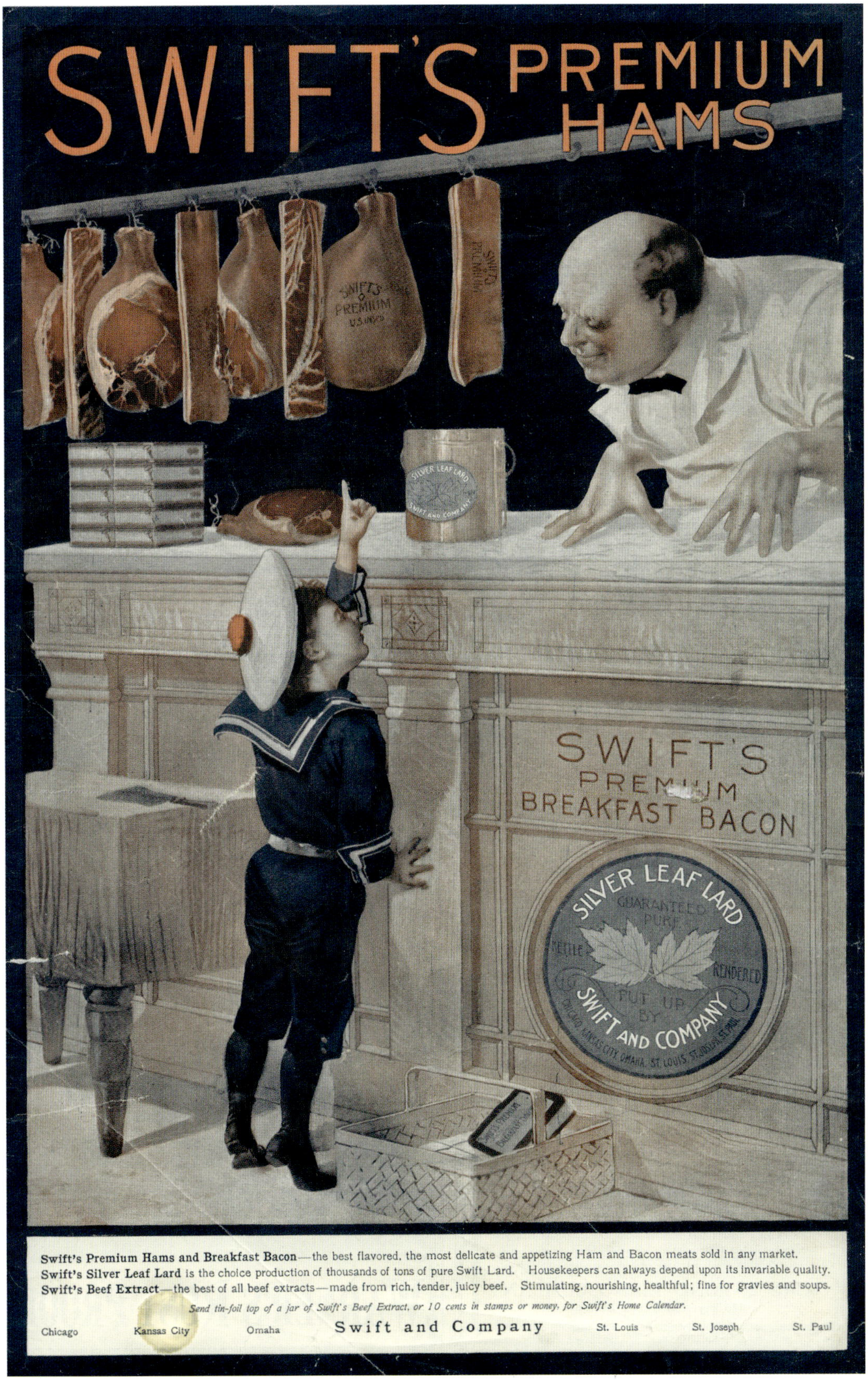

This boy's navy blue sailor suit figures prominently in a back page advertisement. *Ladies' Home Journal*, February 1900.

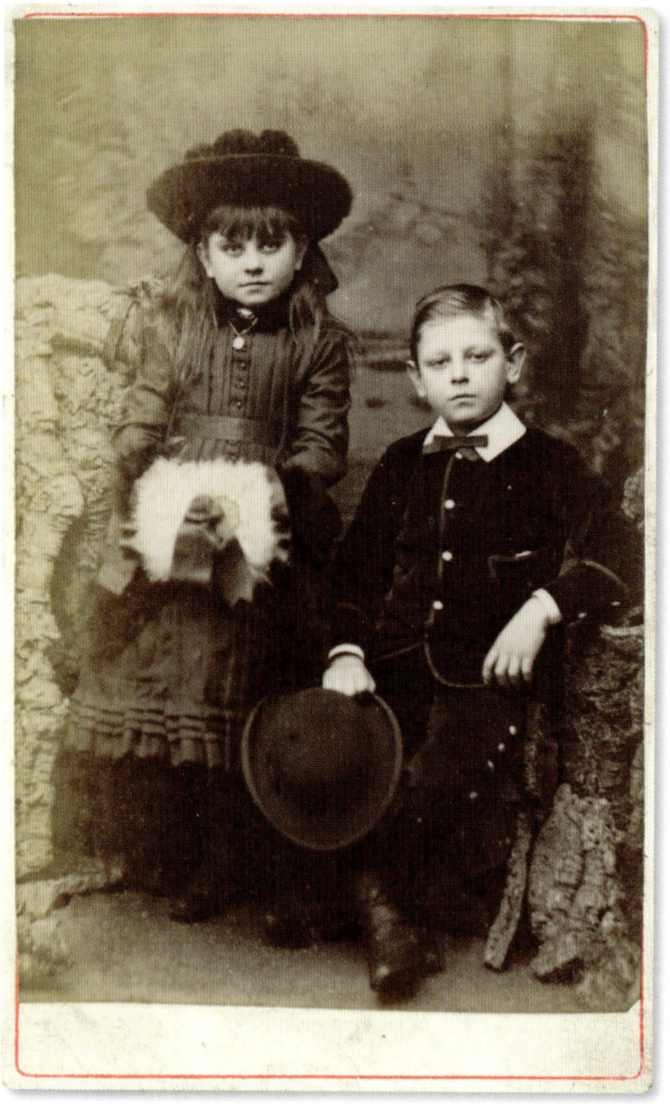

Winter dressing 1890s style. Note the ribbon-trimmed fur muff, the girl's large dark halo hat, and the smartly attired boy's bowler.

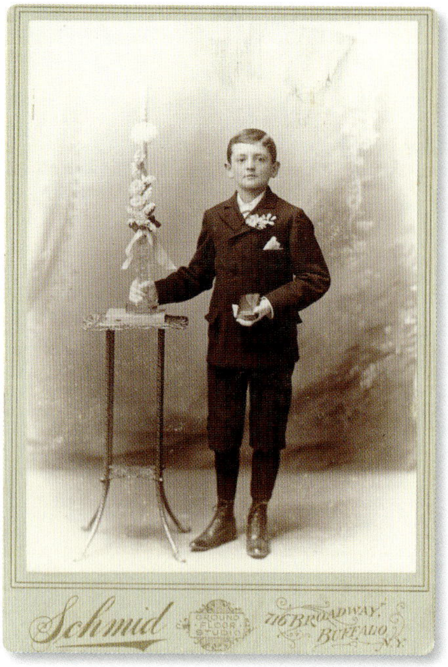

First communion portrait of a boy in a double-breasted knickers suit.

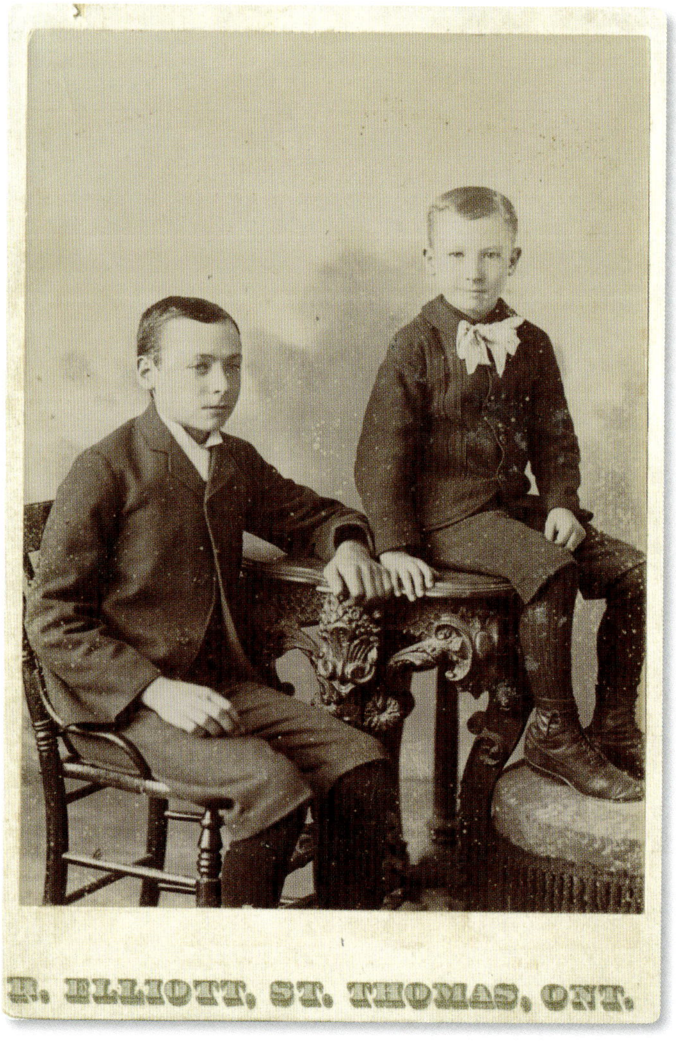

A pair of school-aged boys in knickers suits.

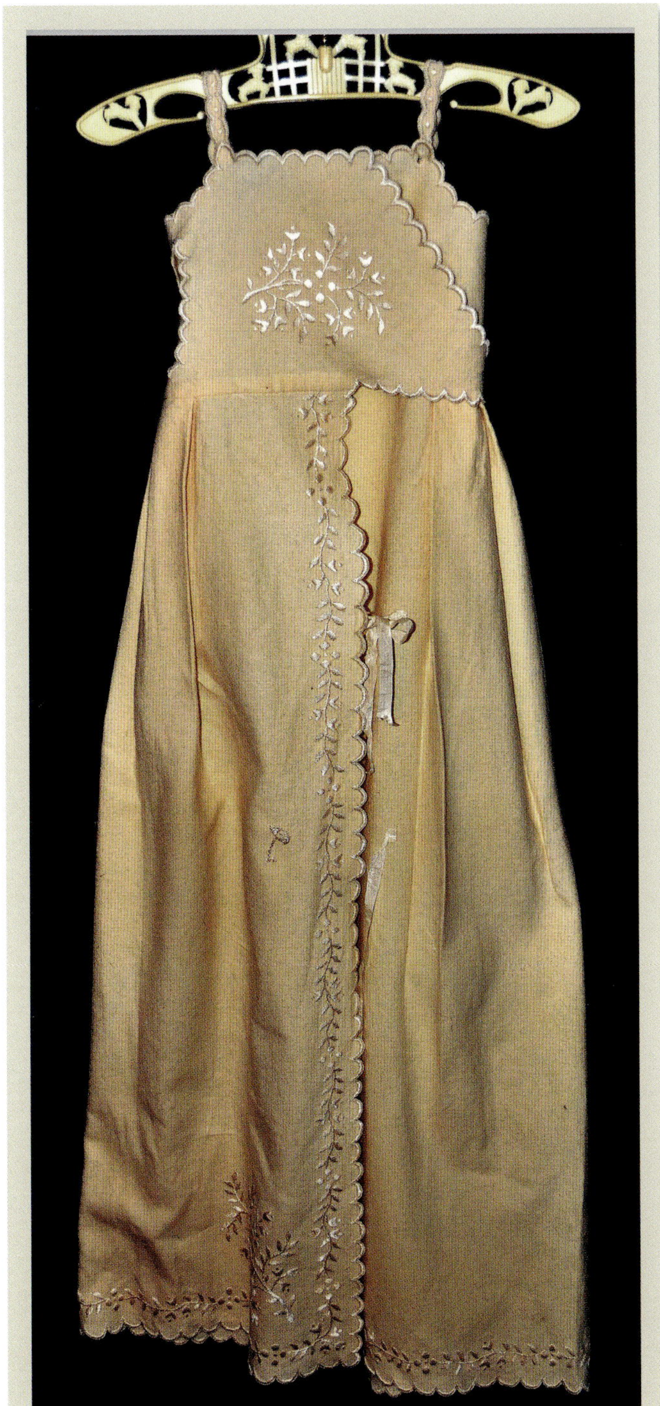

Young child's embroidered cashmere wrap-around jumper with silk ribbon ties.

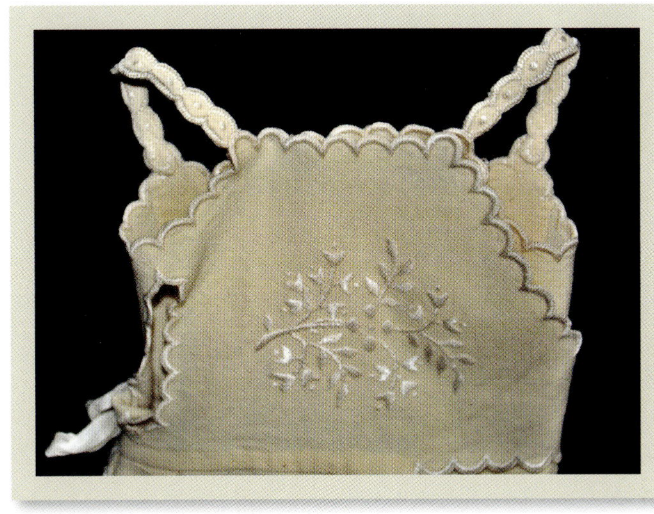

Bodice detail.

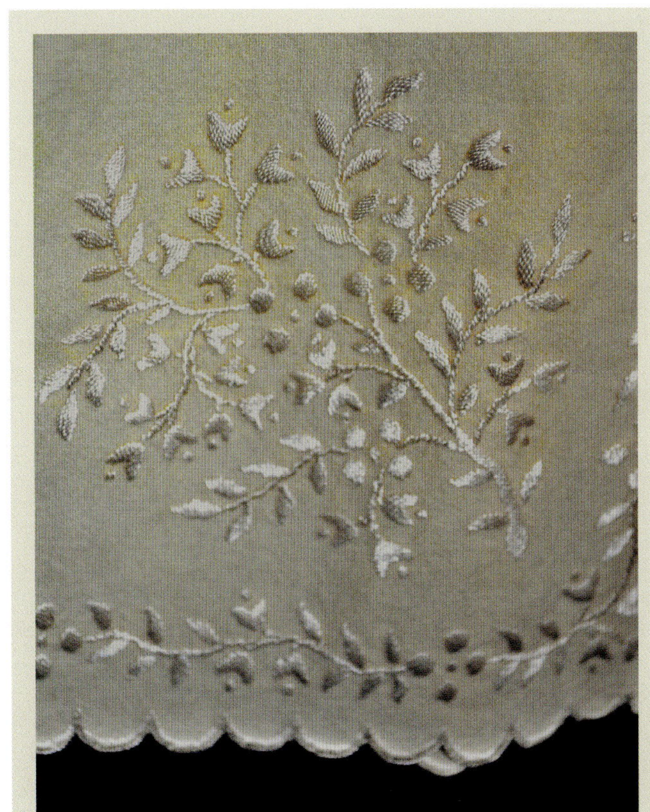

Detail: silk embroidery embellishment at hem.

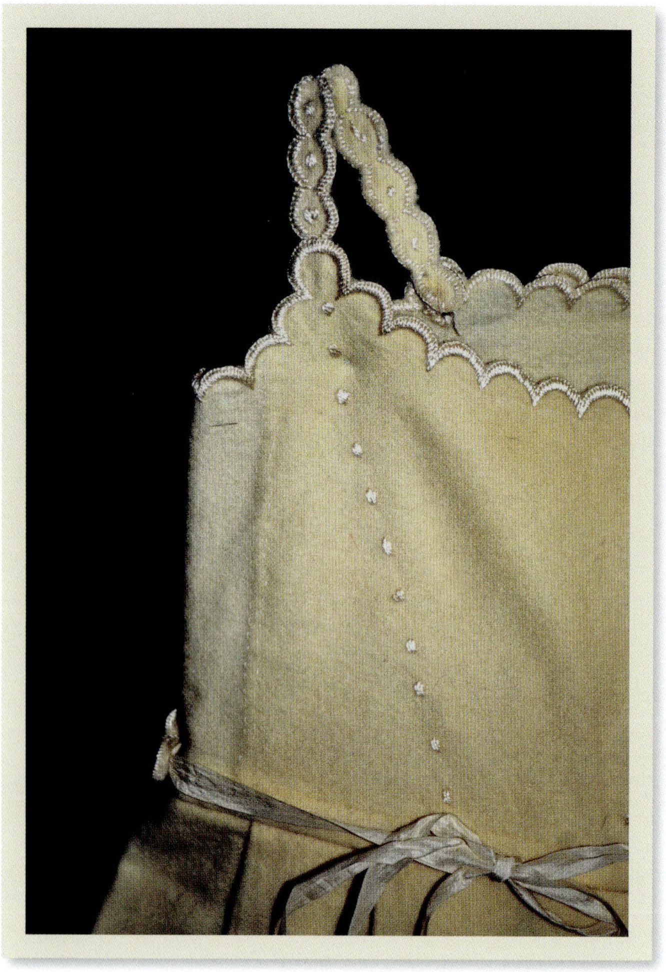

Detail: back bodice.

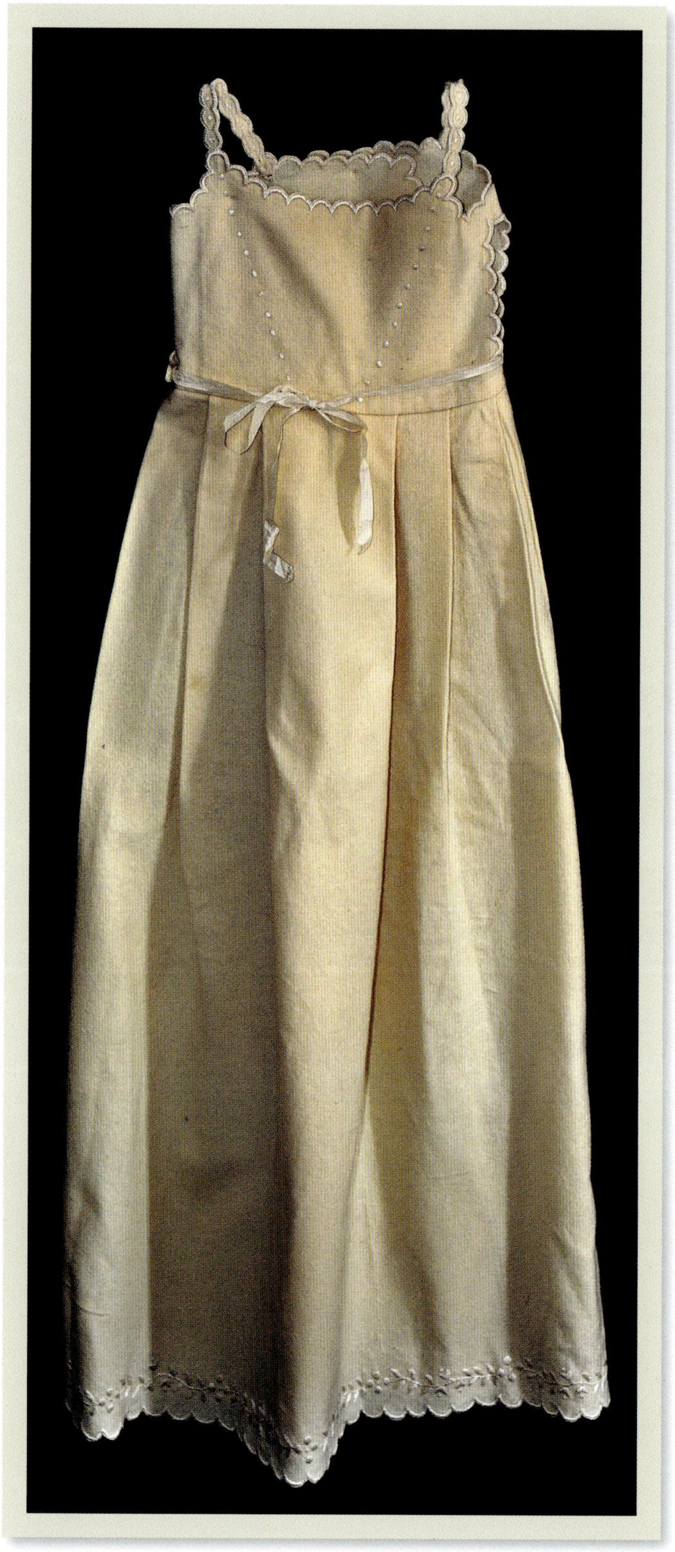

Back view.

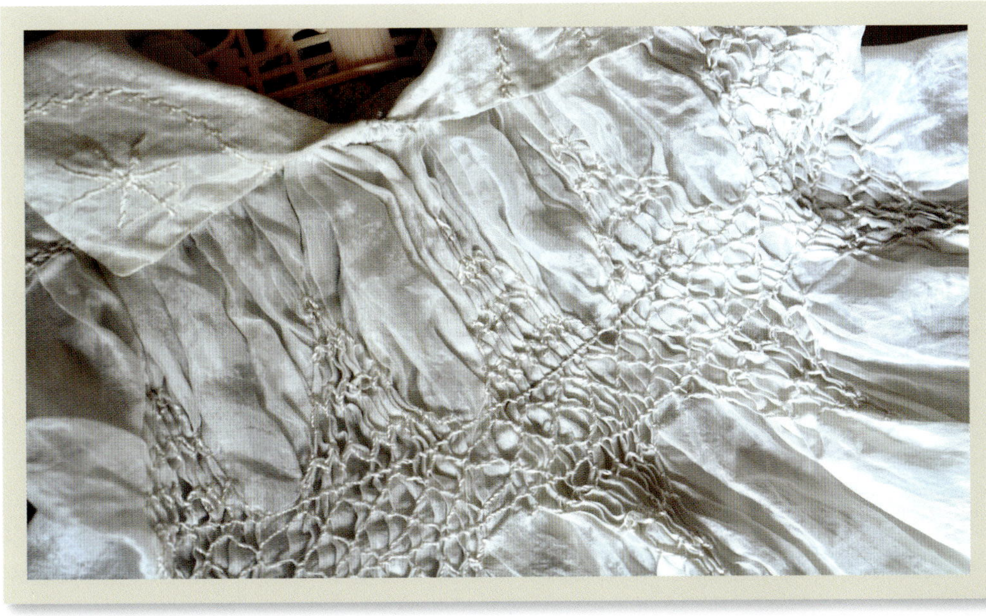

Smocked bodice detail of an infant's white silk dress.

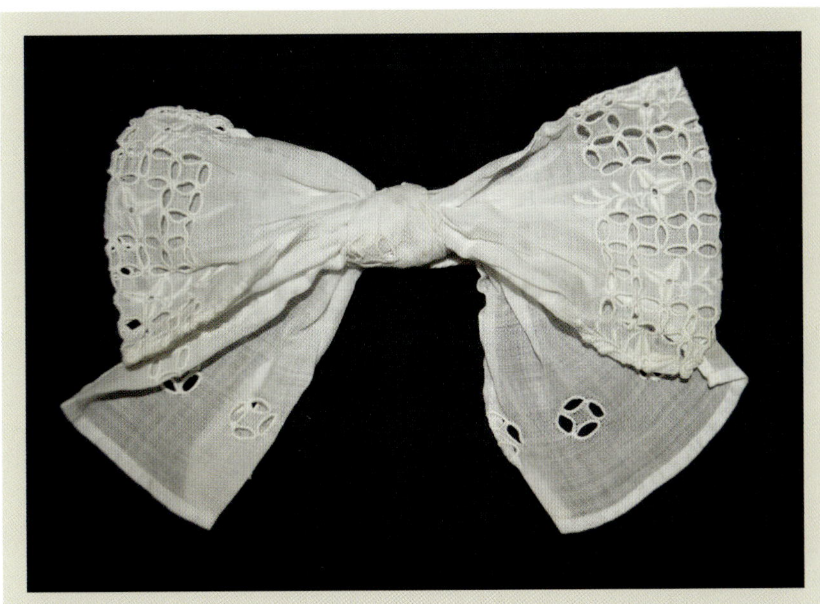

Cotton eyelet hair bow à la Dolly Dingle.

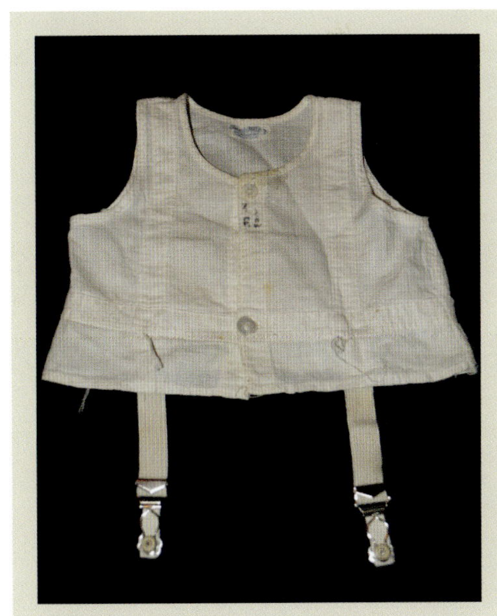

Gender-neutral young child's waist with detachable garters.

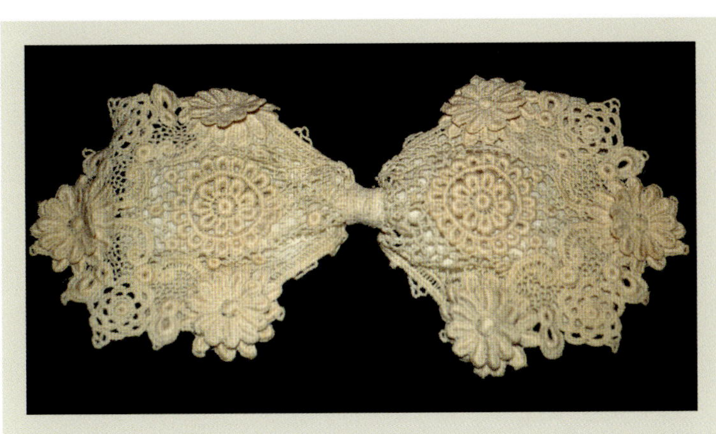

Ultra-feminine floral-patterned lace hair bow.

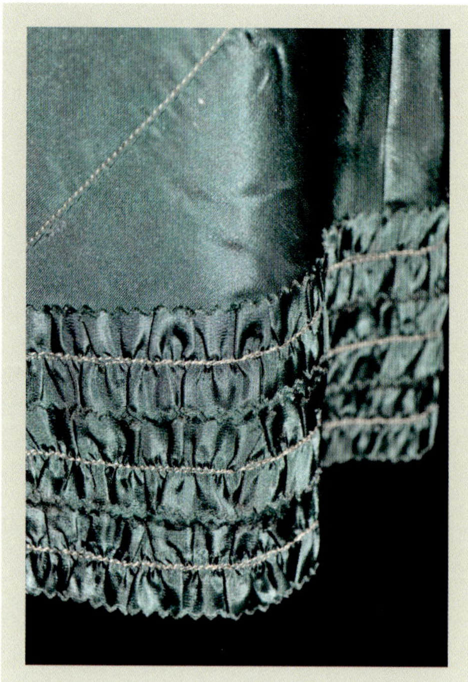

Detail: ruffled hem.

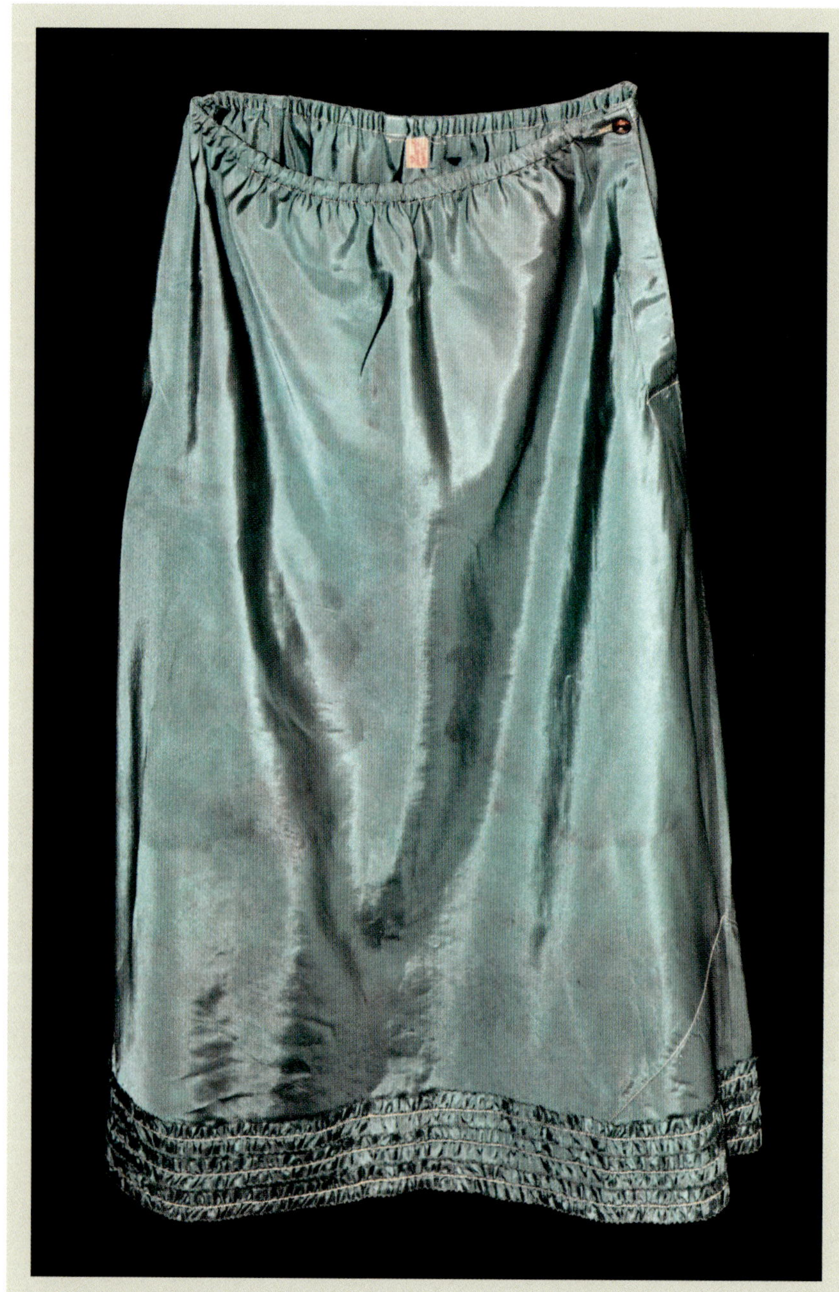

Emerald-green taffeta petticoat gored at the hem for wear with trumpet shaped skirts, c. 1900. Hem flounced with a triple row of self-fabric ruffles. Label: Toronto Petticoat Co.

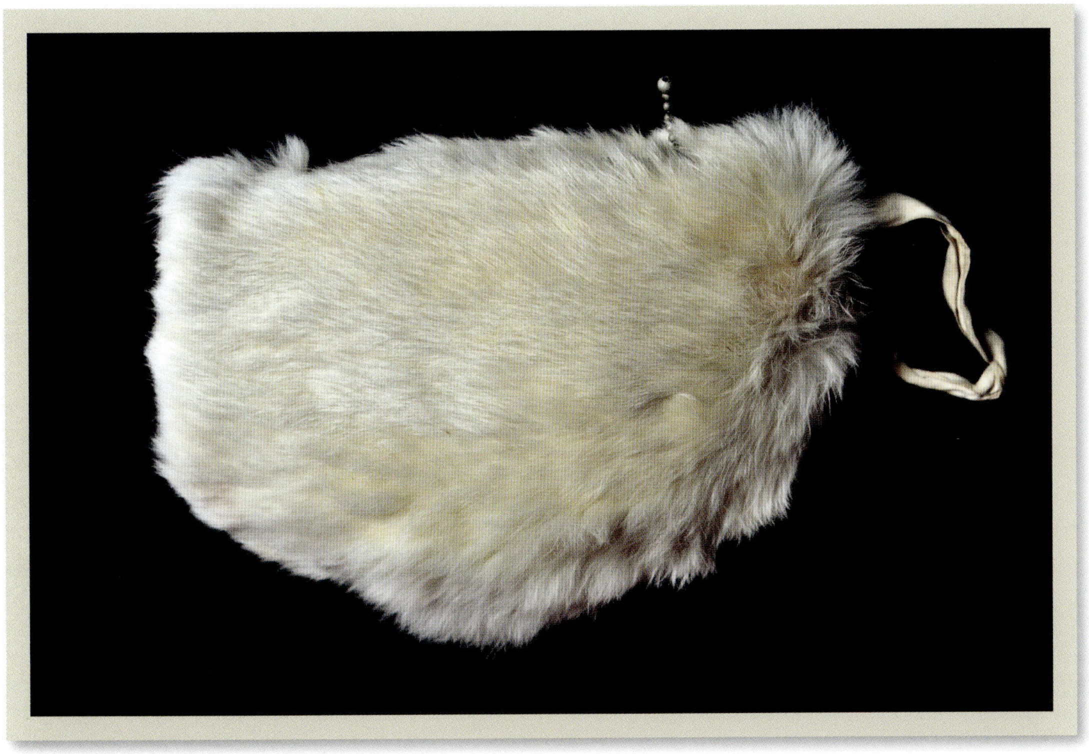

Child's white rabbit fur muff.

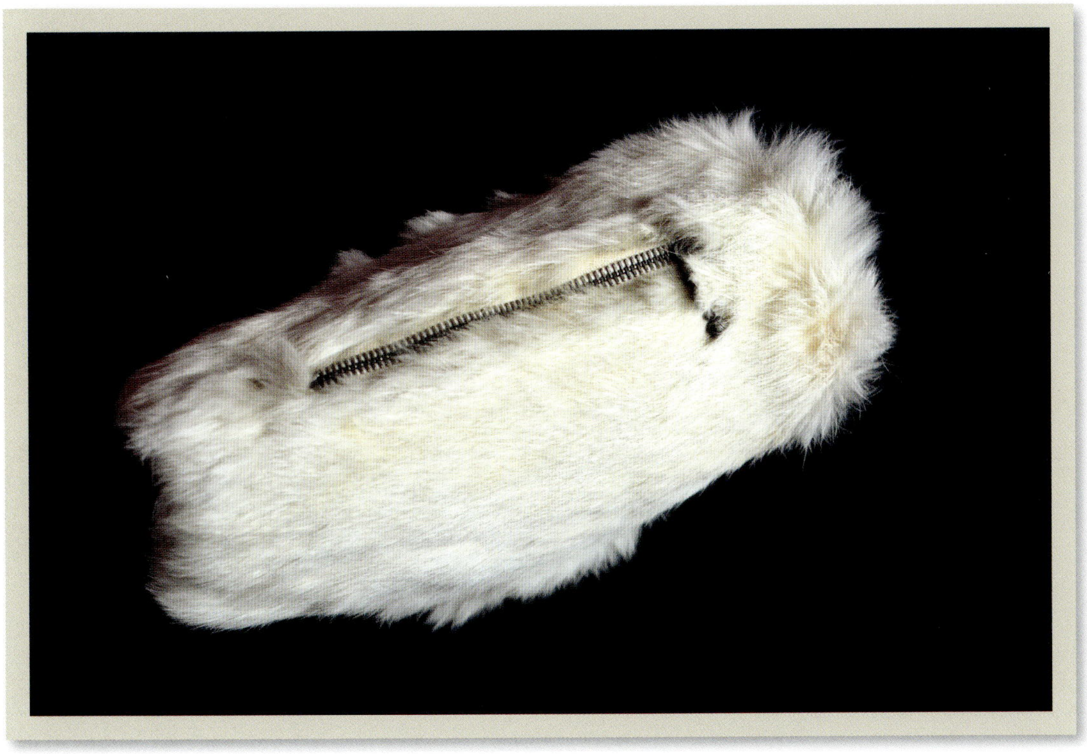

Detail: Zipper pouch for coins.

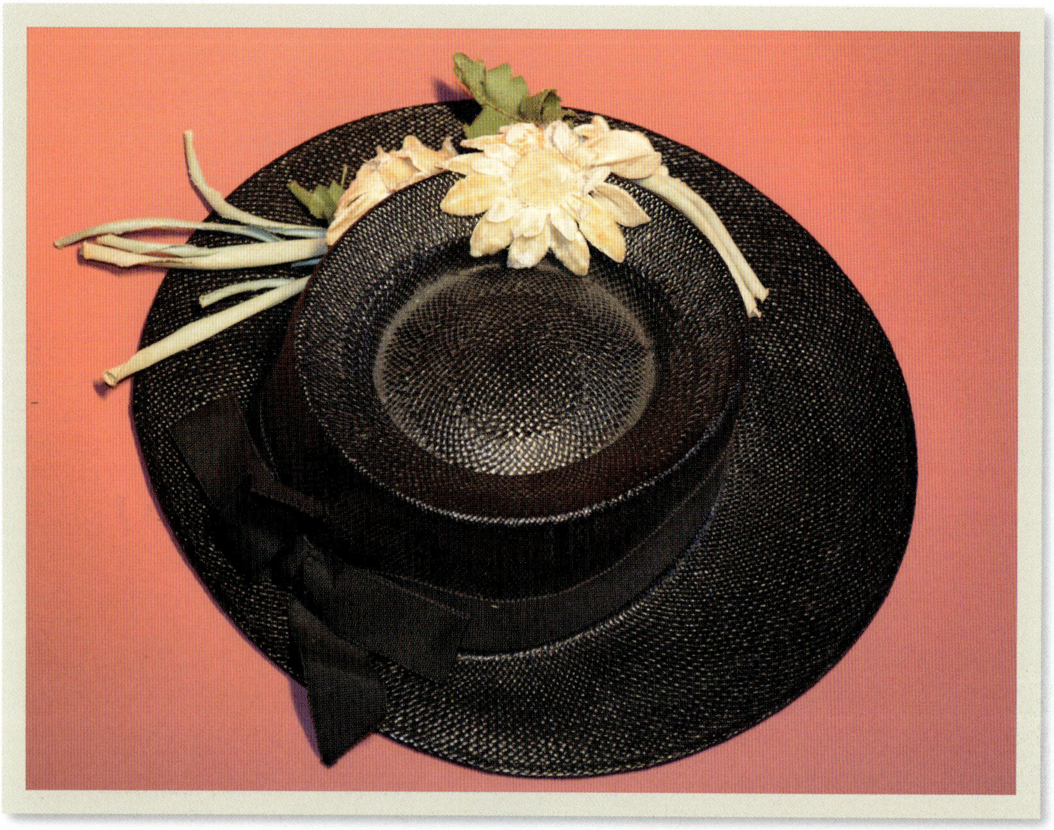

Girl's straw hat with velvet flowers and grosgrain band.

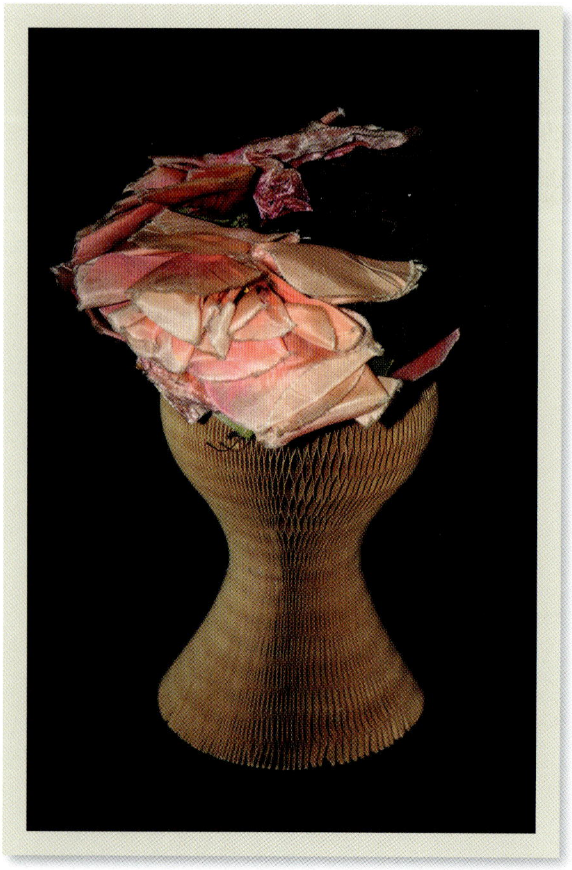

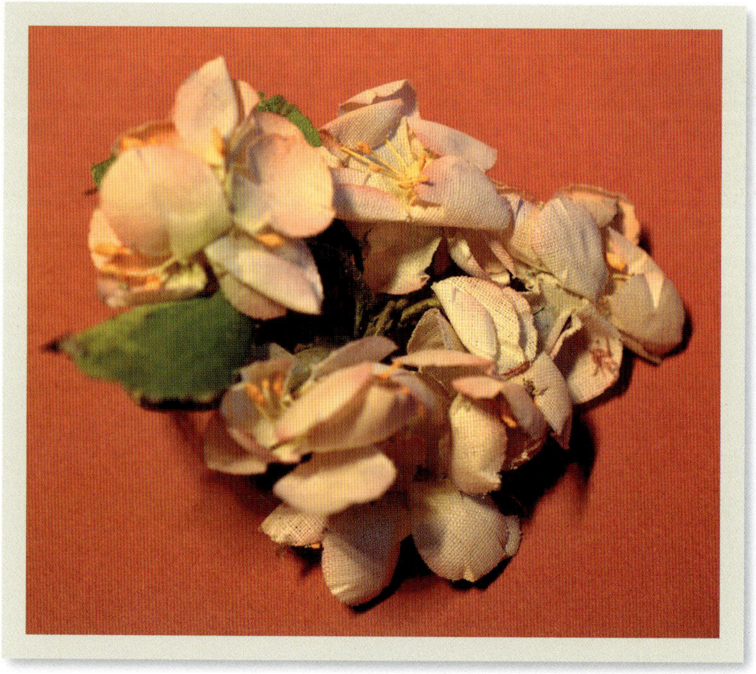

Floral cluster bonnet trim.

Velvet bonnet with fabric flowers.

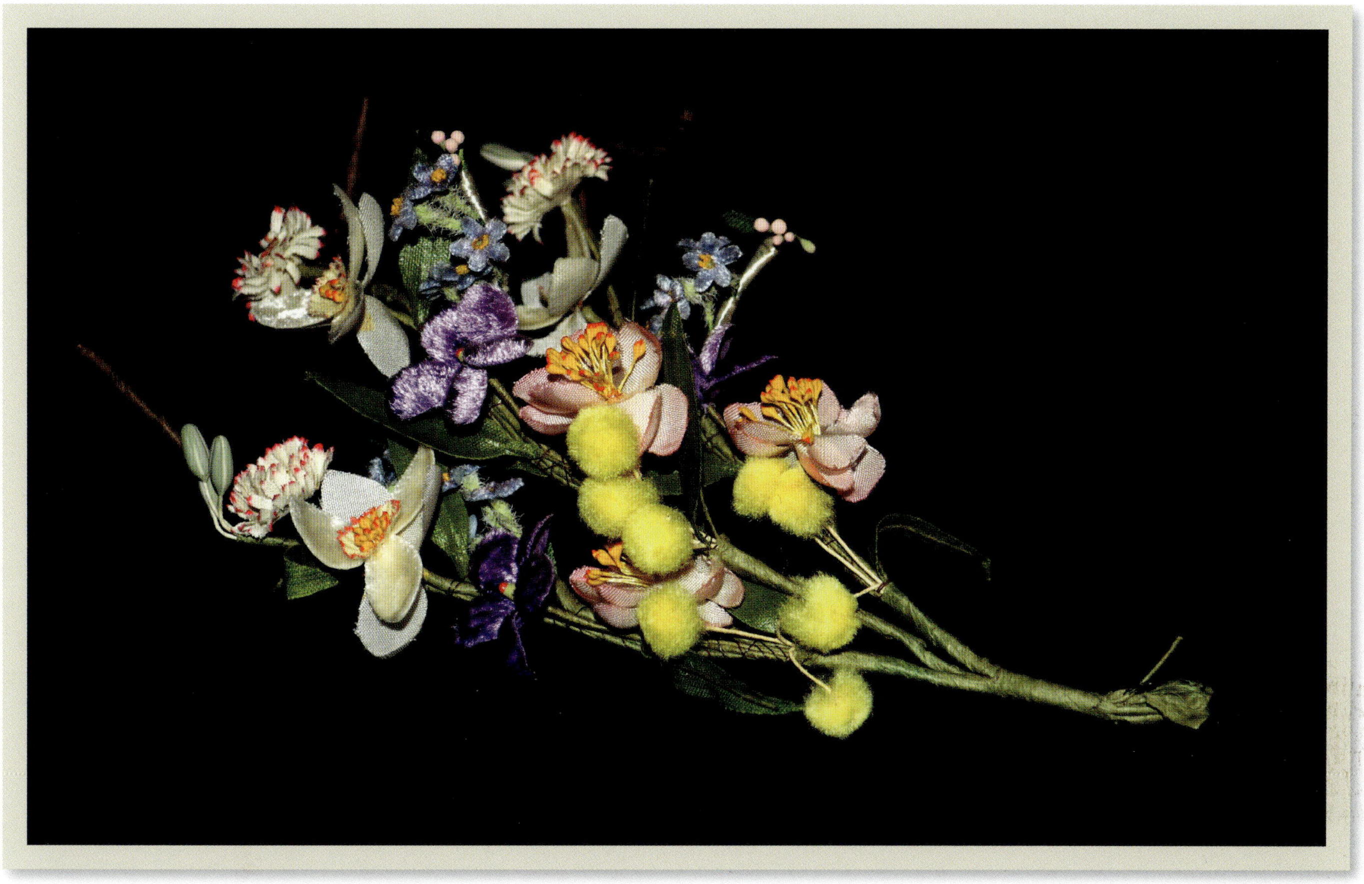

Bonnet trimmings such as this could be purchased at large millinery emporiums and supply houses.

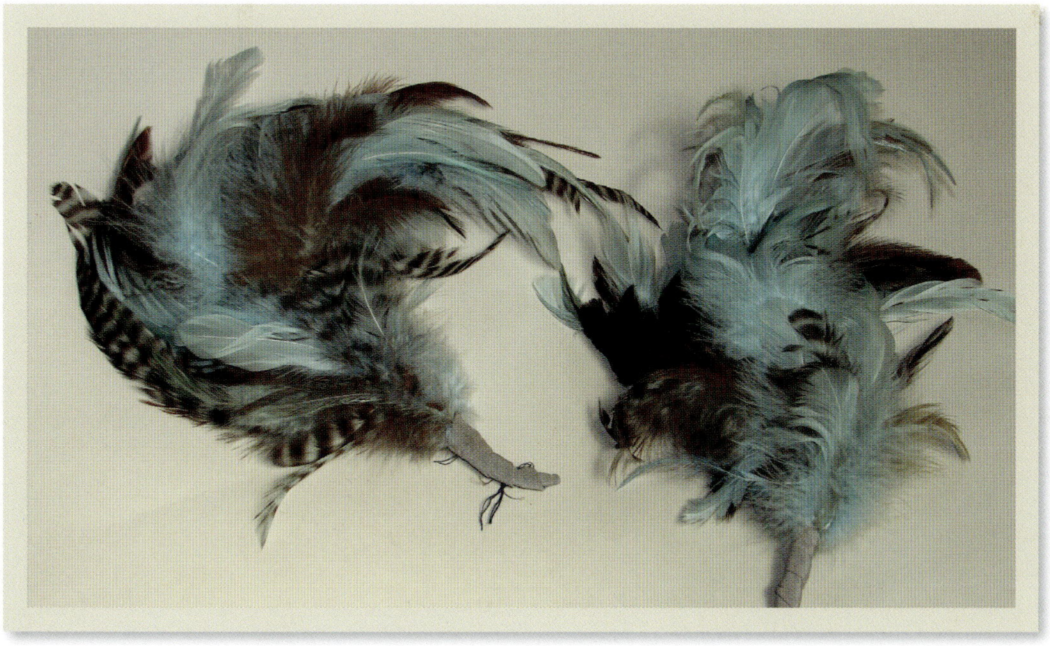

Feather sprays were popular bonnet trimmings for women and children alike.

CHAPTER SIX

Dressed to Excess
1910–1920

"The white wash gown, which we universally call the lingerie frock, is a subject of interest as soon as the warm weather advances on us."—Anne Rittenhouse, New York Times, *May 26, 1912*

Cultural Influences

The second decade of the twentieth century came to be defined by The Great War. The significance of costume as it relates to war is evidenced by the importance placed on inspection rituals, and the fact that a recruit's first assignment was to be kitted out with an appropriate uniform before even acquiring arms. While civilian costume generally reflects social standing, during periods of war, military influences creep into costume design, enabling those at home to demonstrate a solidarity with armed forces personnel.

Sailor suits fashioned after the British naval costume, both dress and informal, had long been popular attire for boys, but with the outbreak of World War I, military influence on children's costume accelerated and diversified. The classic sailor suit showed variations in trim and fabrication, some outfitted smartly with a whistle and lanyard, others adorned with parallel rows of contrast soutache braid.

In decades to come, camouflage print jeans, T-shirts, and caps would provide military inspiration for children's play clothes, but during the early twentieth century, children's soldierly attire derived not only from the fact that the men were engaged in warfare but that the women had taken domestic employment formerly reserved for men. These jobs often necessitated the wearing of uniforms.

As more women settled into the workplace and faced the civilian hardships caused by the war, ease became an imperative for their duties at home. Children's ready-made "washables" remained popular, and embroidered baby dresses could be made up quickly and easily by attaching a length of fabric to a pre-made separate yoke. Separate yokes also served as hasty cover-ups for a dress that baby might have drooled or spit up on.

Although yardage restrictions were put in place during the conflict, militaristic influences such as epaulettes and belts began appearing on clothing manufactured for civilian wear, particularly clothing designed for children.

Shortages of leather due to the war effort changed how mothers shopped for their older children as well. A plethora of canvas-topped boots and shoes hit the market to compete with one-strap, one-button leather styles.

Though militarism was a dominating influence on second-decade twentieth-century fashion, one of the most original cultural innovations to impact fashion was the spectacle known as the *Ballets Russes*. Producer Serge Diaghilev's novel art form was an instant hit when it toured in Paris in 1909. Boldly colored and ethnic-inspired costumes were so visually and texturally intriguing that their impact on style was felt immediately.

The *Ballets Russes* effect was applied to children's clothing through the application of sash belts, shortened skirts, loose jackets, and cuffed trousers. Bloomer knickers that pouched out beneath long Russian jackets were an adaptation of the harem pants seen on *Ballets Russes* dancers.

Style Retrospective

> "There is rarely a time in the average household when some portion of the children's wardrobe is not under consideration."—Harriet Clement Wheeler, *Needlecraft Magazine,* July 1916

Childhood-Specific Designs

The advent of fashion shows to benefit the war effort increased the public's interest in fashion and altered the way designers advertised their wares. One of the most influential designers of children's wear during this period was Jeanne Lanvin. The great designer was a child herself when she embarked on her career in fashion, apprenticing in her teens to Madame Bonni, a Parisian milliner. Many of the decorative techniques Lanvin absorbed while studying the art of hat making served her well in later years.

Whereas previously children were dressed in what amounted to down-sized versions of adult clothing, Lanvin's vision for smartly dressed youth ushered in an era of childhood-specific design. Utilizing her millinery skills, she created coordinated ensembles for girls and *fillettes* that were wonderfully embellished with self-fabric pompoms, felt appliqués, embroidery, sashes, ribbons and bows, lace roundels, fringes, frills, and fabric flowers. Her belief that no costume is complete without the finishing touch of a coordinating chapeau was widely accepted.

With names like *Chérubin, Très Sage, JouJou, Reverie, Robin Hood*, and *Carmillon*, sketches of Lanvin's handmade ensembles charmed readers of the fashion periodicals in which they appeared, driving buyers to her fashion house at 16 rue Boissy d'Anglas, Paris.

By 1909, Lanvin's vision for children's clothing had caught the attention of her socialite clients who wished to dress their own children in her luxurious and romantic confections, prompting her to officially open a children's clothing operation at the site of her millinery atelier. By 1913, when Lanvin's young daughter, Marguerite, appeared in the fashion magazine *Les Modes* wearing a three-quarter-sleeve, drop-waist, lace-trimmed dress with madras sash and hat, she was already a practiced model for her mother's creations.

As Marguerite grew, so too did Lanvin's reputation and the scope of her enterprise; she became known for being able to outfit a girl from infancy to adulthood. The September 15, 1911, issue of *Vogue* declared, "No designer in Paris can excel Jeanne Lanvin in the gowning of the young débutante—

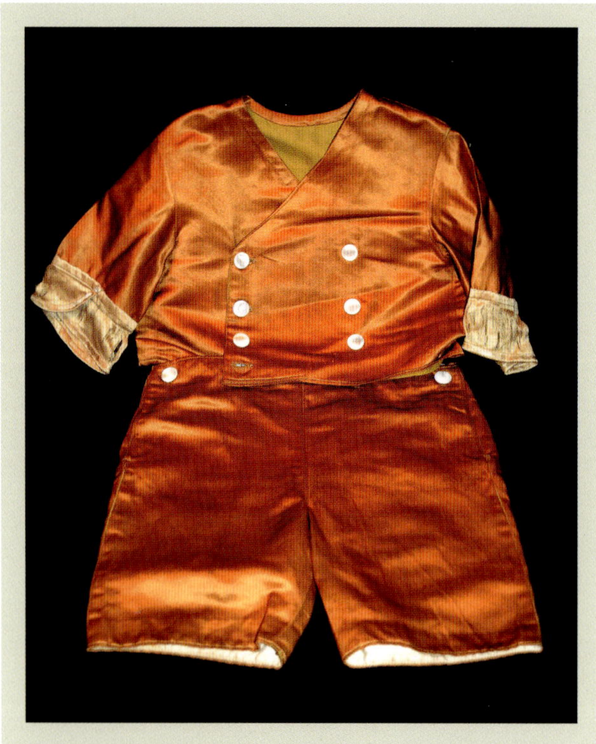

Boy's button-trimmed silk and satin romper.

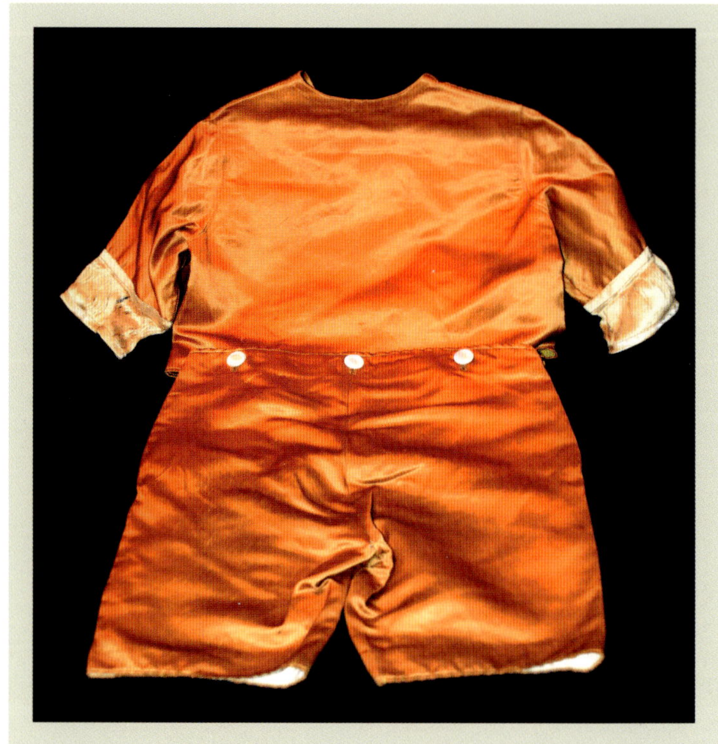

Back view.

slender young figures are adorable in her quaint conceptions." While Lanvin's daughter served as her adored and ever-present muse/model, the great designer was equally skilled at creating romantic and highly sought after boys wear.

A free-spirited approach to design distinguished Lanvin from many of her contemporaries, particularly Poiret, who was known for his replication of ethnic and oriental designs. "My dresses aren't premeditated," explained Lanvin. "I am carried away by feeling, and technical knowledge helps me make my clothes become a reality (Polan 2009." Her technical skill can clearly be seen in the draping of her garments as well as their imaginative surface design.

> "All children just love the quaint little strap aprons, particularly when they have an appliqué decoration of bunnies, chickens, kittens, or other illustration."—Harriet Clement Wheeler, *Needlecraft Magazine*, July 1916

At mid-decade, children's dresses and coats were generally designed to incorporate the use of two contrasting materials. Part of the sewer's joy in making up these garments must have come from the selection of fabric combinations: velvet or satin with wool, stripes and plaids with plain serge or corduroy, cashmere with fur fabrics, or simply a contrast of weaves in the same color. Embroidery, Puerto Rican drawn work, filet crochet, blackwork, and buttonholing were popular needlecraft techniques employed to create or embellish these garments.

Widely banded waists made an appearance in the spring of 1915 whether in coat styles, party wear, or walking suits. Small, tailored collars and plain, narrow sleeves made the scene, at times banded in contrast fabric to match collars or waistbands. Sacque-cut dresses (front and back cut in one length from neck to hem) were shirred at the neck and waist to provide fullness and could be simply made up in a number of soft materials, satisfying the prevailing trend for ease of construction and simplicity in dress.

Many of the dresses for children under eight years of age opened down the center back, a number of them fooling the eye with double tucks at the center front. To allow for growth, some dress skirt designs incorporated contrast hem bands, which could be easily lengthened.

Novelties in construction such as drop shoulders and asymmetric button closures revealed in the spring of 1915 ensured monetary success for pattern makers, as each month revealed new must-have fashion details.

Low-waisted tunics and wrap dresses in contrast fabrics created the appearance of complexity, but in reality were easy to construct.

In November 1915, *Needlecraft Magazine* professed that the belted, patch pocketed boys' Norfolk suit was "undoubtedly the leading favorite" of the day. The boy's Dutch suit was "much preferred for smaller boys" aged two to eight years.

As the decade progressed, belts and hip-level bands supported pouched bodices. Short pants took on a blouson effect as well with knickers morphing into what we would today call bloomers. Dora Douglas, writing in February 1915 for *Needlecraft Magazine* on fashion's progress, reported that due to the conflict in Europe, "garish colors have been banished and vulgar, exaggerated fashions pushed aside in favor of simplicity, dignity and austerity." The large fashion houses were contributing financially to the war effort and many an executive was volunteering personally at hospitals.

The general tendency was toward keeping a flat appearance in the front of skirt designs, which were either gored at the hem, cut circularly, or attached to yokes. Large cordings and tucks were the one nod to ornamentation. The Russian peasant look remained popular for children with the variation that fullness was created at the sides. Some fabric shortages were reported as many of the French mills were in areas of the country most affected by the war.

The use of contrast fabrics remained popular and surplice-fronted dresses were at times worn over a chemisette fitted with an attached collar. Pattern makers responded to the cry for simplicity by creating dress styles in which the yoke and sleeves were cut in one piece. Patterns for rompers were also designed for ease of construction, with each half cut in one piece and button closure applied along the inseam and center back.

> "A man's shirt which is worn around the neckband but otherwise good can be made into rompers for a one-year-old boy by using the buttoned front of the shirt for the back of the rompers, shaping the smaller arm size slanting down to sides of the shirt. Shape the bottom for legs and gather neck into band."—Inez Redding, *The Modern Priscilla Magazine,* May 1910

Boys

Many a young boy approached the second decade of the twentieth century still turned out in what was known as a Russian suit, a long and loose double-breasted jacket with wide collar and low-riding decorative belt worn with a silk tie or bow; the matching elastic "bloomer knickers" barely peeking out below the hem. Although knickers at times were referred to as bloomers during the nineteenth century, by the 1910s there was a definite distinction. Bloomers, worn by both boys and girls, were always gathered at the knee and often hidden or partially hidden beneath a sacque-cut frock, at times being attached to an underwaist. It is unfortunate that the photography of the times was not able to capture color, as many of the examples, whether of tweed or serge, are described as possessing a purple, red, or blue stripe, or all-over blue hue.

While terms like Russian Suits, Oliver Twists, Norway Reefers, and College Ulsters mean little to the average consumer today, these monikers spelled high fashion to the 1910s mother shopping for the latest styles to outfit her sons as stylish little gentlemen.

By the end of the decade, pencil stripes in crisp summer percales, Linene, and Daytona cloth intersected with wide, buckled, waist-level belts on short-pant Russian Suits and Oliver Twists. Boys' sailor suits and Norfolks also presented vertical interest through the placement of box pleats or the smaller knife pleats through which the intersecting buckled or buttoned belt could pass. Boys thirteen to eighteen years of age stood tall and proud in knee-hugging bloomer suits, also belted at the waist, but with peaked lapels befitting their maturity.

Newly fashionable wool knit sweaters in bright navy, red, green, maroon, or brown proved a smart choice for boys, whether hand knit or purchased from retailers. Pull-over styles were typically long-waisted for warmth and featured thick shawl collars that could be pulled up to protect sensitive necks.

Bucket-style hats of tartan or wool check with narrow, flip-up brims kept school-age boys warm in fall or winter. These machine-stitched segmented caps were usually lined with black cotton and banded in remnants of leather. As for footwear, contrast machine stitching was applied to boys' shoes, as were grosgrain ribbon bows.

Girls

At the outset of the decade, girls continued to be dressed in fanciful frocks of featherweight fabrics such as voile and dotted Swiss. Full-skirted dresses in summery sorbet colors sprouted broad collars decorated with flounces, ribbon bows, or embroidery.

Three years into the decade, however, the girls' dresses and coats took on a more streamlined appearance. Low sashes incorporated into the design appeared as visual belts with no cinching of the fabric. Large collars remained and were paired with cuffs in contrasting colors and fabrics.

By mid-decade, following the outbreak of The Great War, girls' costume morphed once more, taking on a more sober appearance. The September 1915 issue of *The Delineator* featured a boy and girl in back-to-school costumes—his a blue sailor costume and hers a short white bloomer dress and pink jacket. While still feminine, the jacket is edged in double bands of dark contrast braid, providing a hint of militarism.

Fall issues of *The Delineator* presented children's styles appropriate for school, and because the periodical was published

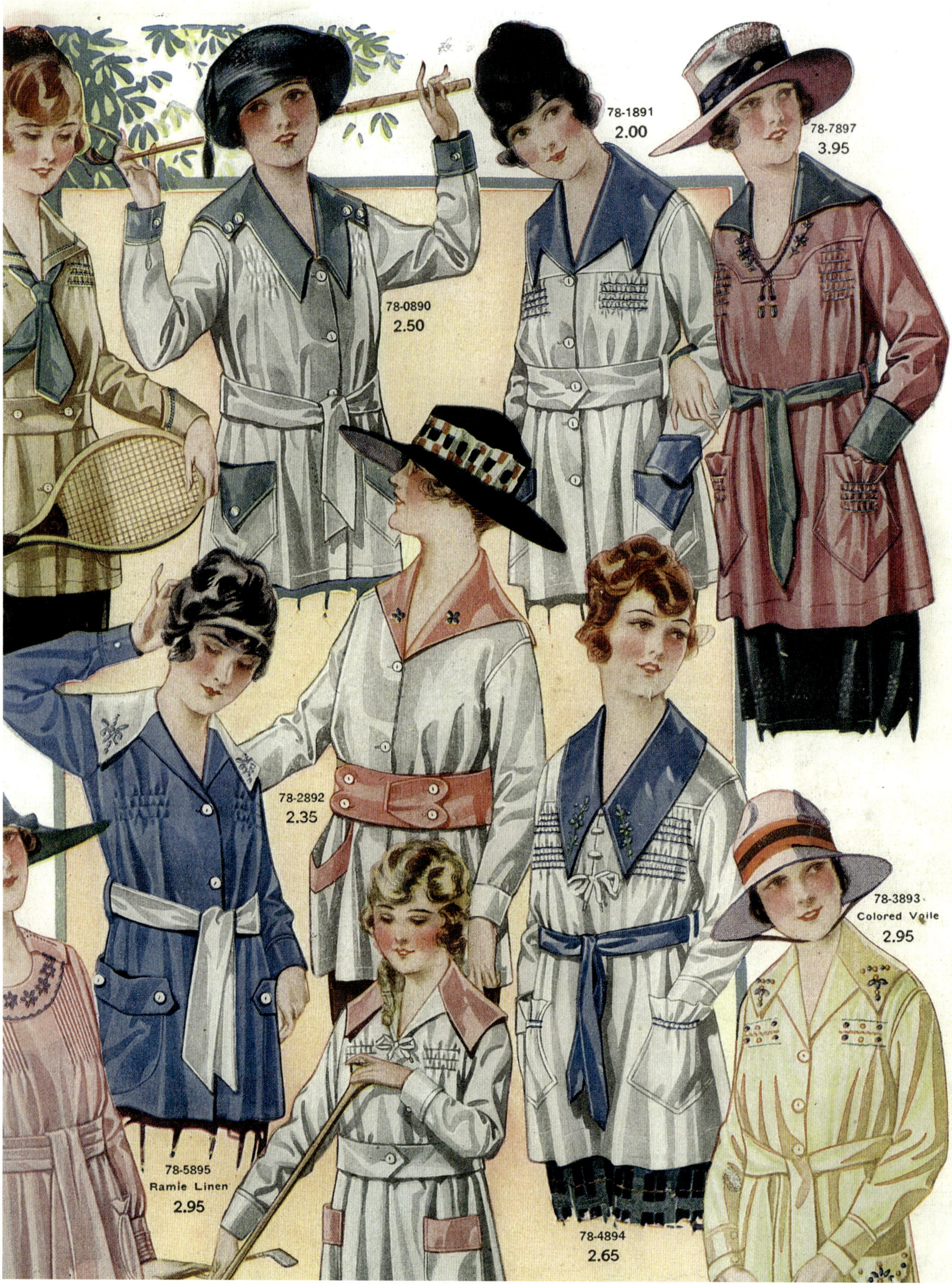
78-1891
2.00
78-7897
3.95
78-0890
2.50
78-2892
2.35
78-3893
Colored Voile
2.95
78-5895
Ramie Linen
2.95
78-4894
2.65

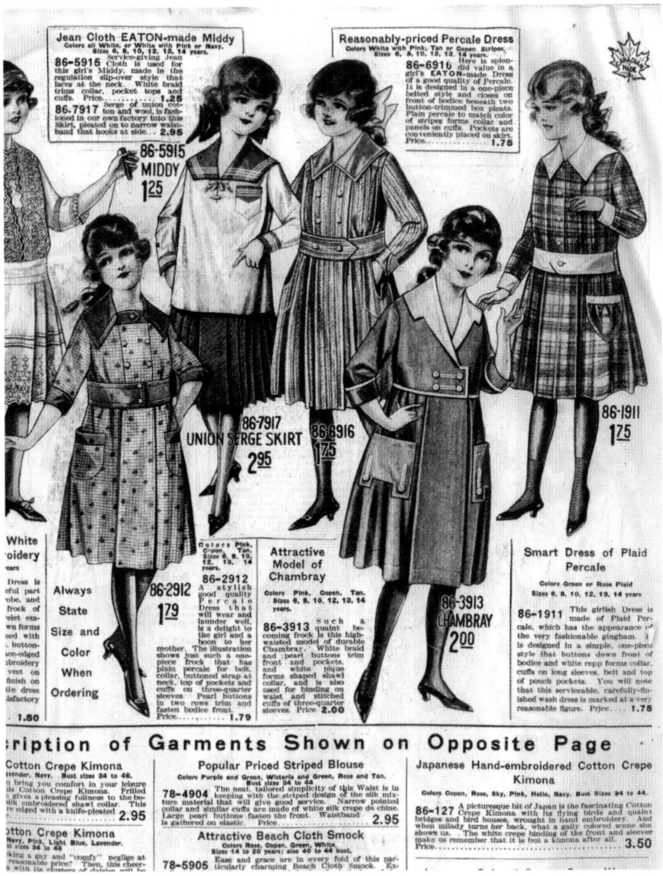

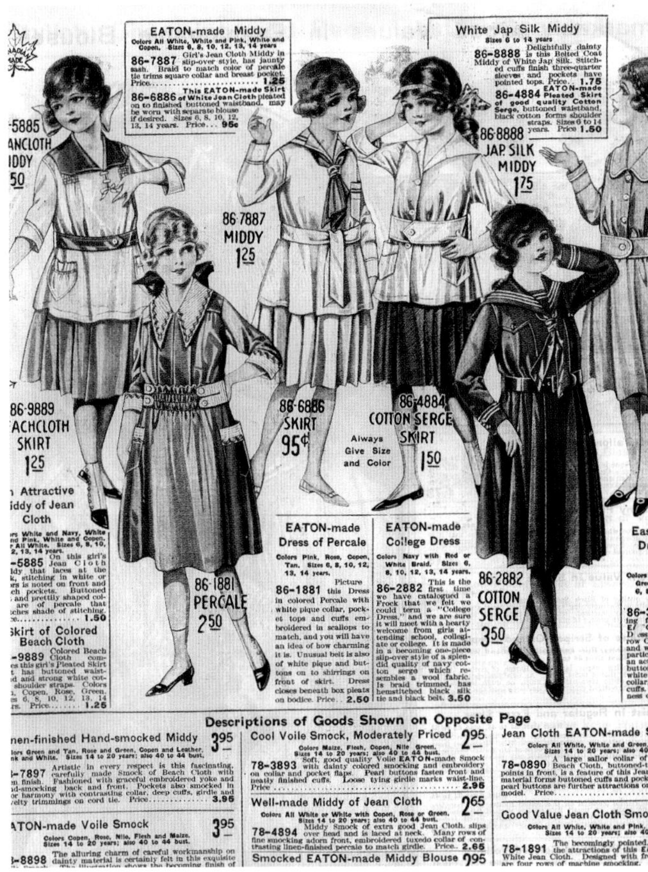

Midi blouses and nautical inspired dresses, suits, and coats for girls six to fourteen years. *Eaton's Spring and Summer Catalogue*, 1919.

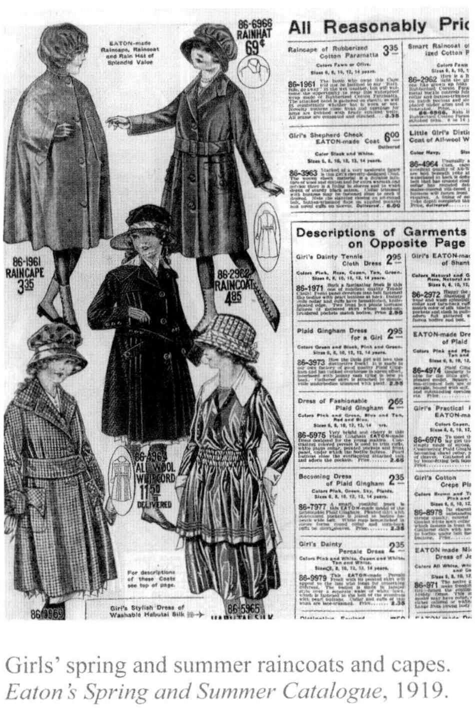

Girls' spring and summer raincoats and capes. *Eaton's Spring and Summer Catalogue*, 1919.

by a pattern company, suggestions were always made for fabric selection. In the August 1911 issue, an interesting distinction is made between textiles suitable for city kids (wash dresses) and those more suited to children living in rural locations: "For children who live in the city," the pattern book stressed, "where there are steam-heated houses and schoolrooms, the smartest materials for their dresses are the linens, poplins, repps, galateas, percales, ginghams, chambrays, and cotton drillings. Of course, for children who live in country districts where furnaces and radiators are unknown, wash dresses in winter are out of the question. They should wear pretty little dresses of serge, flannel, or any good woven material, and washable pinafores and aprons."

With such pronouncements reaching a wide audience of homemakers, it is no wonder that fabric companies seized on the opportunity to advertise their wares directly to home sewers through fashion publications. In April 1919, the Amory, Browne and Co. textile firm promoted their ginghams in *The Delineator* through a charming sketch of three tots, each dressed in tri-color gingham play suits. *The Sears Roebuck*

Catalogue for the same year showed girls' dresses in a variety of checks and stripes, each frock falling loosely from the shoulders to the knee, but banded horizontally at the waist.

Not everyone, of course, was outfitting their children in couture garments or applying their foot to the sewing machine treadle. Many a parent enjoyed the economy, convenience, and availability of ready-to-wear children's garments. Distinctive clothing for the newly identified adolescent cohort was also widely available.

Lingerie Dresses

Lingerie dresses were a staple in an Edwardian woman's wardrobe and that of many a girl. These thin, white fashion fantasies required an under-dress—often a brightly colored silk—because of their transparent quality. New versions were introduced each season according to the prevailing style and many were accessorized with a matching lingerie parasol.

During the teens, many young girls' lingerie dresses resembled a full front and back apron or pinafore style, though fashioned of lace, silk net, or cotton eyelet. As delicate and intricate as many of these afternoon or special occasion gowns were, they could be made at home following a fashion magazine sewing pattern adapted from such leading designers as the Boué sisters. Their delicate aesthetic of signature hand-made laces, feminine ribbon work, and appreciation for metallic embellishments were widely copied for girls and young women during the teens and 1920s. The intricacy of the Boué sisters' vision can be seen in a number of US patent applications for corset cover, night dress, and jacket patterns.

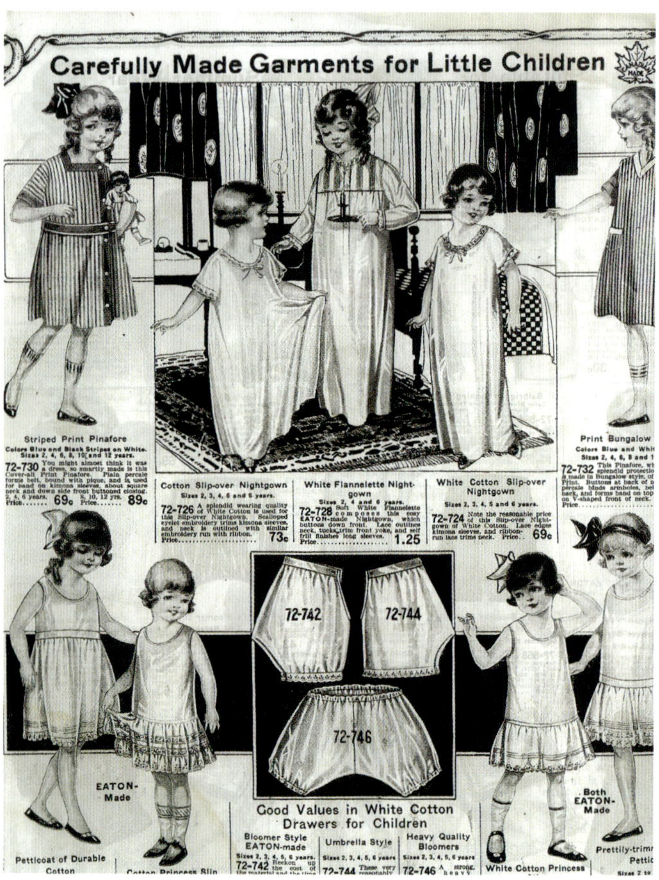

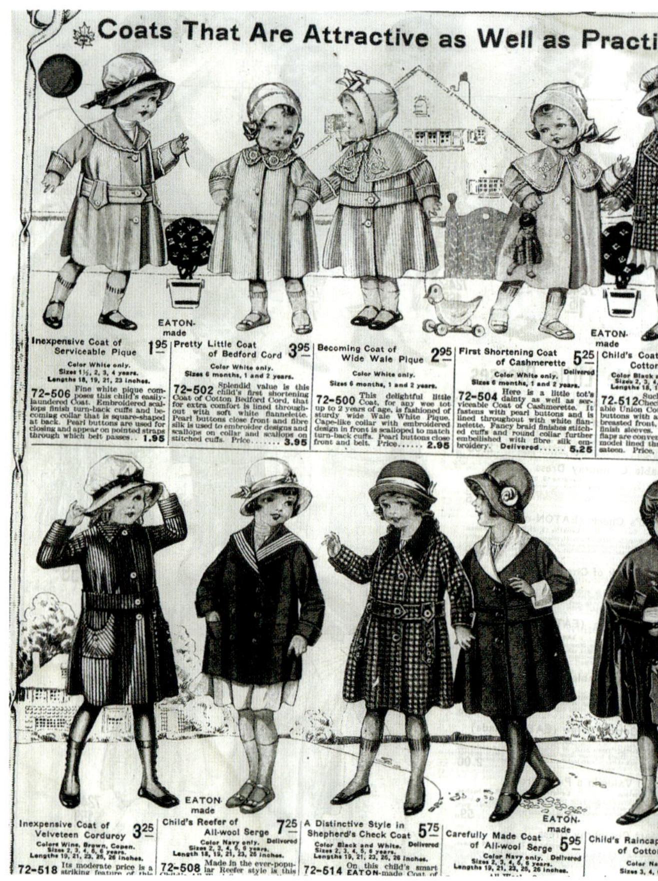

Inner and outer garments for the younger child. *Eaton's Spring and Summer Catalogue*, 1919.

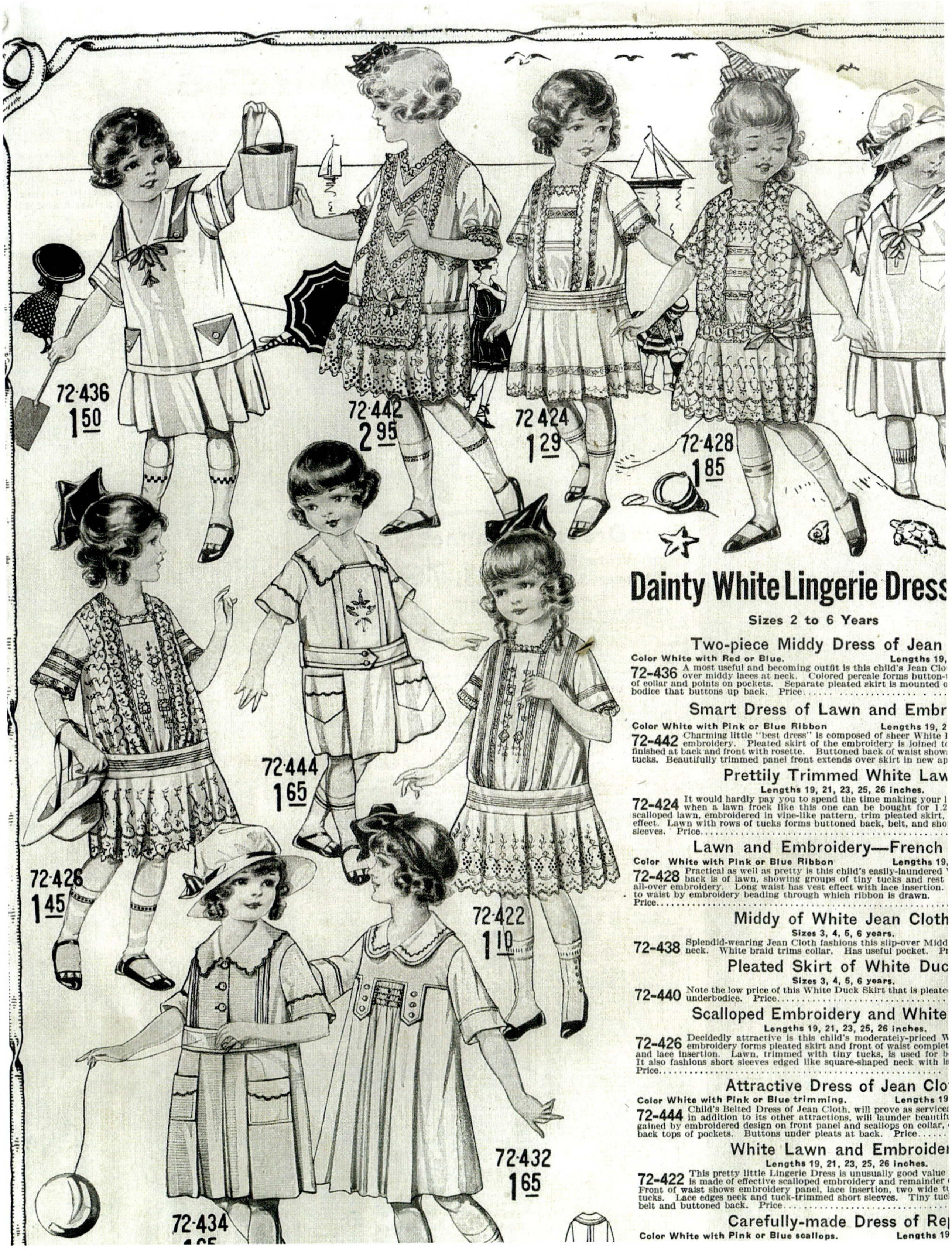
72·436
1 50
72·442
2 95
72 424
1 29
72·428
1 85
72·444
1 65
72·426
1 45
72·422
1 10
72·432
1 65
72·434
Dainty White Lingerie Dress
Sizes 2 to 6 Years
Two-piece Middy Dress of Jean
Color White with Red or Blue. Lengths 19,
72-436 A most useful and becoming outfit is this child's Jean Clo
over middy laces at neck. Colored percale forms button-
of collar and points on pockets. Separate pleated skirt is mounted c
bodice that buttons up back. Price
Smart Dress of Lawn and Embr
Color White with Pink or Blue Ribbon Lengths 19, 2
72-442 Charming little "best dress" is composed of sheer White
embroidery. Pleated skirt of the embroidery is joined t
finished at back and front with rosette. Buttoned back of waist show
tucks. Beautifully trimmed panel front extends over skirt in new ap
Prettily Trimmed White Law
Lengths 19, 21, 23, 25, 26 inches.
72-424 It would hardly pay you to spend the time making your
when a lawn frock like this one can be bought for 1.2
scalloped lawn, embroidered in vine-like pattern, trim pleated skirt,
effect. Lawn with rows of tucks forms buttoned back, belt, and sho
sleeves. Price
Lawn and Embroidery—French
Color White with Pink or Blue Ribbon Lengths 19,
72-428 Practical as well as pretty is this child's easily-laundered
back is of lawn, showing groups of tiny tucks and rest
all-over embroidery. Long waist has vest effect with lace insertion.
to waist by embroidery beading through which ribbon is drawn.
Price
Middy of White Jean Cloth
Sizes 3, 4, 5, 6 years.
72-438 Splendid-wearing Jean Cloth fashions this slip-over Midd
neck. White braid trims collar. Has useful pocket. Pr
Pleated Skirt of White Duc
Sizes 3, 4, 5, 6 years.
72-440 Note the low price of this White Duck Skirt that is pleate
underbodice. Price
Scalloped Embroidery and White
Lengths 19, 21, 23, 25, 26 inches.
72-426 Decidedly attractive is this child's moderately-priced W
embroidery forms pleated skirt and front of waist complet
and lace insertion. Lawn, trimmed with tiny tucks, is used for b
It also fashions short sleeves edged like square-shaped neck with la
Price
Attractive Dress of Jean Clo
Color White with Pink or Blue trimming. Lengths 19
72-444 Child's Belted Dress of Jean Cloth, will prove as service
in addition to its other attractions, will launder beautif
gained by embroidered design on front panel and scallops on collar,
back tops of pockets. Buttons under pleats at back. Price
White Lawn and Embroider
Lengths 19, 21, 23, 25, 26 inches.
72-422 This pretty little Lingerie Dress is unusually good value
is made of effective scalloped embroidery and remainder
Front of waist shows embroidery panel, lace insertion, two wide tu
tucks. Lace edges neck and tuck-trimmed short sleeves. Tiny tuc
belt and buttoned back. Price
Carefully-made Dress of Re
Color White with Pink or Blue scallops. Lengths 19

Midi and lingerie dresses for pre-schoolers. *Eaton's Spring and Summer Catalogue*, 1919.

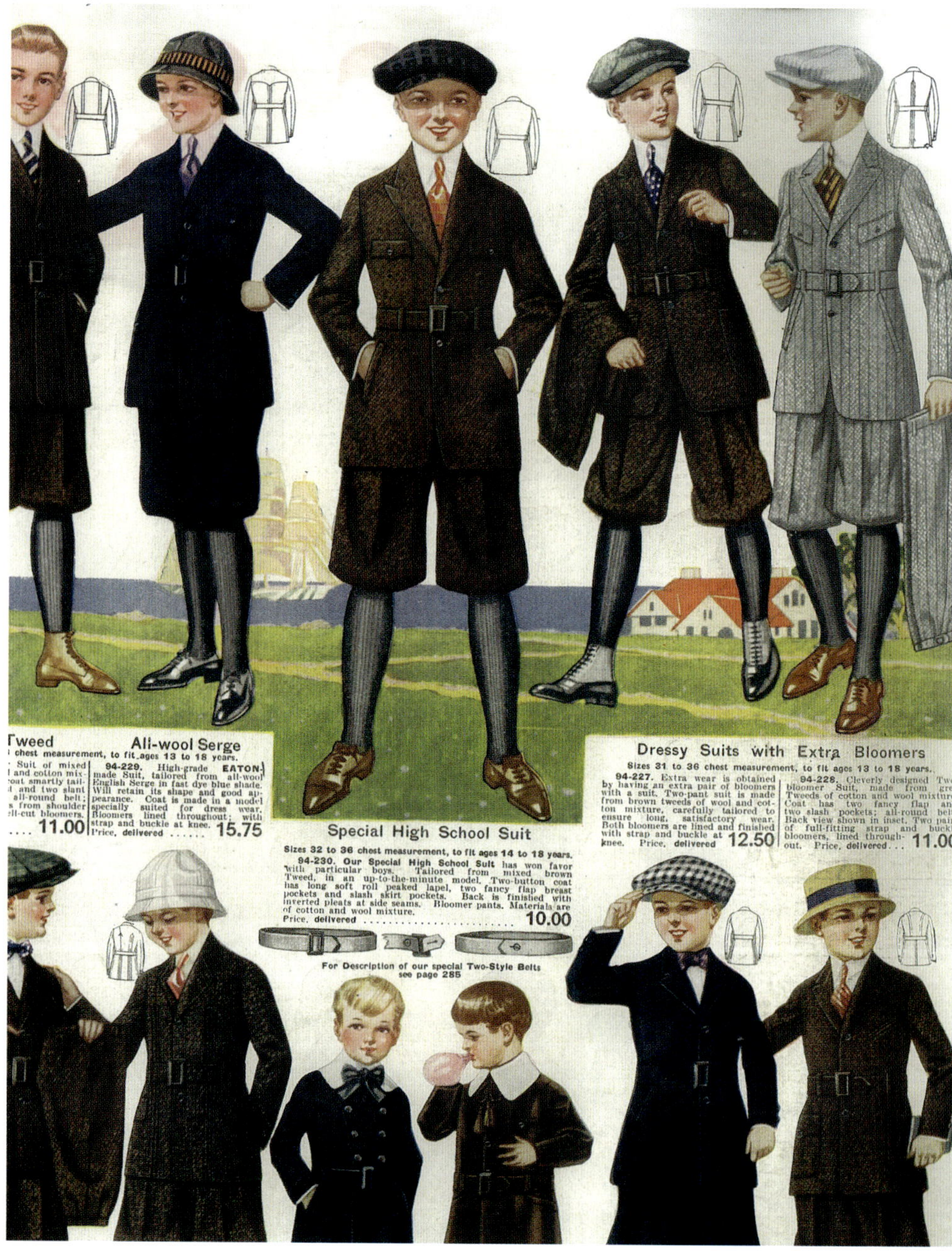

Boys' Russian suits, Oliver Twists, Norfolks, and rompers. *Eaton's Spring and Summer Catalogue*, 1919.

Millinery

Capes, hoods, and tams covered girls' heads in winter, while boaters and chopping bowl confections shaded young faces in the warmer seasons. The importance of hats during the teen years cannot be understated. A report out of Addergoole, Ireland, records the story of a young *Titanic* survivor, Delia McDermott, who—although she was one of the first to find a lifeboat after the fated ship struck ice—returned to her cabin to fetch the new hat she had made a special trip to purchase prior to the voyage. By the time she got back to the lifeboat, the famous passenger liner was sideways in the water, but hat in hand, McDermott managed to jump to safety from a suspended rope ladder.

While some may wonder what makes Edwardian fashion worth risking one's life for, period costume collectors recognize the special appeal of this spectacular fashion era, traveling great distances at times to acquire new pieces. Similarly, throughout the early twentieth century, many North American socialites relied on European couturiers for their own pieces as well as those of their children.

Period Care and Cleaning of Edwardian Accessories

"To wash China silk, rub lightly in a lather made from a good laundry soap, rinse in lukewarm water to which a little ammonia has been added."—Mrs. Garrett Webster, *Ladies' Home Journal,* September 1899

"A silver chatelaine to be worn at the waist is an acceptable gift for a girl of seventeen."—Elizabeth Robinson Scovil, *Ladies' Home Journal,* April 1898

The following methods were used to maintain accessories and trimmings in good condition:

• Umbrellas were to be wiped dry as soon as possible using a piece of soft black silk, and placed to dry with the ferrule up.

• Steel buckles and buttons could be kept in a box of powdered starch or wrapped in tissue paper when not in use.

• To clean beading of jet, a flannel cloth soaked in equal parts alcohol and water was recommended.

• White straw hats could be cleaned by scrubbing with a nailbrush soaked in lemon juice and flowers of sulphur.

• For gold lace, *Ladies' Home Journal* columnist Emma M. Hooper recommended the following: "prepare one ounce of stale bread grated into fine crumbs, a quarter of an ounce of magnesia, and half an ounce of cream of tartar. This can be made into a paste with spirits of wine and applied to the lace with an old toothbrush. When perfectly dry, the crumbs should be dusted off and the lace itself rubbed gently with chamois leather (October 1896)."

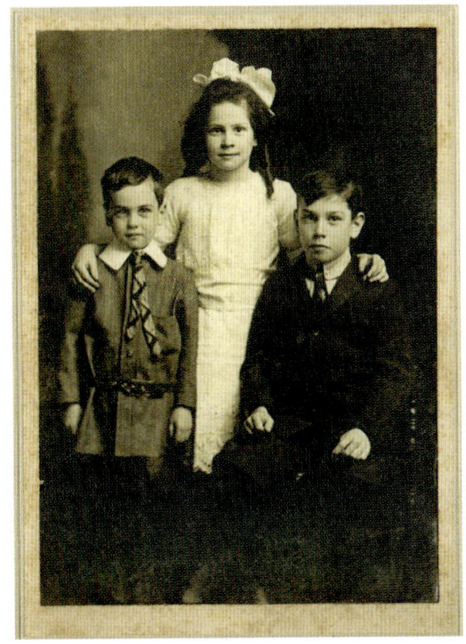

A ringletted young miss in a crisp banded white summer frock and hair bow is flanked by two smartly attired boys, the youngest of which is outfitted in a low-belted Norfolk suit with collar and necktie. The older lad sports a tailored suit with high collar and tie.

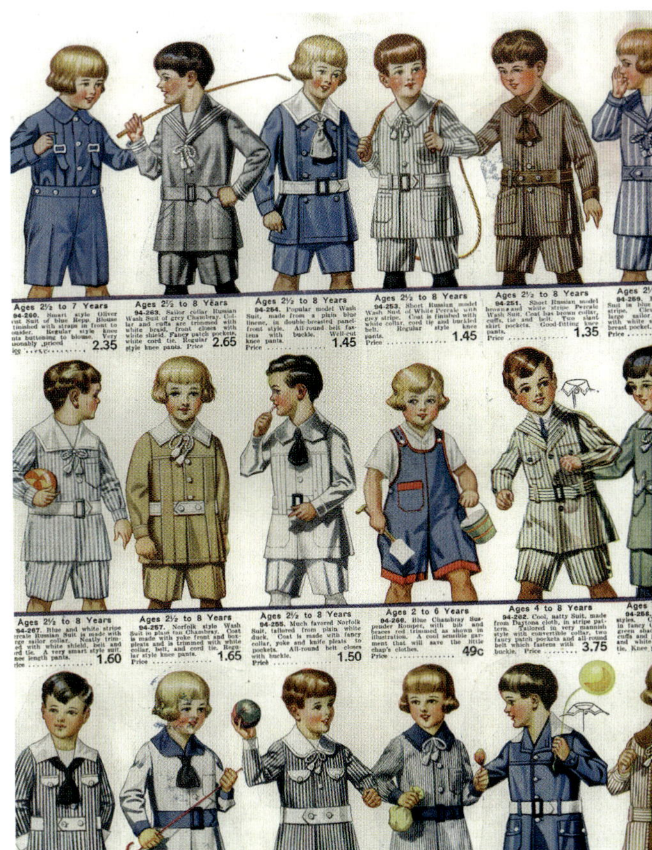

Boys' Russian suits, Oliver Twists, Norfolks, and rompers. *Eaton's Spring and Summer Catalogue*, 1919.

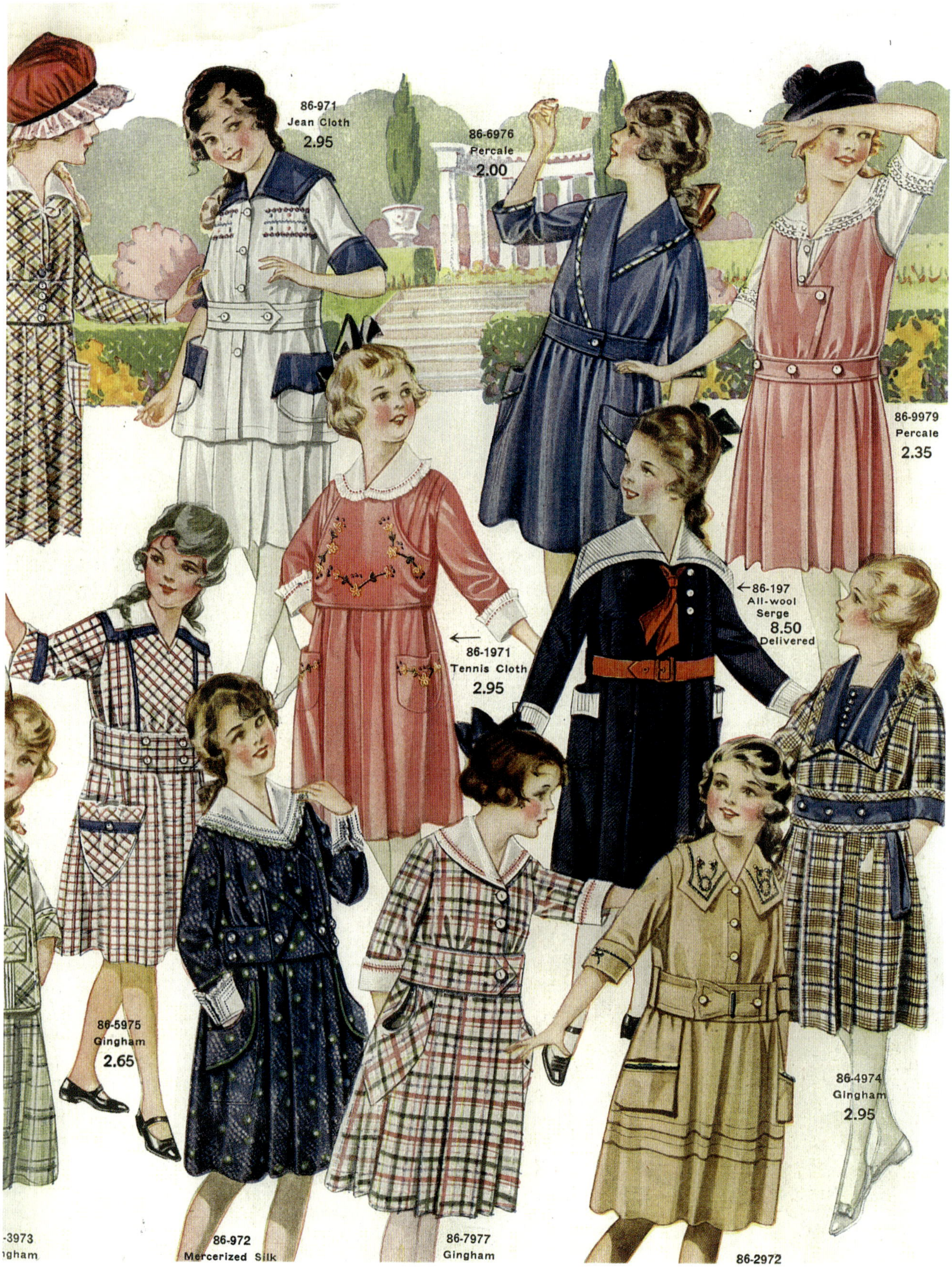

Department store sections for young misses. *Eaton's Spring and Summer Catalogue*, 1919.

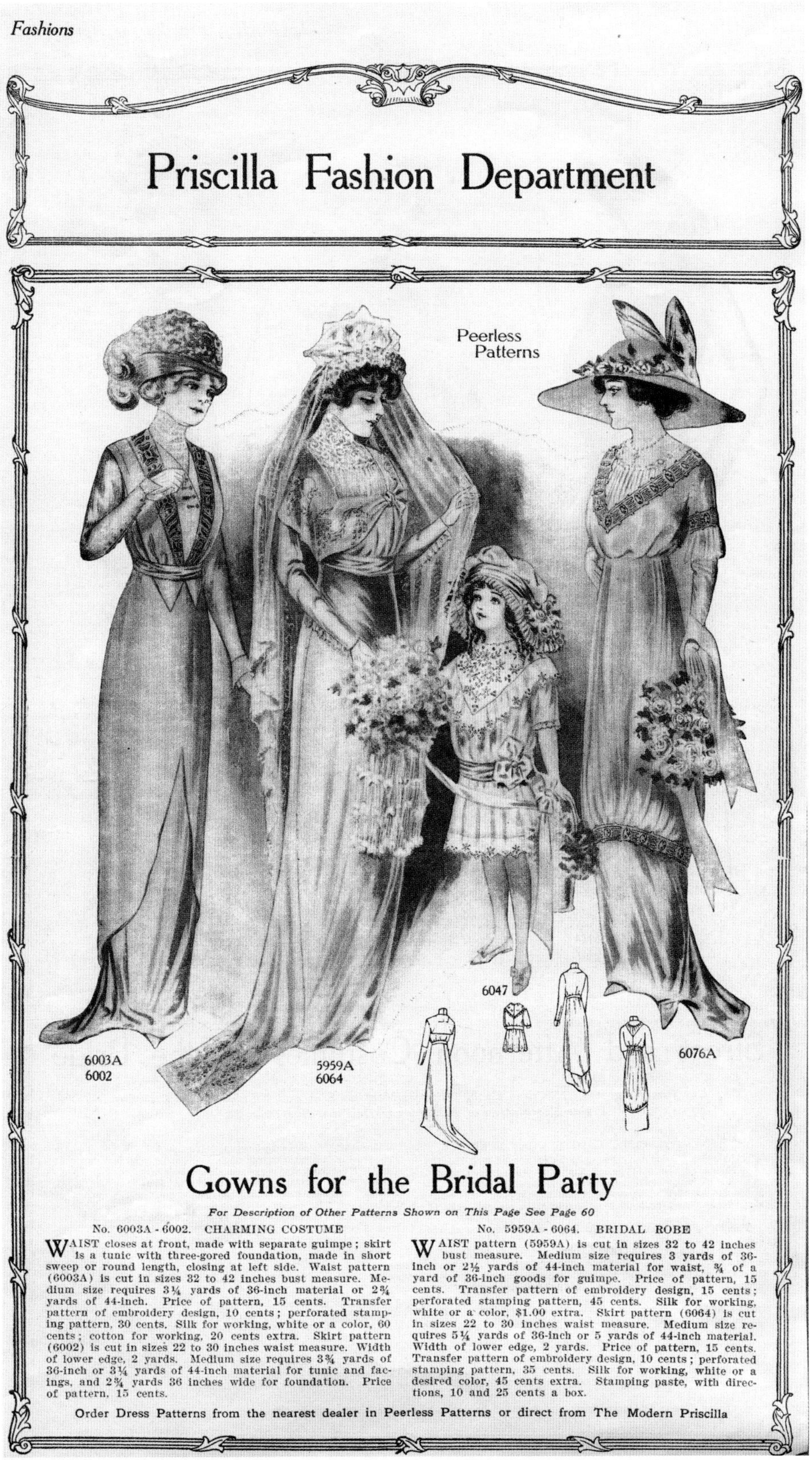

Fashions

Priscilla Fashion Department

Peerless Patterns

6003A
6002

5959A
6064

6047

6076A

Gowns for the Bridal Party

For Description of Other Patterns Shown on This Page See Page 60

No. 6003A - 6002. CHARMING COSTUME

WAIST closes at front, made with separate guimpe; skirt is a tunic with three-gored foundation, made in short sweep or round length, closing at left side. Waist pattern (6003A) is cut in sizes 32 to 42 inches bust measure. Medium size requires 3¼ yards of 36-inch material or 2¾ yards of 44-inch. Price of pattern, 15 cents. Transfer pattern of embroidery design, 10 cents; perforated stamping pattern, 30 cents. Silk for working, white or a color, 60 cents; cotton for working, 20 cents extra. Skirt pattern (6002) is cut in sizes 22 to 30 inches waist measure. Width of lower edge, 2 yards. Medium size requires 3¾ yards of 36-inch or 3¼ yards of 44-inch material for tunic and facings, and 2¾ yards 36 inches wide for foundation. Price of pattern, 15 cents.

No. 5959A - 6064. BRIDAL ROBE

WAIST pattern (5959A) is cut in sizes 32 to 42 inches bust measure. Medium size requires 3 yards of 36-inch or 2½ yards of 44-inch material for waist, ¾ of a yard of 36-inch goods for guimpe. Price of pattern, 15 cents. Transfer pattern of embroidery design, 15 cents; perforated stamping pattern, 45 cents. Silk for working, white or a color, $1.00 extra. Skirt pattern (6064) is cut in sizes 22 to 30 inches waist measure. Medium size requires 5¼ yards of 36-inch or 5 yards of 44-inch material. Width of lower edge, 2 yards. Price of pattern, 15 cents. Transfer pattern of embroidery design, 10 cents; perforated stamping pattern, 35 cents. Silk for working, white or a desired color, 45 cents extra. Stamping paste, with directions, 10 and 25 cents a box.

Order Dress Patterns from the nearest dealer in Peerless Patterns or direct from The Modern Priscilla

These pattern sketches for formal wedding attire include one for a banded, knee-length flower girl's frock. *The Modern Pricilla*, April 1913.

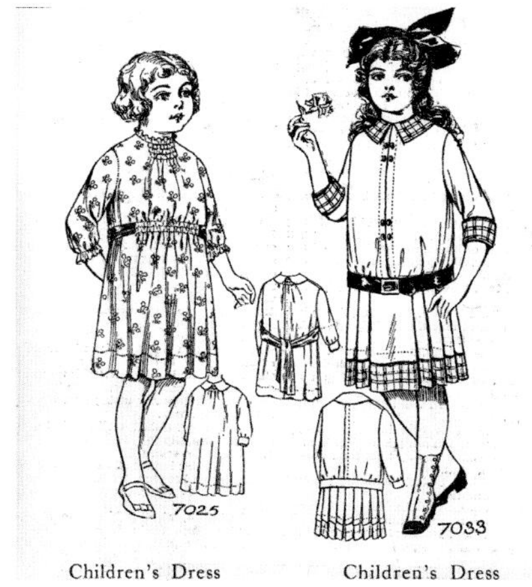
7025
7033
Children's Dress
Children's Dress

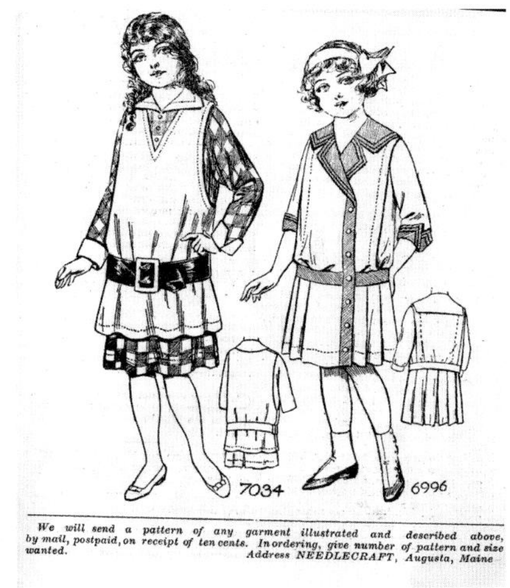
7034
6996
We will send a pattern of any garment illustrated and described above, by mail, postpaid, on receipt of ten cents. In ordering, give number of pattern and size wanted.
Address NEEDLECRAFT, Augusta, Maine

Patterns for these frocks for juniors featured in the February 1915 issue of *Needlecraft Magazine* could be obtained for ten cents by writing to the magazine.

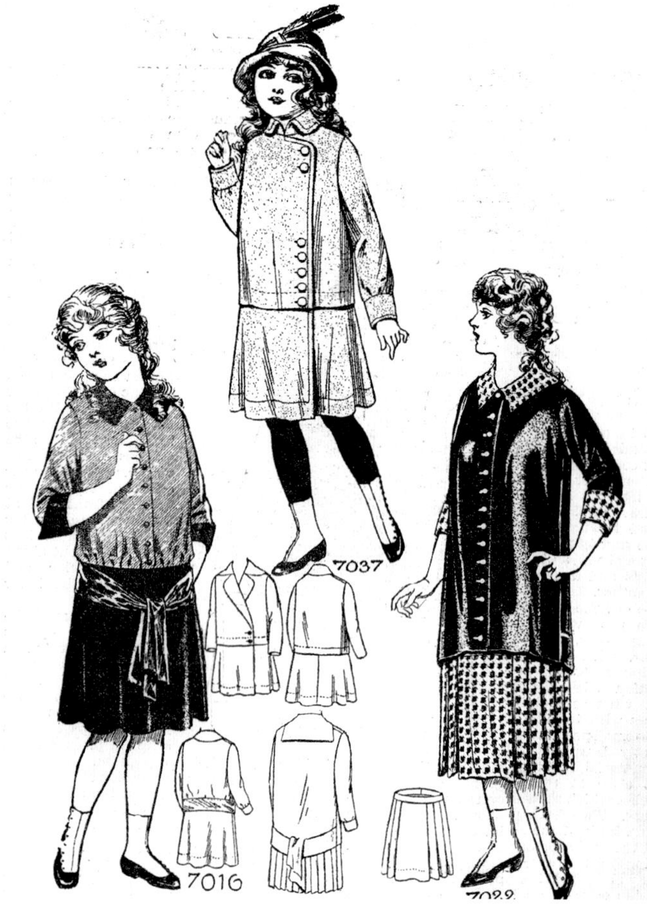

Low-waisted, tunic-style frocks and coat patterns. *Needlecraft Magazine*, February 1915.

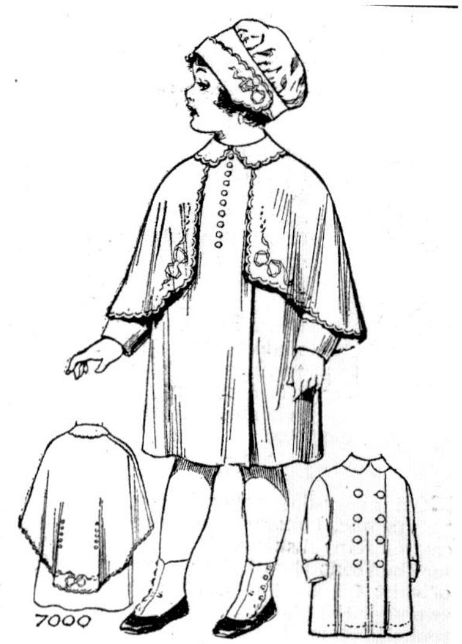

Coat and hat pattern for a very young child. This style with attached or detachable ornamental cape in cashmere was easy to make and extremely popular for both boys and girls. *Needlecraft Magazine*, February 1915.

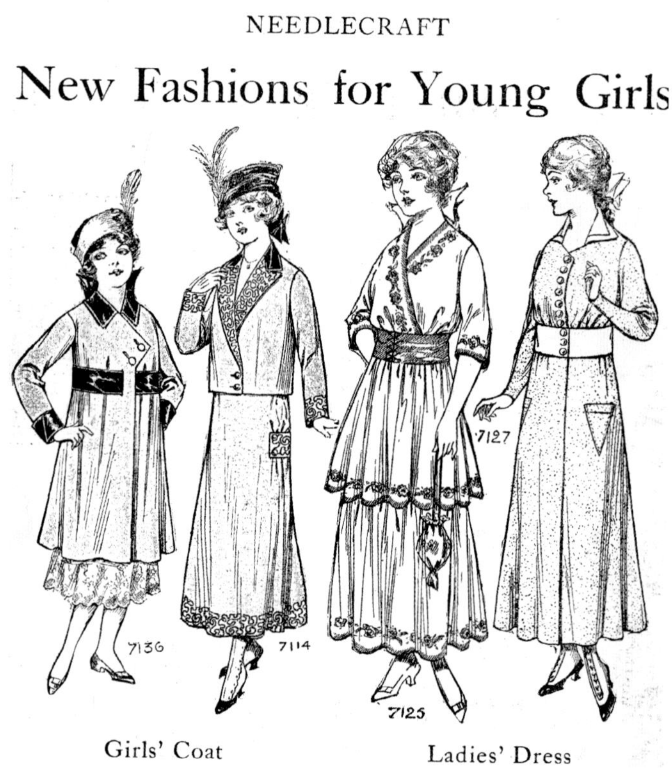

Fashions for young girls with descriptions for making up at home are presented in *Needlecraft Magazine*, April 1915.

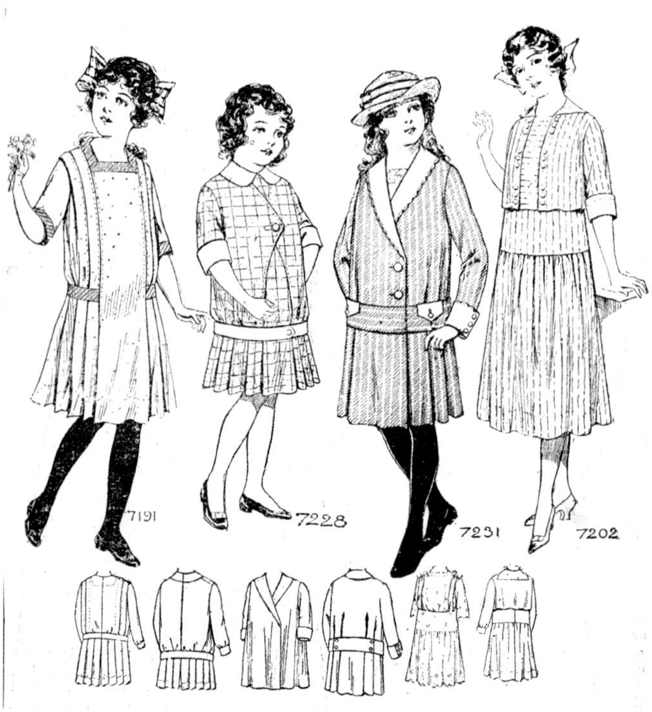

Under the heading, "Novelties for Little Men and Women," the May 1915 issue of *Needlecraft Magazine* presented this sashed bolero dress and empire coat for girls ages six to twelve.

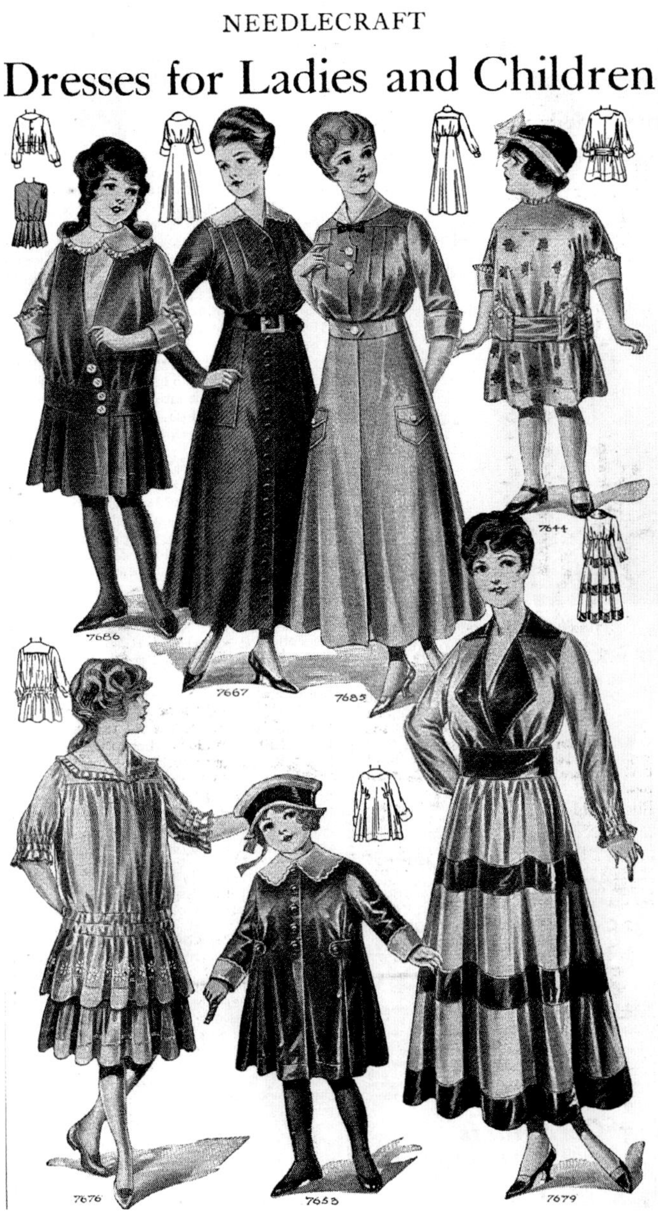

These dresses and coat for girls ages six to fourteen illustrate a number of style features current at the time, including box pleats, low-slung faux belts, ornamental pockets, and deeply cuffed sleeves, not to mention the trendy bolero jacket. The dresses are simpler to make than they appear, as they open at the back. *Needlecraft Magazine*, June 1915.

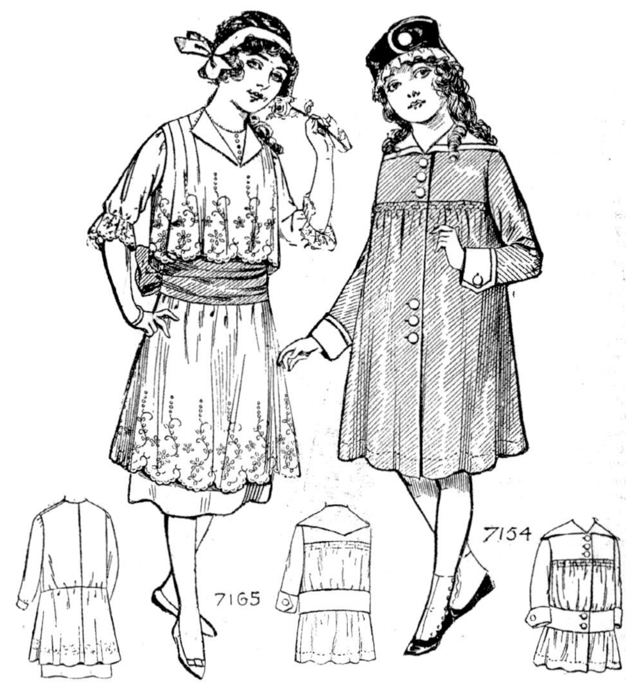

Under the heading, "Novelties for Little Men and Women," the May 1915 issue of *Needlecraft Magazine* presented this sashed bolero dress and empire coat for girls ages six to twelve.

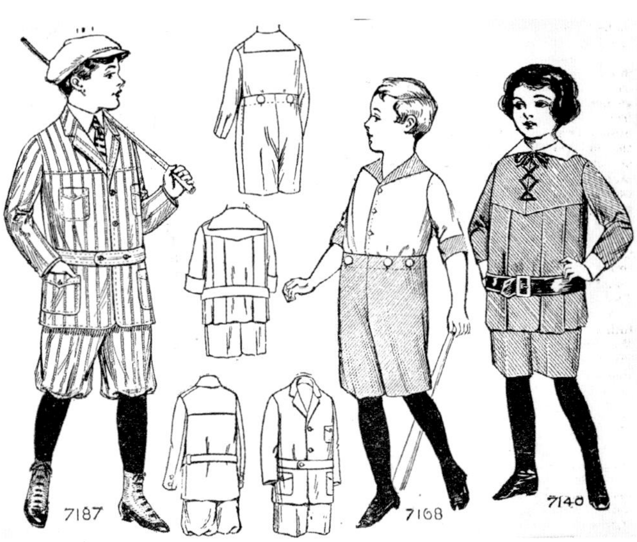

A trio of boys' fashionable outfits: the Norfolk, the Dutch suit, and the low-belted knickers suit. *Needlecraft Magazine*, May 1915.

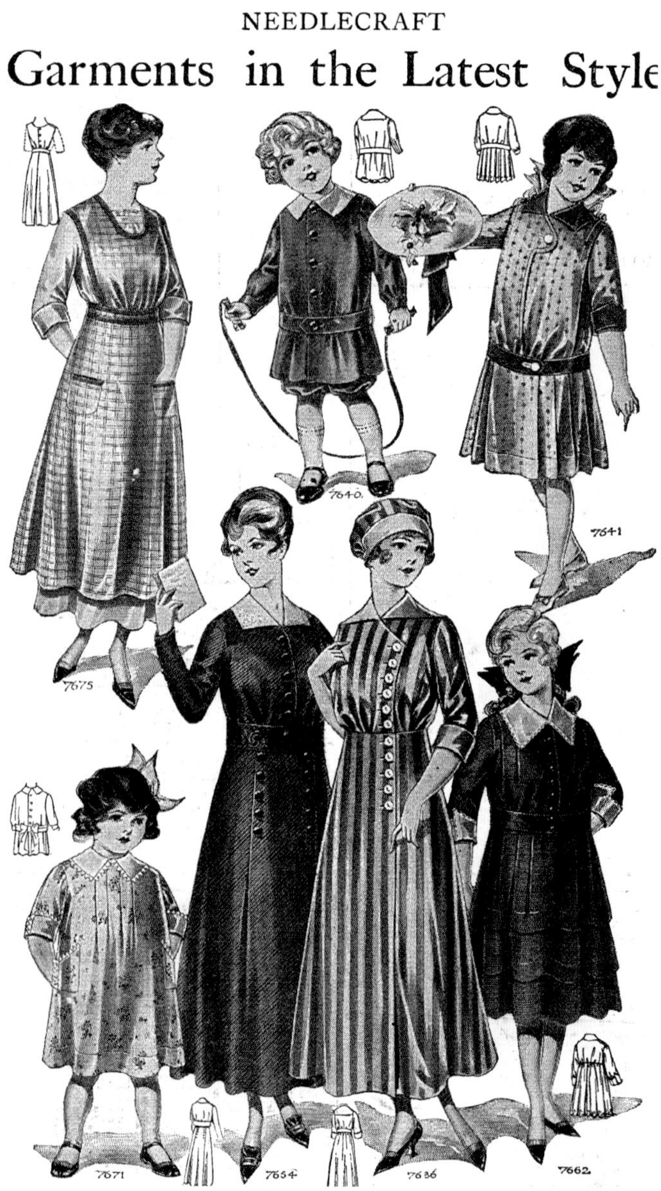

Spring, 1916: Low-belted, loose-fitting frocks for children are shown with the latest styles for Mother. *Needlecraft Magazine*, April 1916.

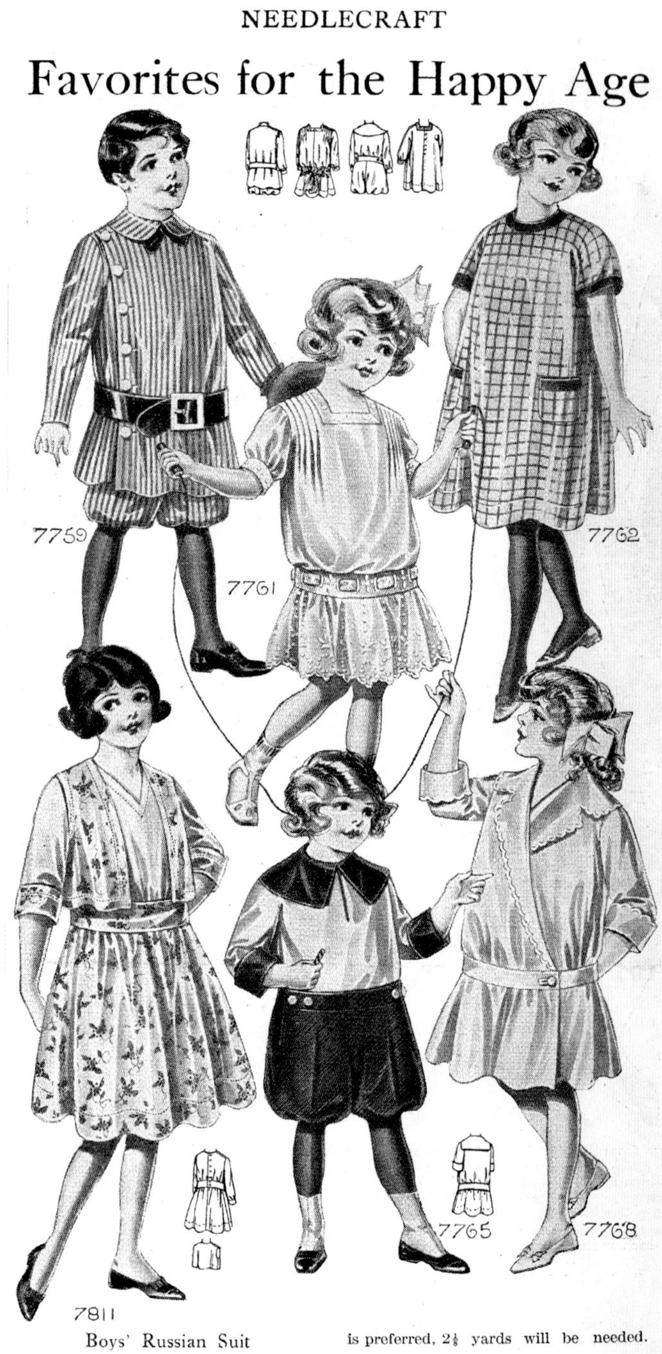

Pattern illustrations for rompers, knickers suits, and dresses. *Needlecraft Magazine*, July 1916.

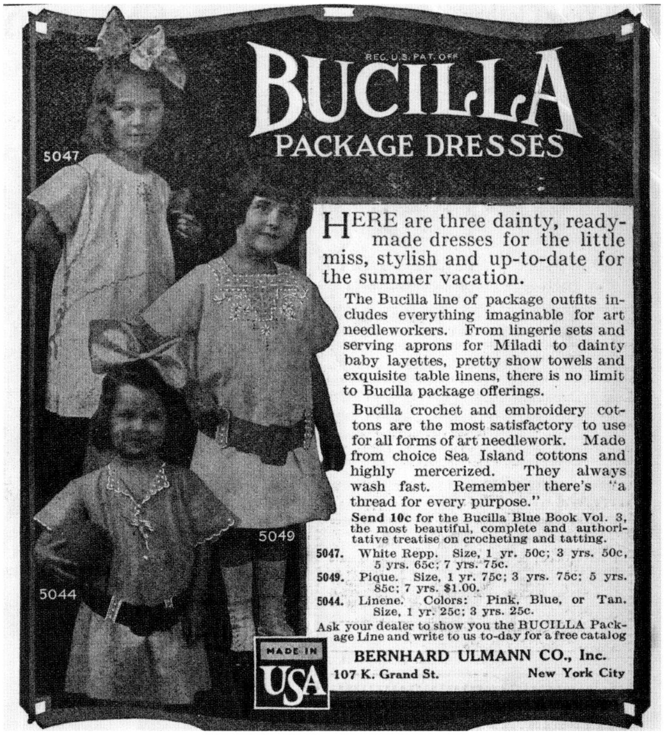

An advertisement for three ready-made dresses for little girls. *Needlecraft Magazine*, April 1916.

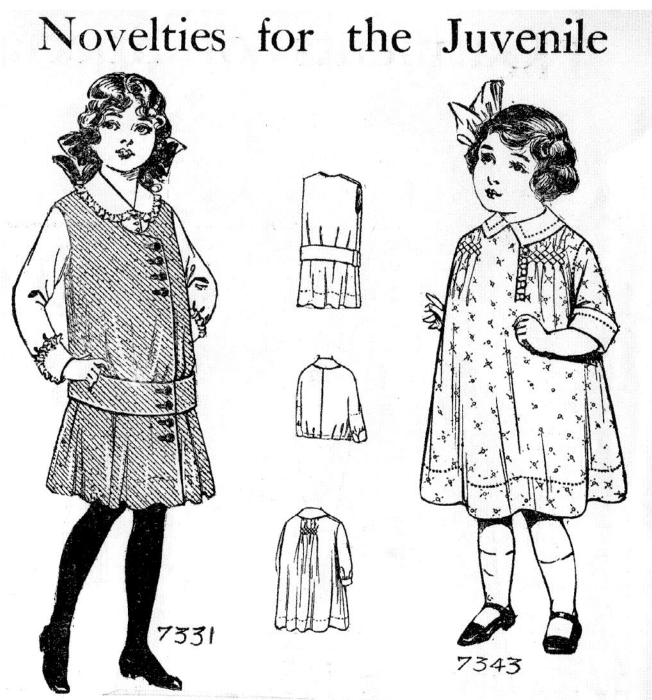

A pair of girl's dress patterns from fall 1915. The first reveals a novelty for asymmetric front button closure; the second falls in straight lines from shoulder to hem with fullness held in place with hand smocking. *Needlecraft Magazine*, September 1915.

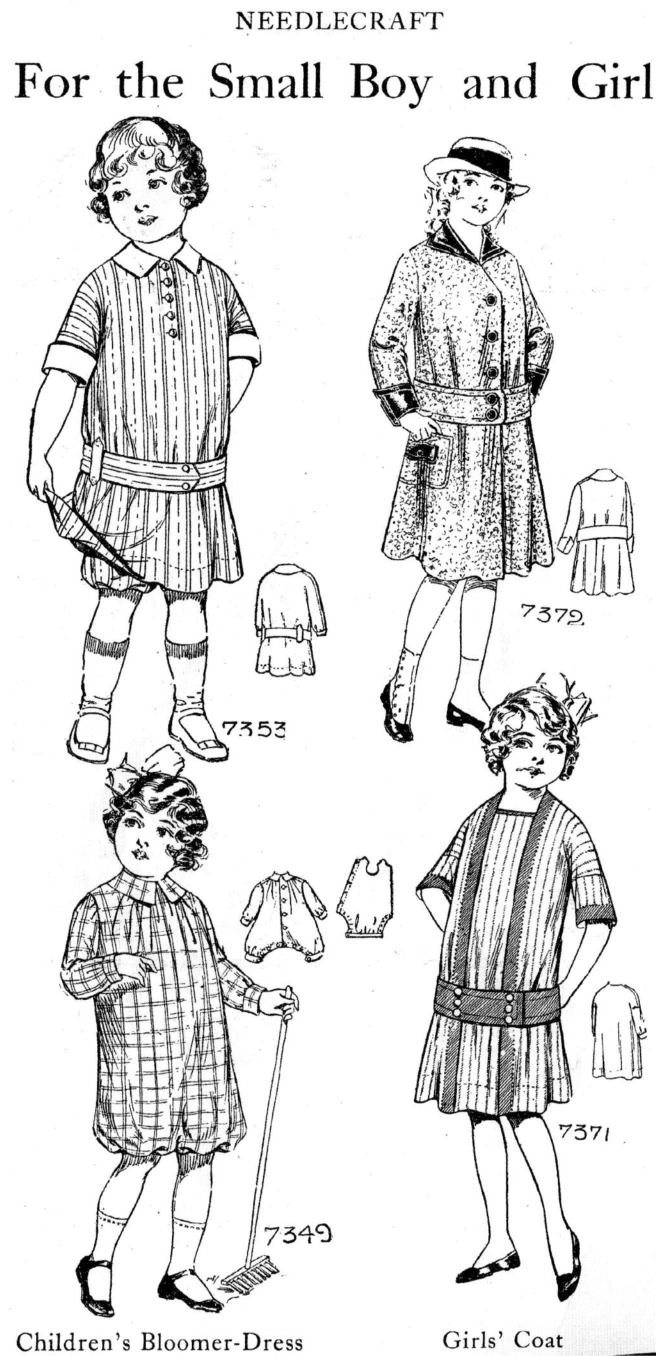

Summer, 1916: Low-waisted styles for boys and girls. *Needlecraft Magazine*, June 1916.

A pattern for a simple-to-construct set of clothing for a small boy or girl. *Needlecraft Magazine*, September 1915.

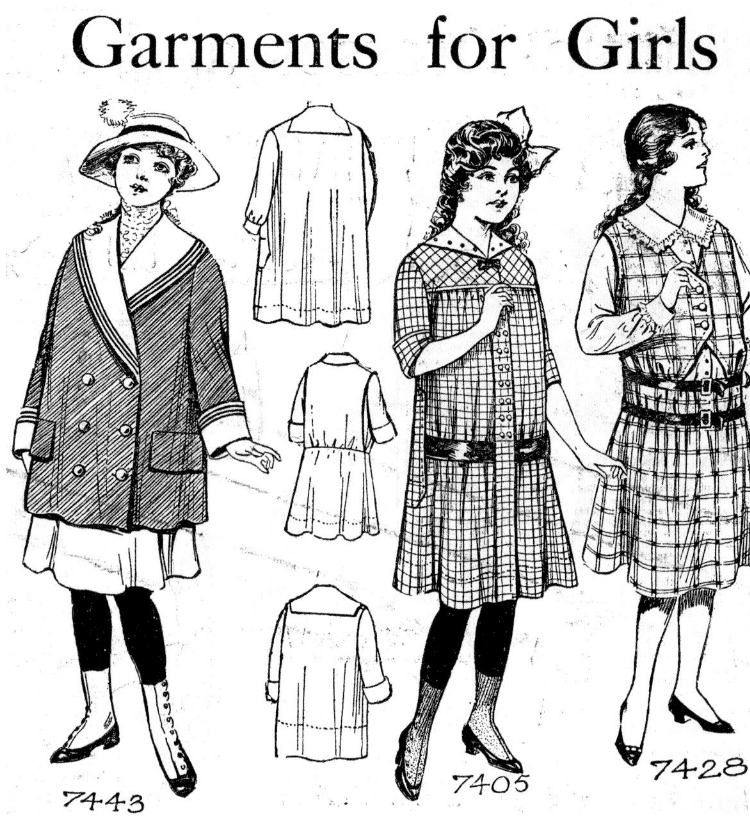

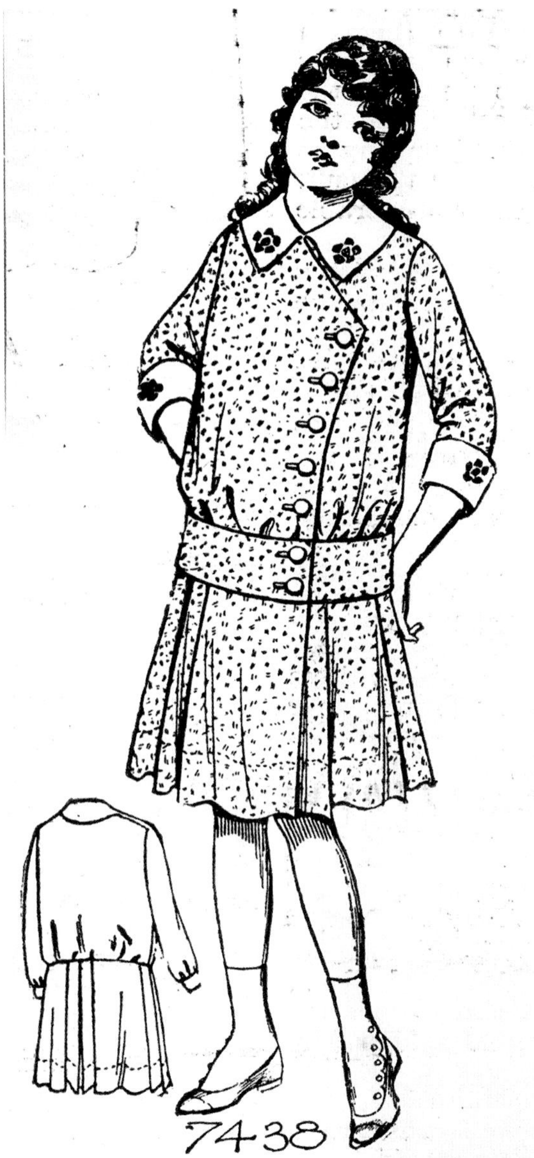

A young girl's wrap dress buttoned left of center. *Needlecraft Magazine*, November 1915.

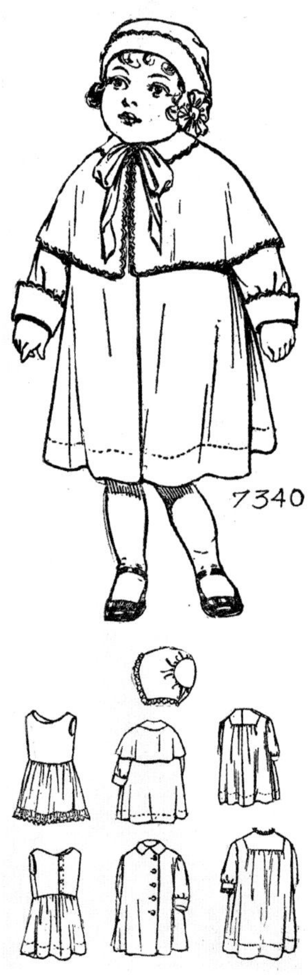

Illustrations from the November 1915 issue of *Needlecraft Magazine* show dresses and coats to be made at home. Each is loose-fitting with attention drawn to the hip area.

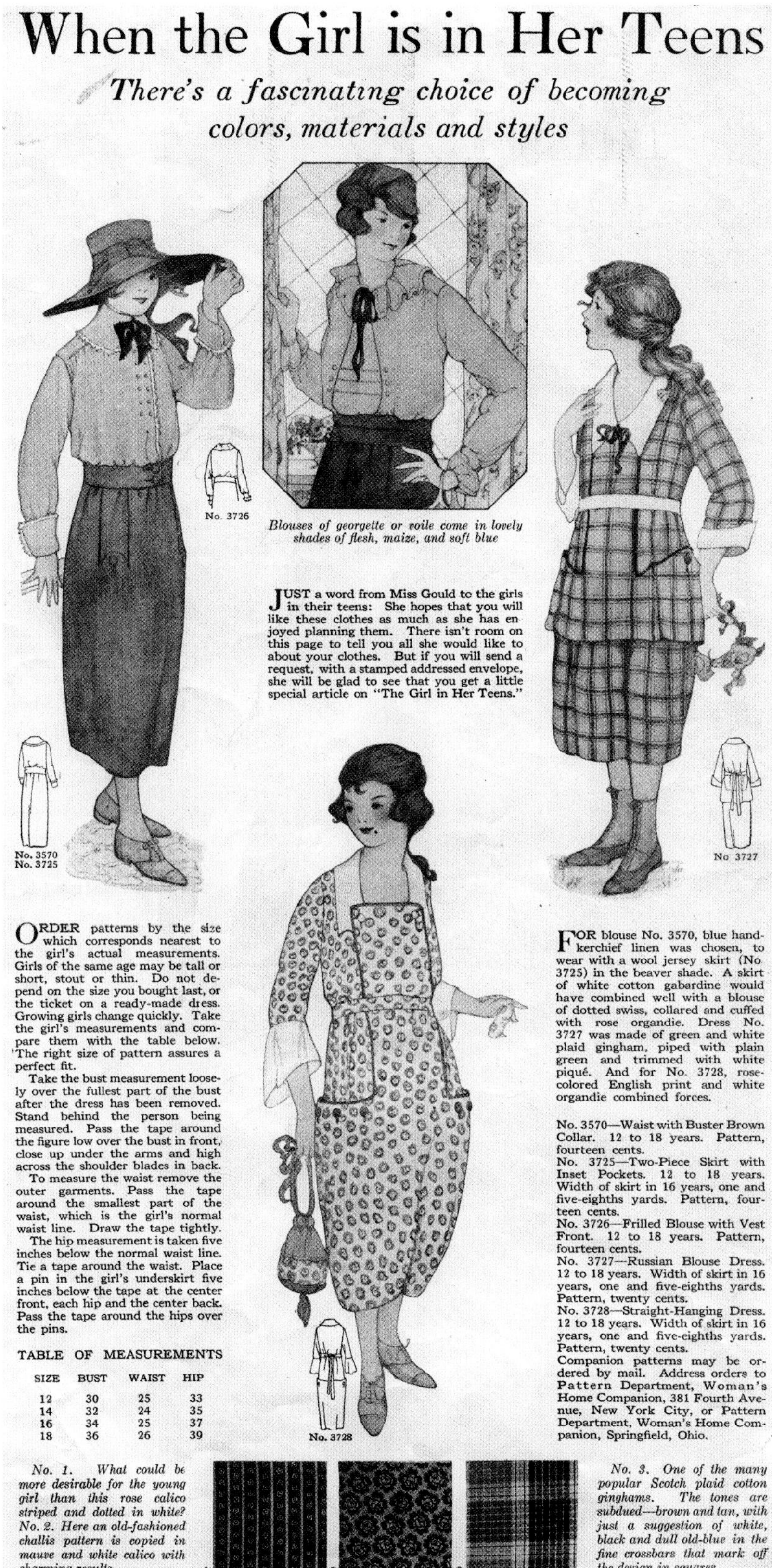

When the Girl is in Her Teens

There's a fascinating choice of becoming colors, materials and styles

No. 3726

Blouses of georgette or voile come in lovely shades of flesh, maize, and soft blue

JUST a word from Miss Gould to the girls in their teens: She hopes that you will like these clothes as much as she has enjoyed planning them. There isn't room on this page to tell you all she would like to about your clothes. But if you will send a request, with a stamped addressed envelope, she will be glad to see that you get a little special article on "The Girl in Her Teens."

No. 3570
No. 3725

No 3727

ORDER patterns by the size which corresponds nearest to the girl's actual measurements. Girls of the same age may be tall or short, stout or thin. Do not depend on the size you bought last, or the ticket on a ready-made dress. Growing girls change quickly. Take the girl's measurements and compare them with the table below. The right size of pattern assures a perfect fit.

Take the bust measurement loosely over the fullest part of the bust after the dress has been removed. Stand behind the person being measured. Pass the tape around the figure low over the bust in front, close up under the arms and high across the shoulder blades in back.

To measure the waist remove the outer garments. Pass the tape around the smallest part of the waist, which is the girl's normal waist line. Draw the tape tightly.

The hip measurement is taken five inches below the normal waist line. Tie a tape around the waist. Place a pin in the girl's underskirt five inches below the tape at the center front, each hip and the center back. Pass the tape around the hips over the pins.

TABLE OF MEASUREMENTS

SIZE	BUST	WAIST	HIP
12	30	25	33
14	32	24	35
16	34	25	37
18	36	26	39

No. 3728

FOR blouse No. 3570, blue handkerchief linen was chosen, to wear with a wool jersey skirt (No 3725) in the beaver shade. A skirt of white cotton gabardine would have combined well with a blouse of dotted swiss, collared and cuffed with rose organdie. Dress No. 3727 was made of green and white plaid gingham, piped with plain green and trimmed with white piqué. And for No. 3728, rose-colored English print and white organdie combined forces.

No. 3570—Waist with Buster Brown Collar. 12 to 18 years. Pattern, fourteen cents.
No. 3725—Two-Piece Skirt with Inset Pockets. 12 to 18 years. Width of skirt in 16 years, one and five-eighths yards. Pattern, fourteen cents.
No. 3726—Frilled Blouse with Vest Front. 12 to 18 years. Pattern, fourteen cents.
No. 3727—Russian Blouse Dress. 12 to 18 years. Width of skirt in 16 years, one and five-eighths yards. Pattern, twenty cents.
No. 3728—Straight-Hanging Dress. 12 to 18 years. Width of skirt in 16 years, one and five-eighths yards. Pattern, twenty cents.
Companion patterns may be ordered by mail. Address orders to Pattern Department, Woman's Home Companion, 381 Fourth Avenue, New York City, or Pattern Department, Woman's Home Companion, Springfield, Ohio.

No. 1. What could be more desirable for the young girl than this rose calico striped and dotted in white? No. 2. Here an old-fashioned challis pattern is copied in mauve and white calico with charming results.

1 2 3

No. 3. One of the many popular Scotch plaid cotton ginghams. The tones are subdued—brown and tan, with just a suggestion of white, black and dull old-blue in the fine crossbars that mark off the design in squares.

These pattern illustrations for teens from June 1919 herald the boyish styles of the coming flapper era. *Woman's Home Companion*, June 1919.

Novelties for Little Girls

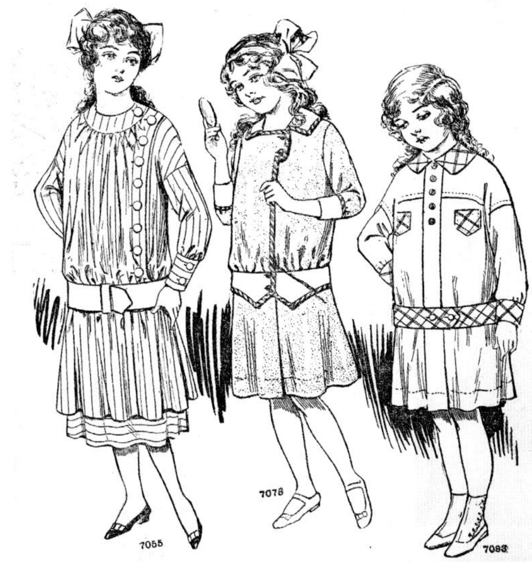

A trio of loose-fitting, low-slung dresses for young girls, the third described as a Norfolk dress. *Needlecraft Magazine*, August 1915.

The Very Latest for All Ages

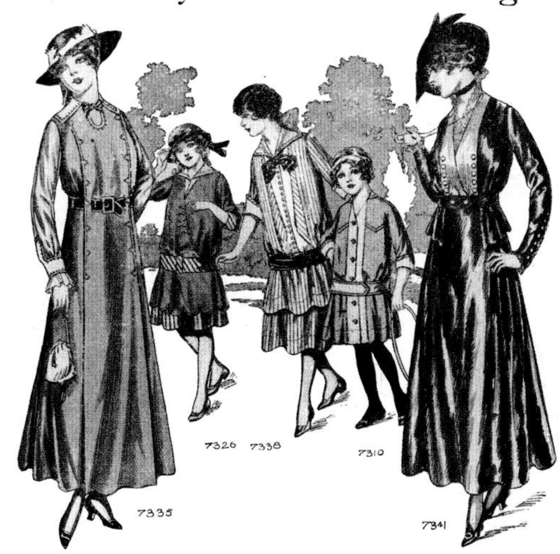

The heading says it all; these patterns reveal subtle changes in the low-belted styles for girls. The dress on the left reveals drop shoulders and far left front button closure, while the other two dresses show attached skirts without added fullness. *Needlecraft Magazine*, March 1915.

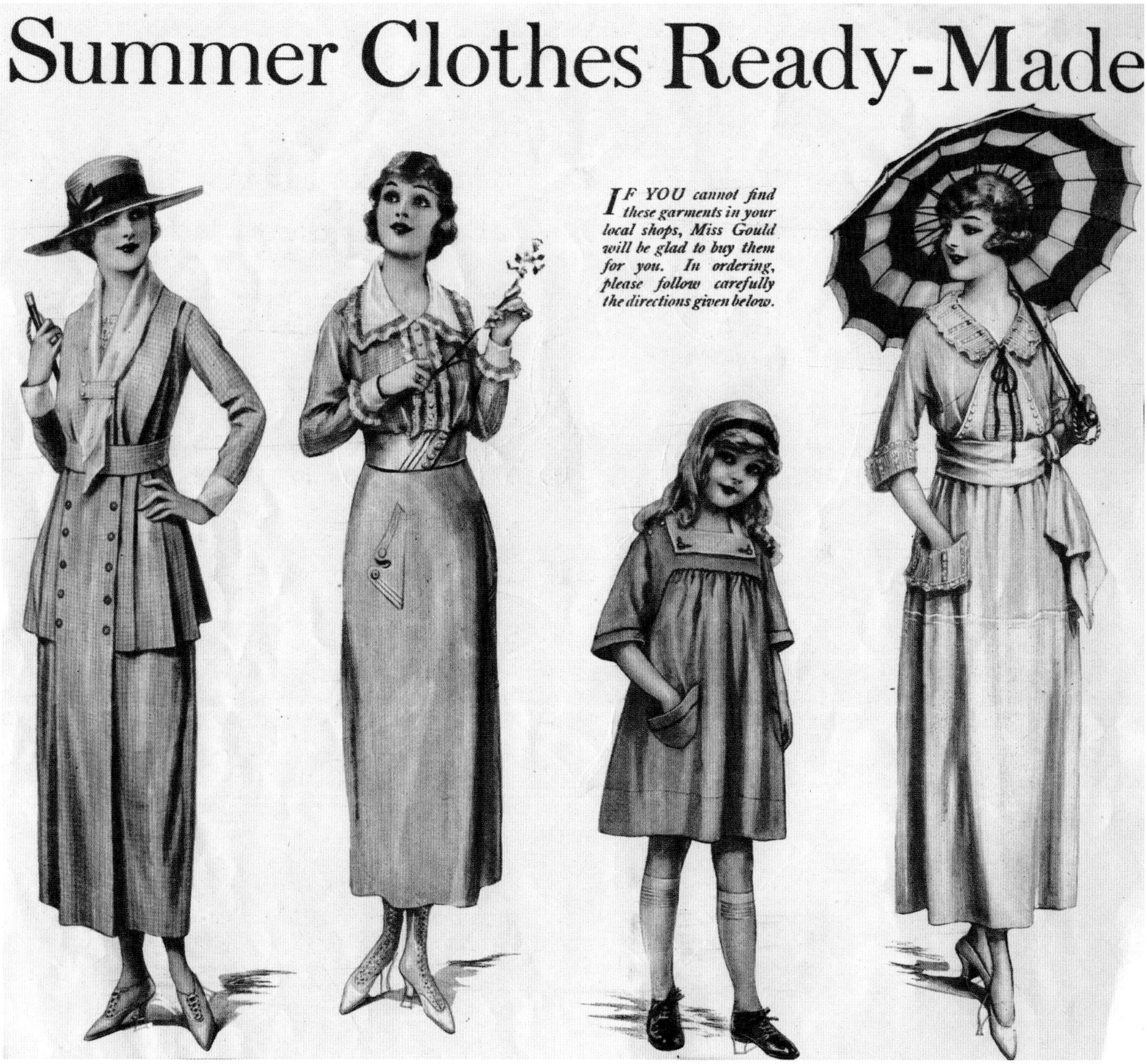
Summer Clothes Ready-Made
IF YOU cannot find these garments in your local shops, Miss Gould will be glad to buy them for you. In ordering, please follow carefully the directions given below.

This ready-made child's dress of gold, green, and lavender or pink chambrette with a batiste collar could be purchased in sizes six to ten years for $4.95. The contrast between this and the illustrations styled for women is a harbinger of the coming shift to clothing styles more distinctly designed for children. *Ladies Home Companion*, June 1919.

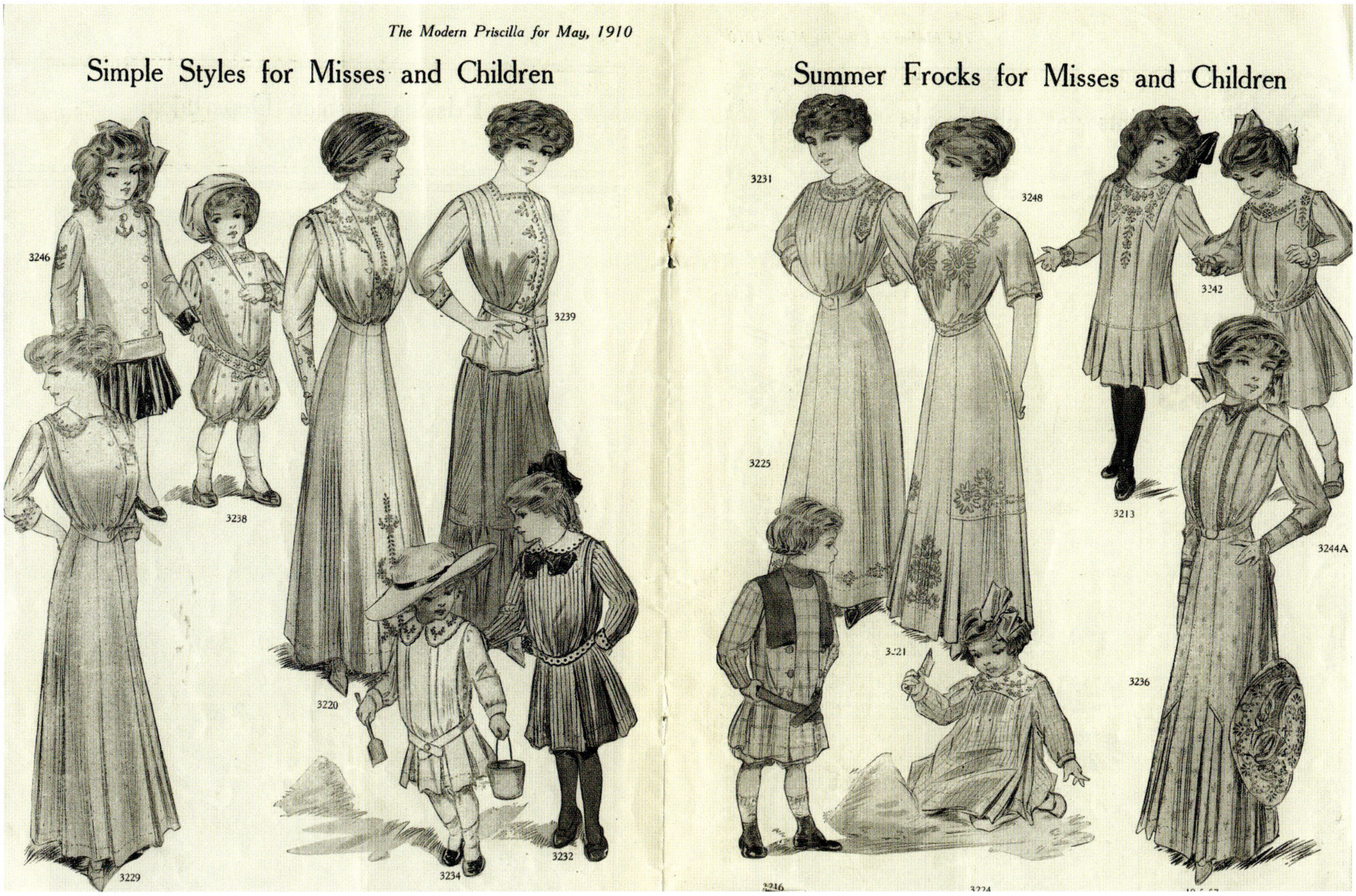

Pattern illustrations for a variety of children's dresses: a middy suit, rompers, and Russian suit, shown with a number of styles for misses and ladies age thirteen years and up. *The Modern Priscilla*, May 1910.

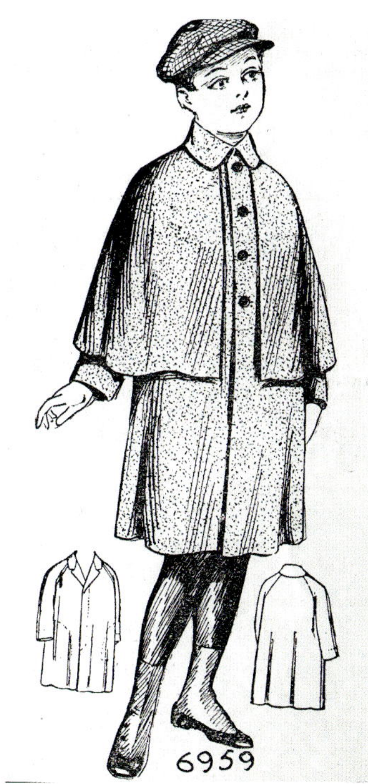

Sketch of a boy's serviceable overcoat with detachable cape for severe weather. *Needlecraft Magazine*, January 1915.

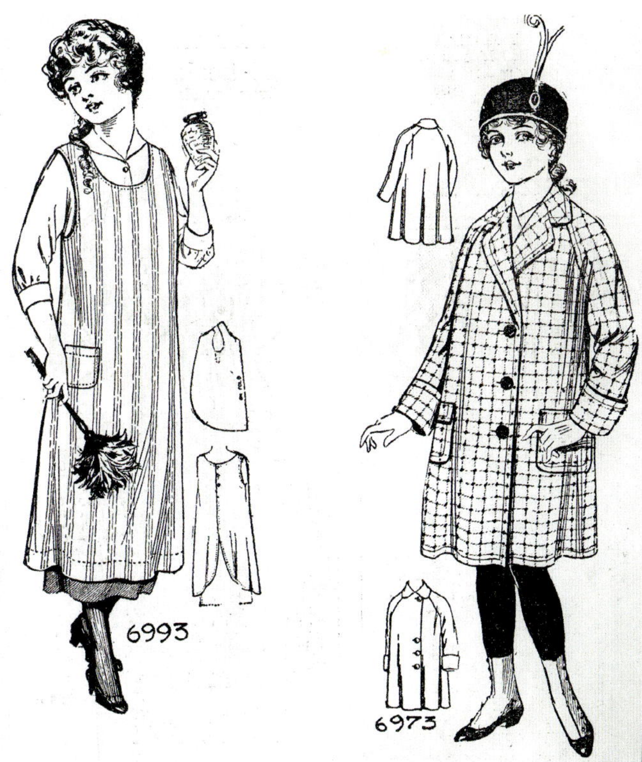

Simple-to-construct apron and overcoat for a young girl. *Needlecraft Magazine*, January, 1915.

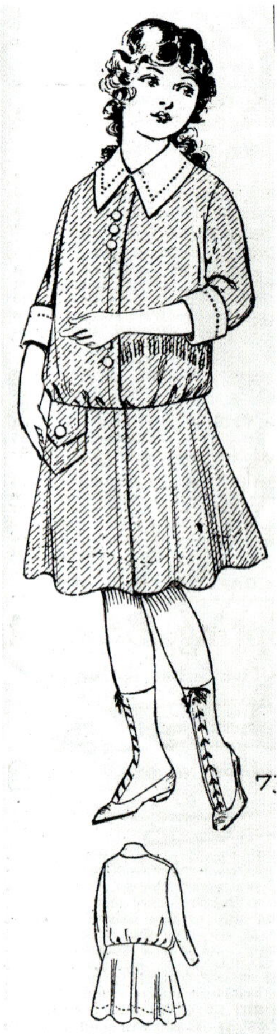

Pattern illustration for a young girl's serviceable dress. *Needlecraft Magazine*, October, 1915.

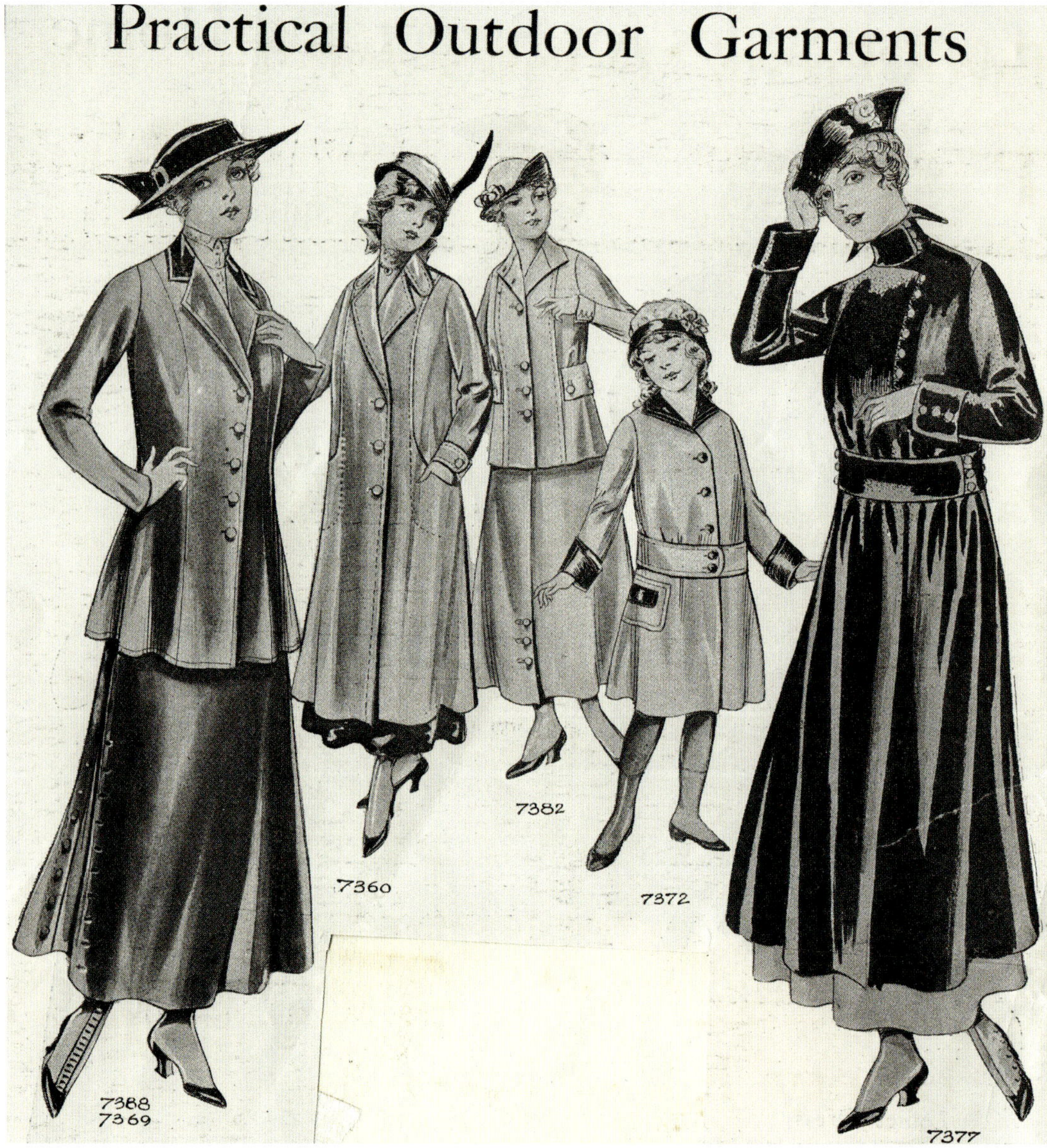

This November 1915 pattern sketch from *Needlecraft Magazine* demonstrates a child's coat in keeping with the latest styles for women. Fabrics such as gabardine, corduroy, tweed, velvet, and krimmer were popular options for such a garment.

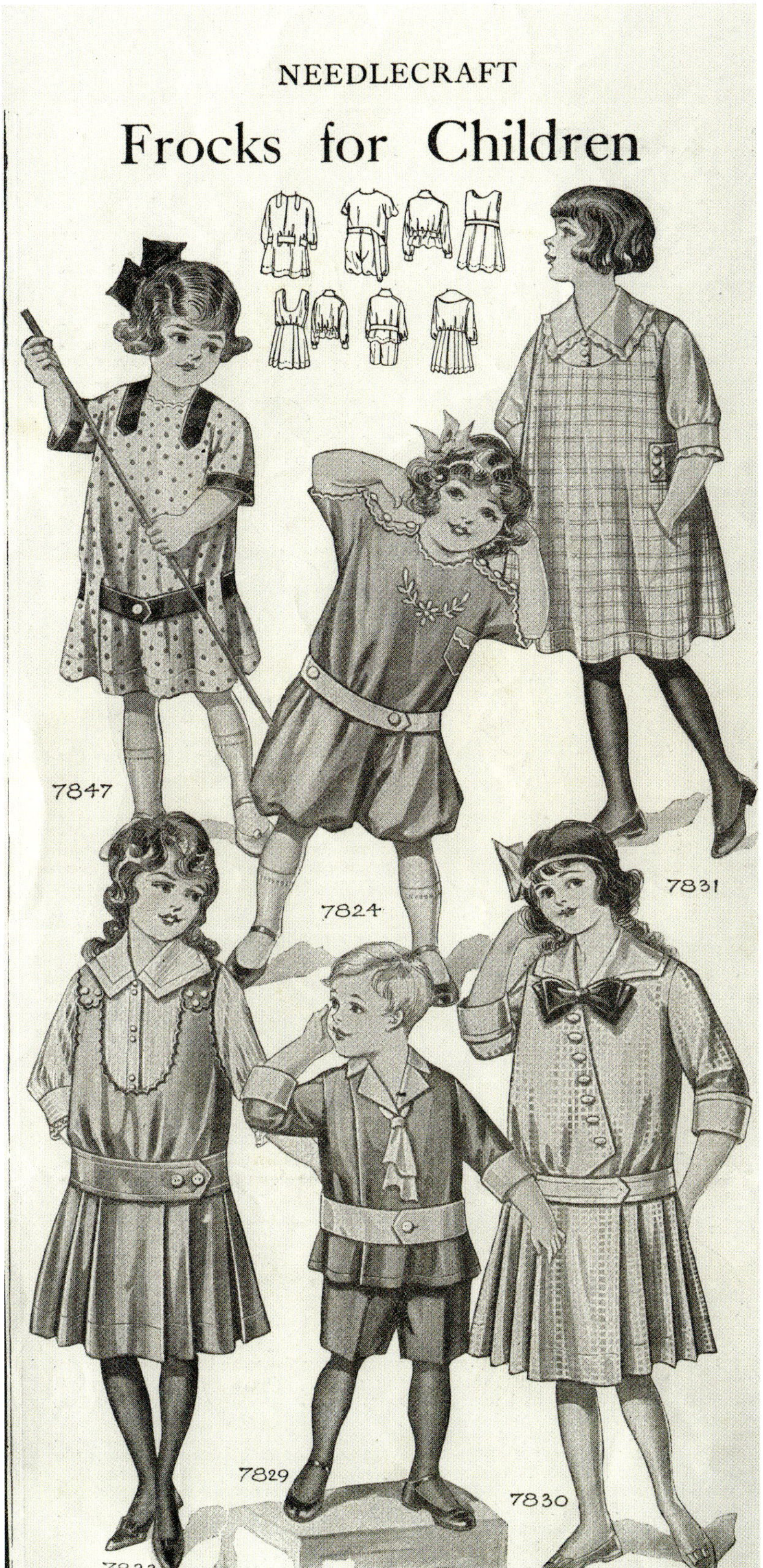

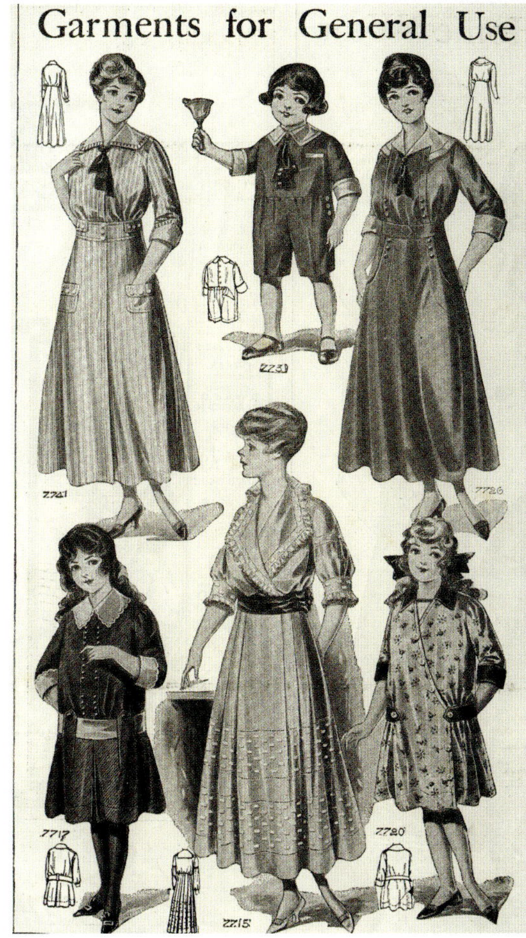

Three children's garments: a boy's suit, a belted dress, and a half-belted dress deemed suitable for general use. *Needlecraft Magazine*, May 1915.

A selection of patterns for girls' dresses, full coverage apron, and classic middy blouse. *Needlecraft Magazine*, February 1916.

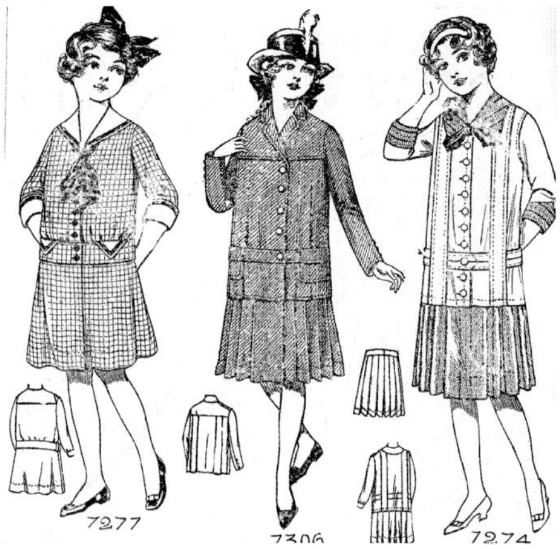

This pattern illustration reveals the trend toward button trimming. The lines of the dresses mimic the drape of women's skirts of that era. *Needlecraft Magazine*, February 1916.

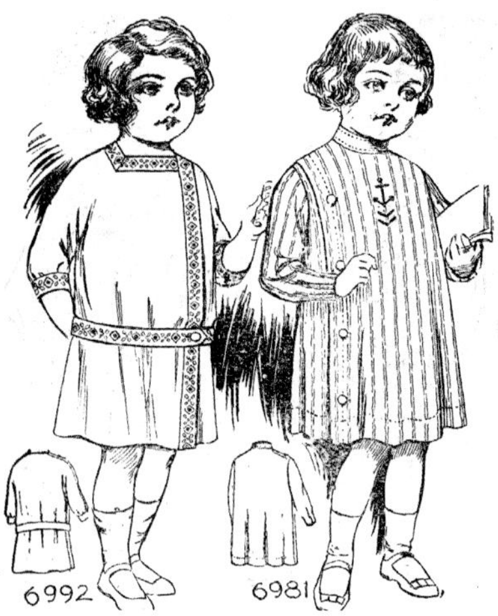

Easy to make slip-on garments with plenty of charm, featured in *Needlecraft Magazine*, January 1915.

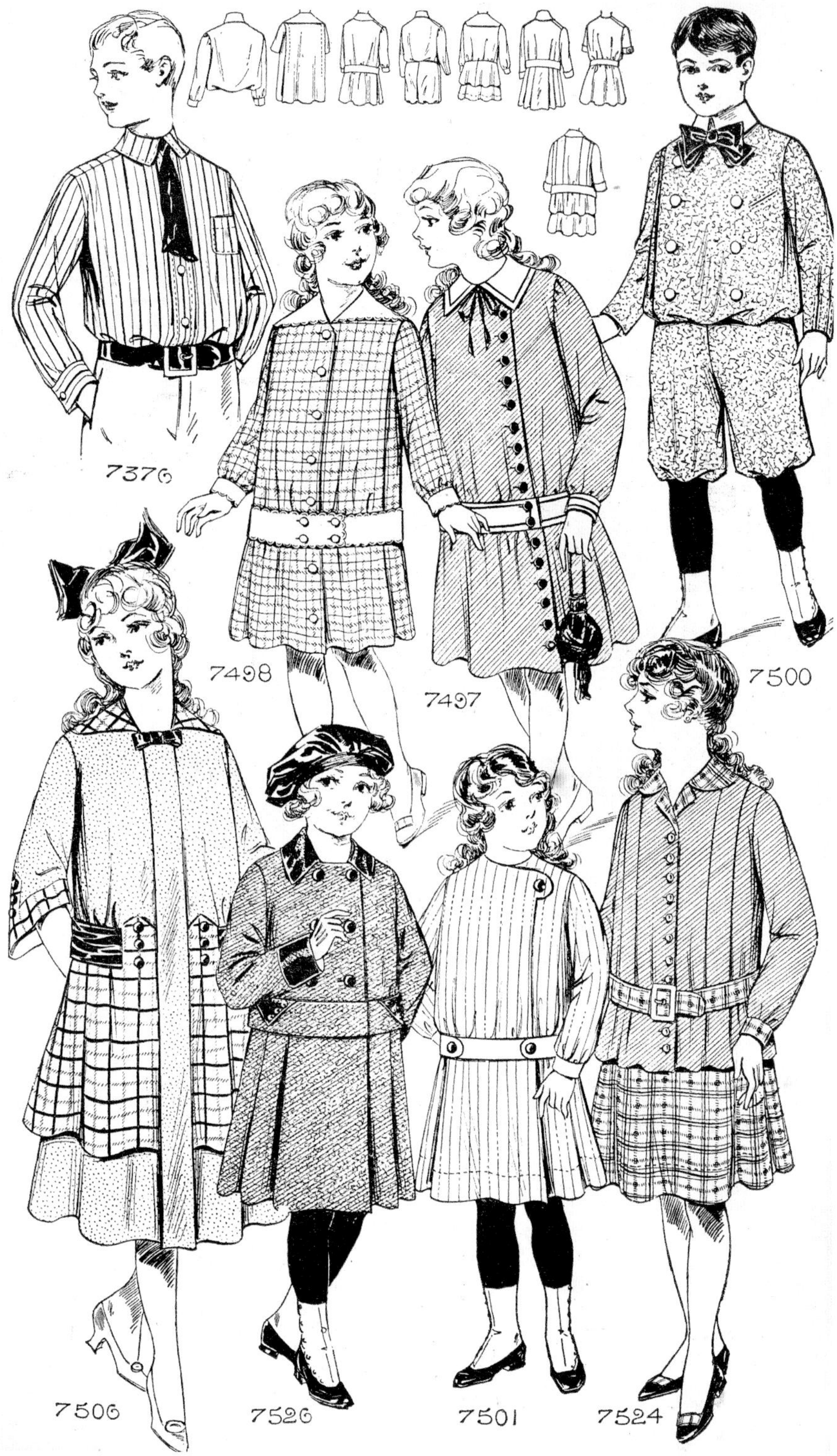

Under the heading "Novel Designs for Boys and Girls," this illustration shows the regulation blouse worn by boys before graduation into the plain man's shirt. The dresses are described as being simple to make and appropriate for school. Khaki, serge, and tweed are suggested for the boy's knickers ensemble, suitable for constant wear. The girls' coats follow the same lines as the dresses. *Needlecraft Magazine*, January 1916.

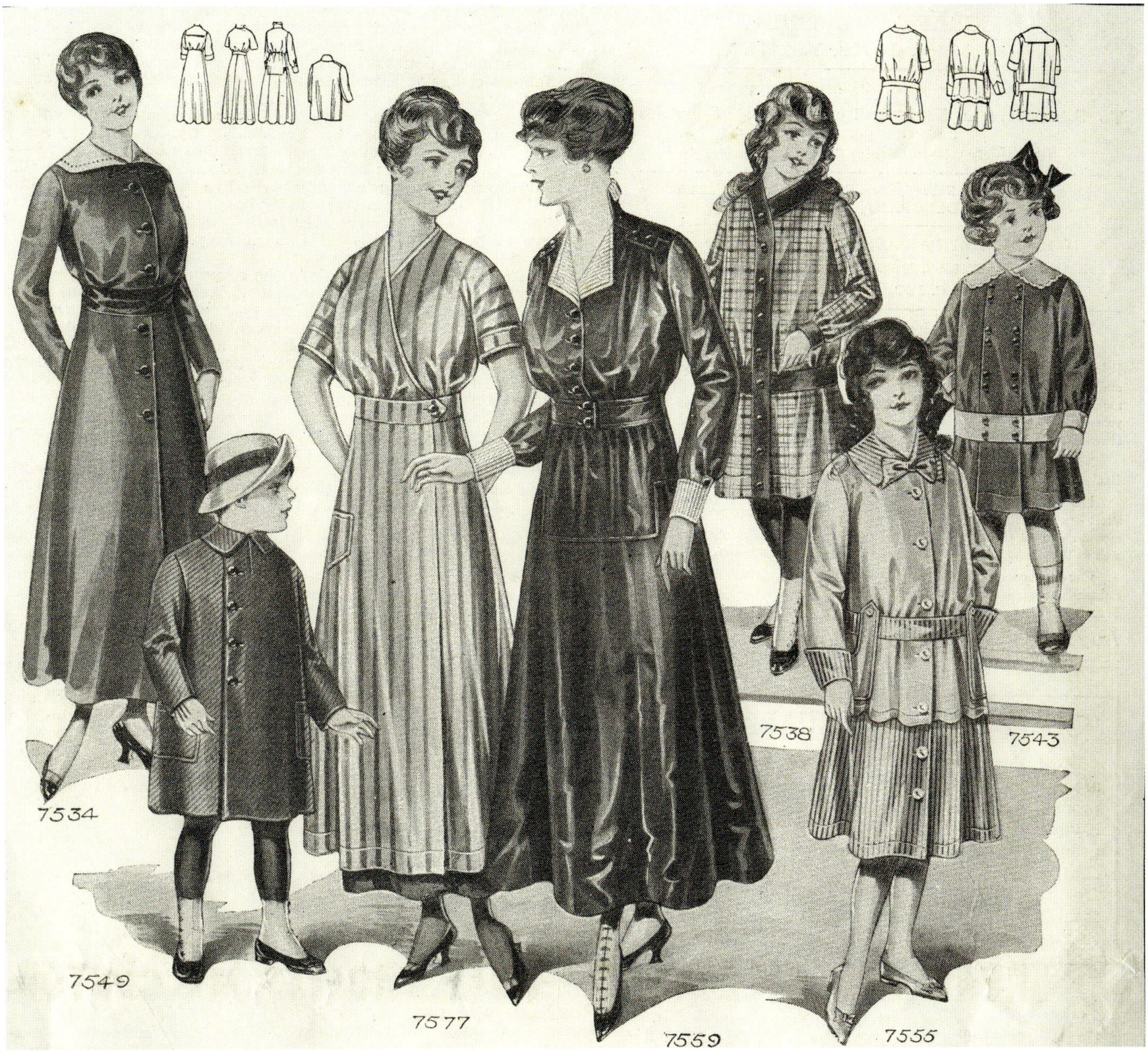

Ease of construction and simple lines are the order of the day c. 1916, as evidenced in this illustration of women's and children's clothing. Clean lines are achieved through a lack of embellishment and buttons colored to match the fabrics. *Needlecraft Magazine*, February 1916.

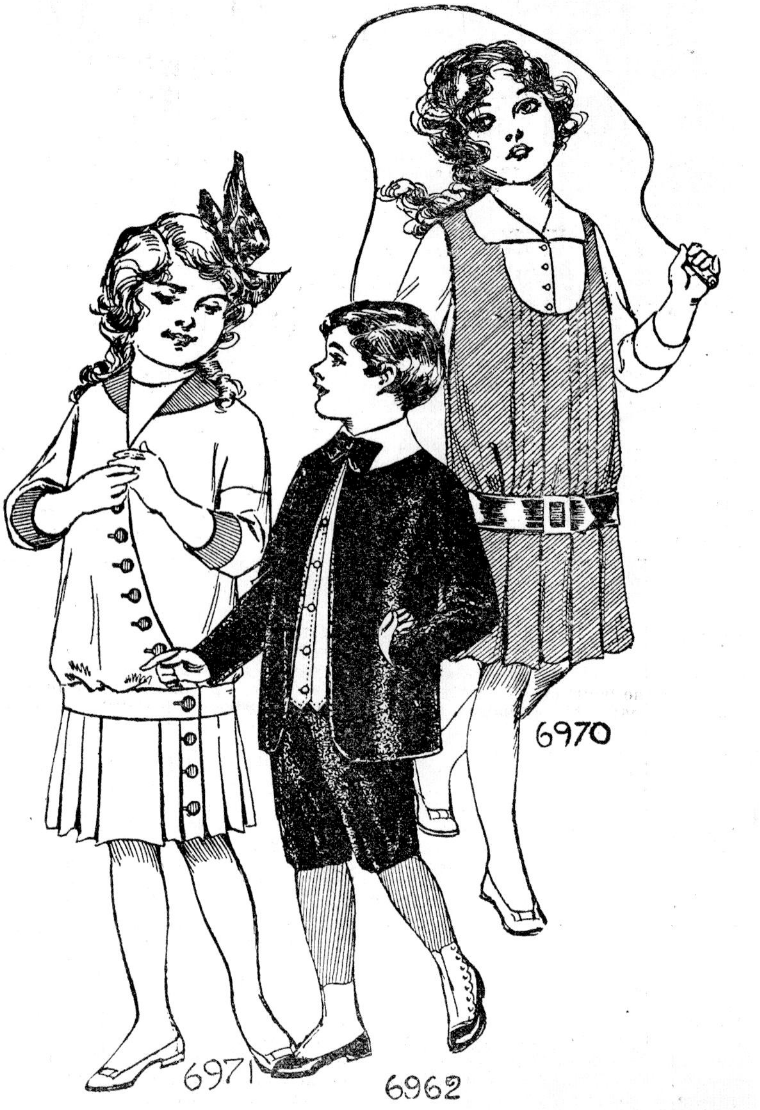

A trio of play clothes for young children from *Needlecraft Magazine*, January 1915.

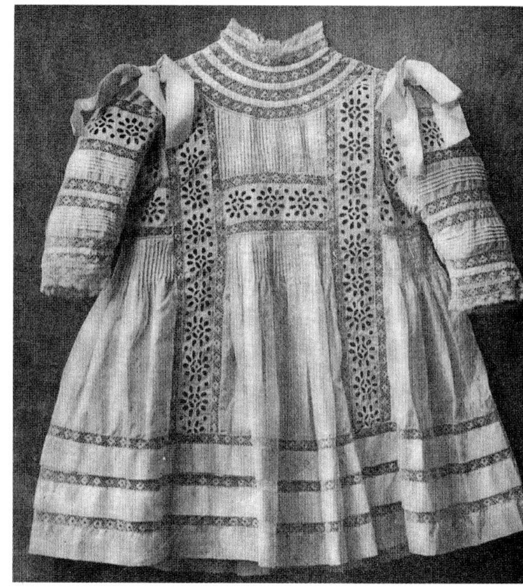

The pattern for this child's dress could be ordered, complete with stamping paste, and features lace and embroidered insertions. *The Modern Priscilla Magazine*, May 1910.

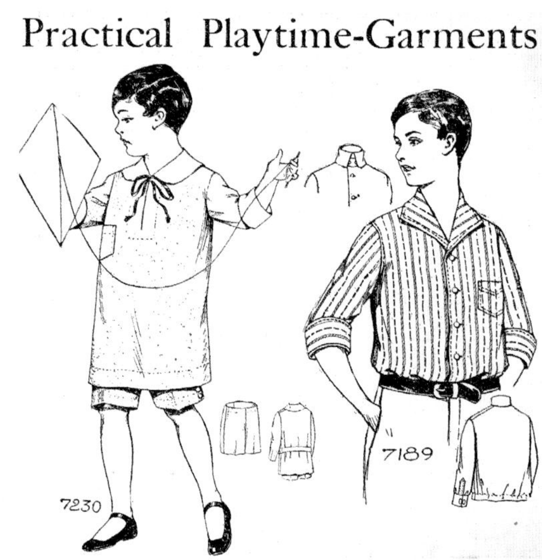

This pattern for a boy's middy suit (left) is easily made, as it slips over the head. The short pants don't have a fly and are straight-edged at the knee. The blouse (right) was described as "the last word in styles for growing boys." The convertible collar could be worn open or buttoned high at the neck. *Needlecraft Magazine*, June 1915.

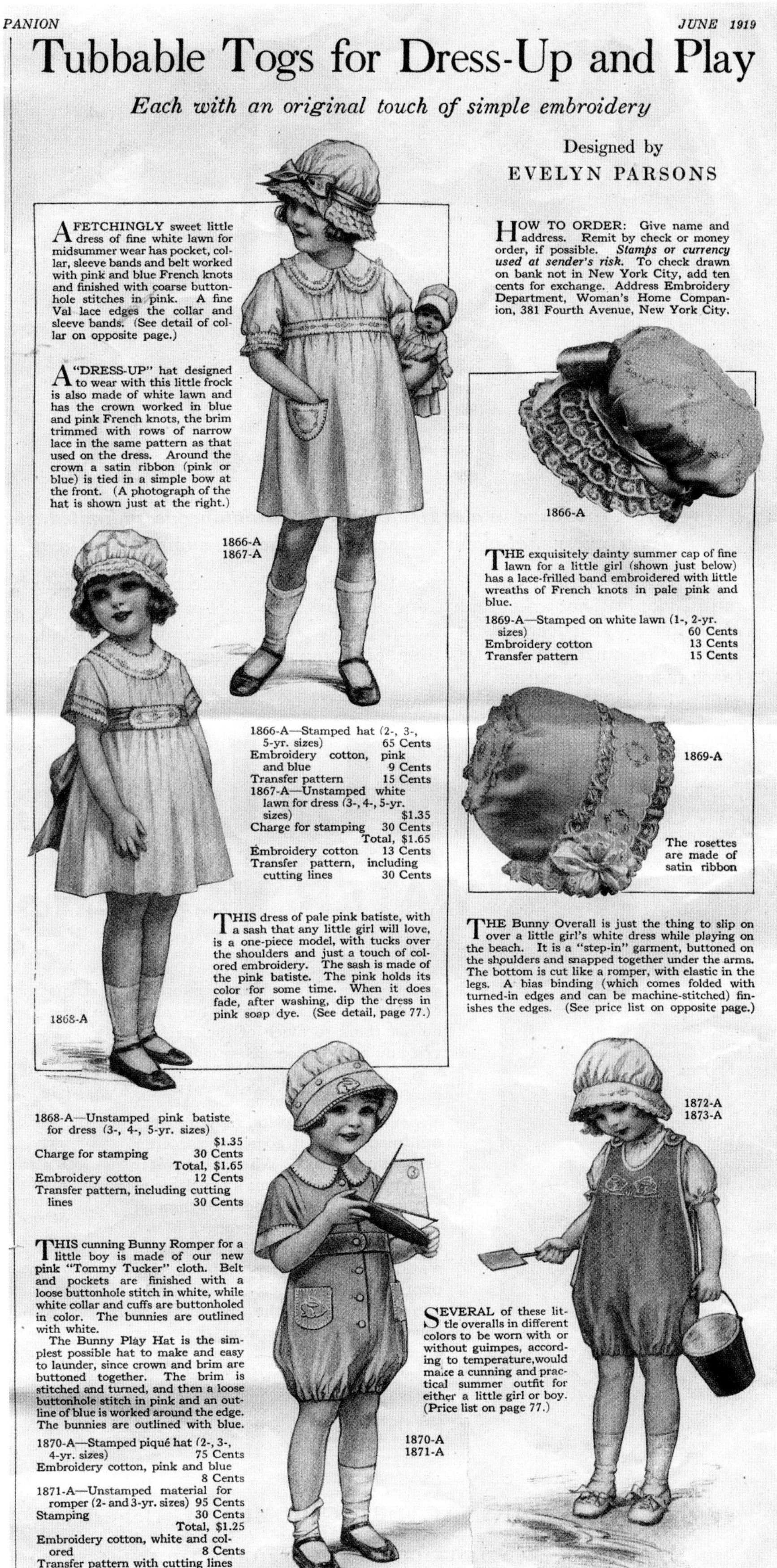

PANION JUNE 1919

Tubbable Togs for Dress-Up and Play

Each with an original touch of simple embroidery

Designed by
EVELYN PARSONS

A FETCHINGLY sweet little dress of fine white lawn for midsummer wear has pocket, collar, sleeve bands and belt worked with pink and blue French knots and finished with coarse buttonhole stitches in pink. A fine Val lace edges the collar and sleeve bands. (See detail of collar on opposite page.)

A "DRESS-UP" hat designed to wear with this little frock is also made of white lawn and has the crown worked in blue and pink French knots, the brim trimmed with rows of narrow lace in the same pattern as that used on the dress. Around the crown a satin ribbon (pink or blue) is tied in a simple bow at the front. (A photograph of the hat is shown just at the right.)

HOW TO ORDER: Give name and address. Remit by check or money order, if possible. *Stamps or currency used at sender's risk.* To check drawn on bank not in New York City, add ten cents for exchange. Address Embroidery Department, Woman's Home Companion, 381 Fourth Avenue, New York City.

1866-A

1866-A
1867-A

THE exquisitely dainty summer cap of fine lawn for a little girl (shown just below) has a lace-frilled band embroidered with little wreaths of French knots in pale pink and blue.

1869-A—Stamped on white lawn (1-, 2-yr. sizes)	60 Cents
Embroidery cotton	13 Cents
Transfer pattern	15 Cents

1866-A—Stamped hat (2-, 3-, 5-yr. sizes)	65 Cents
Embroidery cotton, pink and blue	9 Cents
Transfer pattern	15 Cents
1867-A—Unstamped white lawn for dress (3-, 4-, 5-yr. sizes)	$1.35
Charge for stamping	30 Cents
	Total, $1.65
Embroidery cotton	13 Cents
Transfer pattern, including cutting lines	30 Cents

1869-A

The rosettes are made of satin ribbon

THIS dress of pale pink batiste, with a sash that any little girl will love, is a one-piece model, with tucks over the shoulders and just a touch of colored embroidery. The sash is made of the pink batiste. The pink holds its color for some time. When it does fade, after washing, dip the dress in pink soap dye. (See detail, page 77.)

THE Bunny Overall is just the thing to slip on over a little girl's white dress while playing on the beach. It is a "step-in" garment, buttoned on the shoulders and snapped together under the arms. The bottom is cut like a romper, with elastic in the legs. A bias binding (which comes folded with turned-in edges and can be machine-stitched) finishes the edges. (See price list on opposite page.)

1868-A

1868-A—Unstamped pink batiste for dress (3-, 4-, 5-yr. sizes)	$1.35
Charge for stamping	30 Cents
	Total, $1.65
Embroidery cotton	12 Cents
Transfer pattern, including cutting lines	30 Cents

1872-A
1873-A

THIS cunning Bunny Romper for a little boy is made of our new pink "Tommy Tucker" cloth. Belt and pockets are finished with a loose buttonhole stitch in white, while white collar and cuffs are buttonholed in color. The bunnies are outlined with white.

The Bunny Play Hat is the simplest possible hat to make and easy to launder, since crown and brim are buttoned together. The brim is stitched and turned, and then a loose buttonhole stitch in pink and an outline of blue is worked around the edge. The bunnies are outlined with blue.

1870-A—Stamped piqué hat (2-, 3-, 4-yr. sizes)	75 Cents
Embroidery cotton, pink and blue	8 Cents
1871-A—Unstamped material for romper (2- and 3-yr. sizes)	95 Cents
Stamping	30 Cents
	Total, $1.25
Embroidery cotton, white and colored	8 Cents
Transfer pattern with cutting lines given	30 Cents

SEVERAL of these little overalls in different colors to be worn with or without guimpes, according to temperature, would make a cunning and practical summer outfit for either a little girl or boy. (Price list on page 77.)

1870-A
1871-A

This pattern advertisement from *Woman's Home Companion*, June 1919, presents four above-the-knee styles for young children that can easily be made up and personalized with embroidery. The romper and overalls at bottom are suitable for either gender. Fabric caps ensure a unified silhouette and protection from the sun.

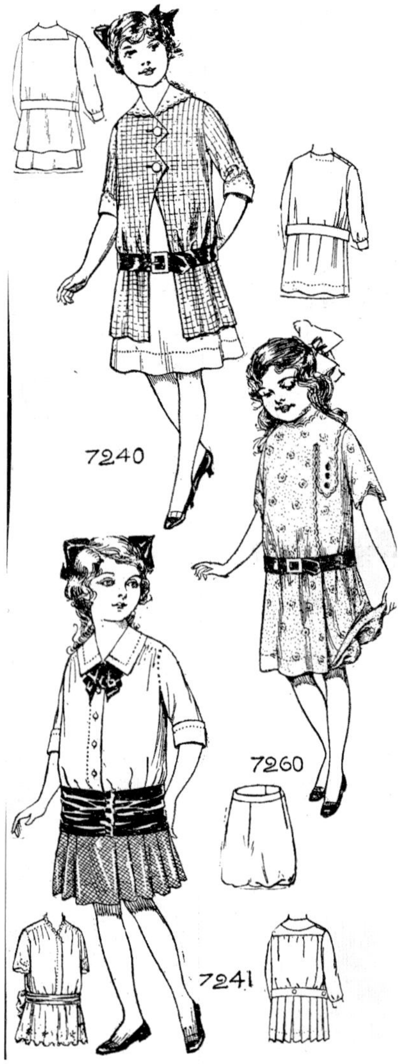

Girls' smart and practical dress patterns, suitable for vacation attire. *Needlecraft Magazine*, August 1915.

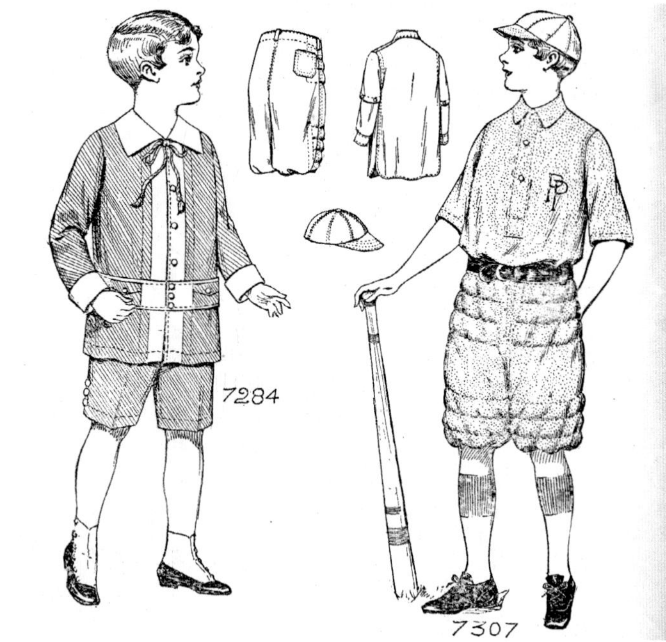

Illustration of home sewing patterns for a boy's knickers suit and baseball ensemble, fashionable sporting attire being a novel concept at the time. *Needlecraft Magazine*, August 1915.

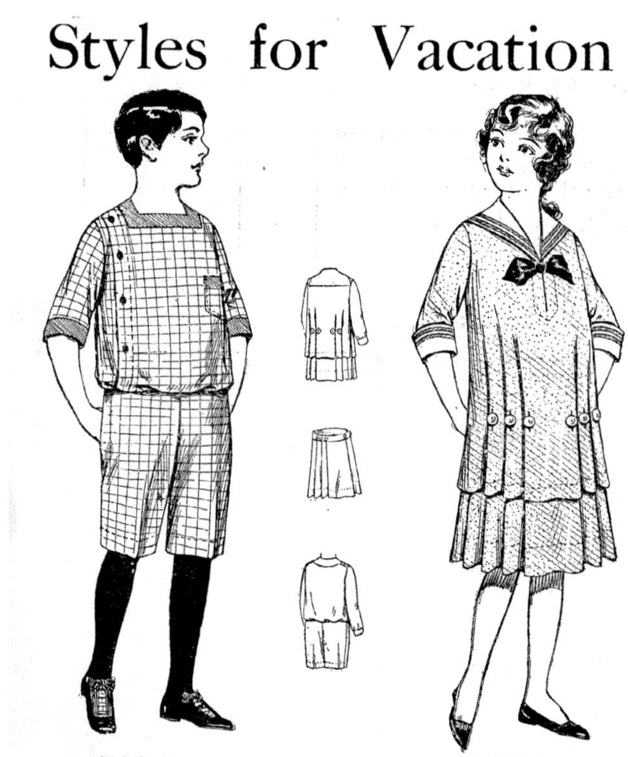

Sewing pattern illustration for a boy's summer suit and a girl's middy dress described as strictly up to date in a summer 1915 issue of *Needlecraft Magazine*.

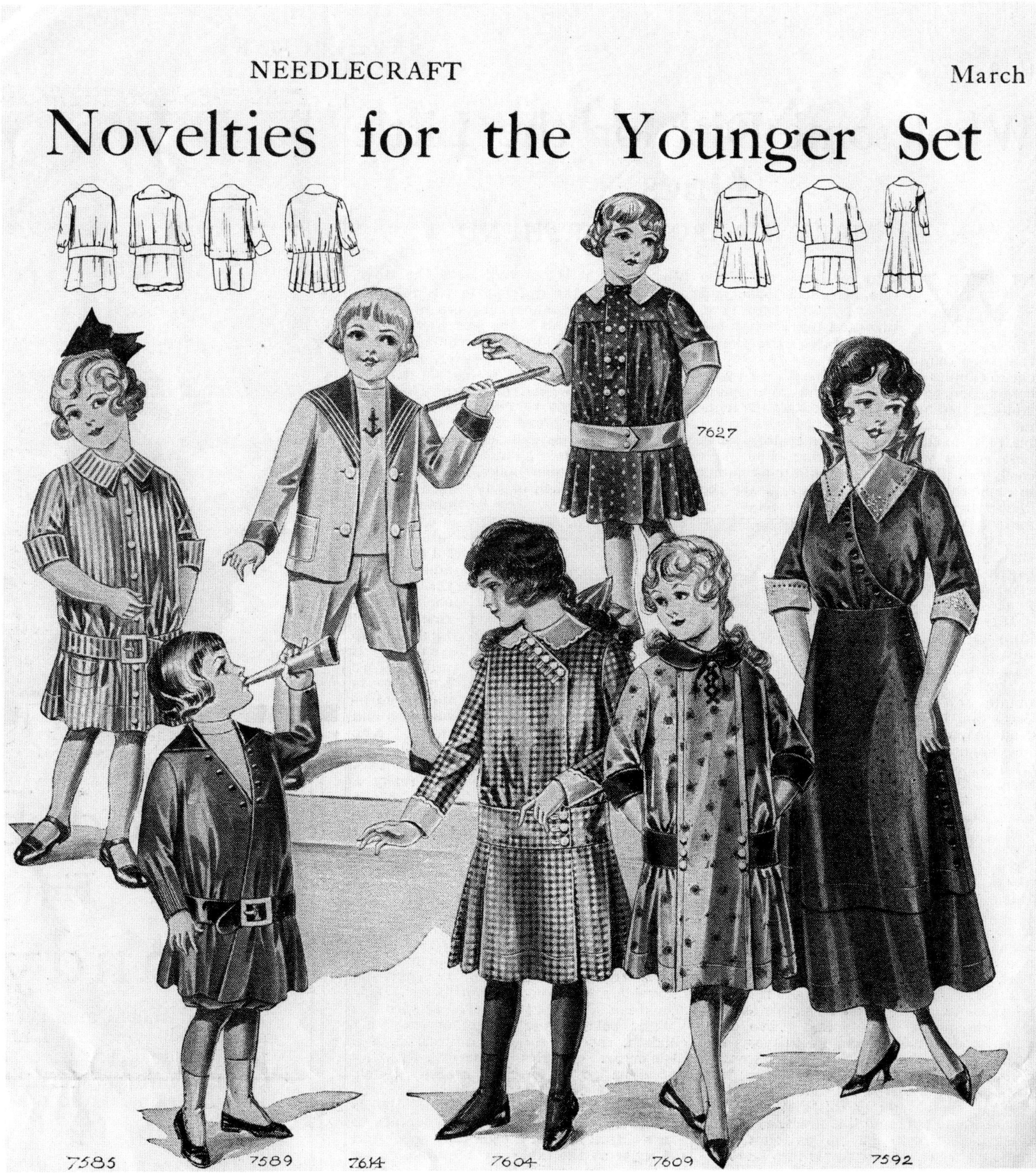

An illustration of children's garments including (top left) a children's frock with hidden underwaist and attached bloomers, and (bottom left) a boys' Russian suit with bloomers that peek out beneath a belted, long-sleeved blouse. *Needlecraft Magazine*, March 1916.

A boy's baby blue woollen sweater.

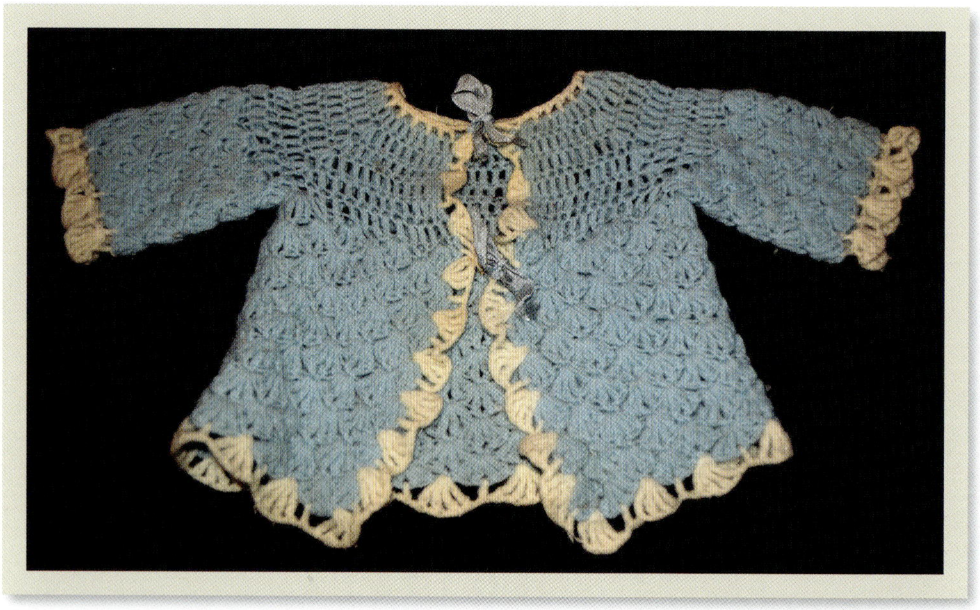

A young child's Valentine-themed celluloid fan.

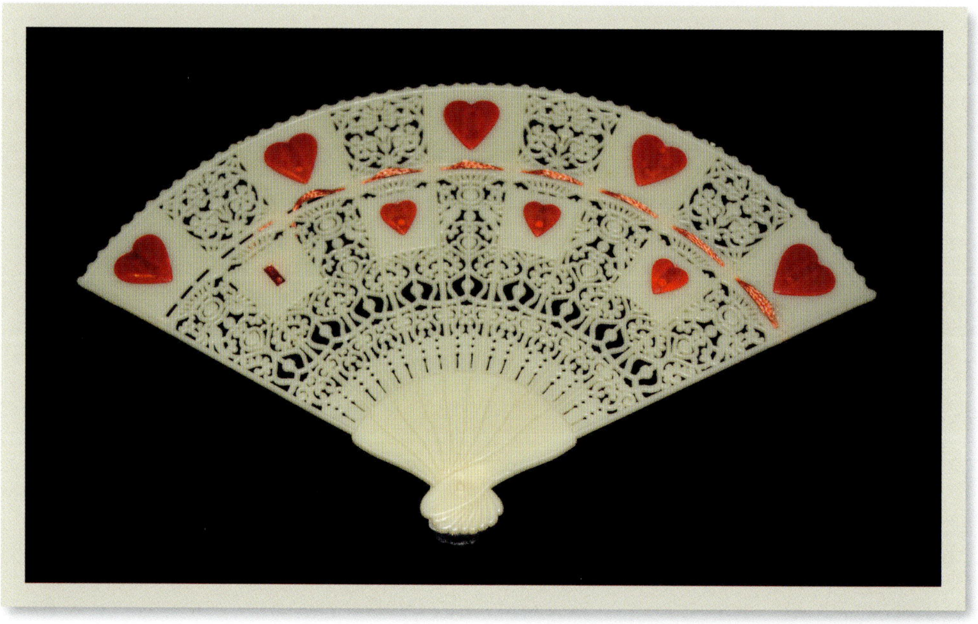

Cotton eyelet separate bodice for hasty cover-ups.

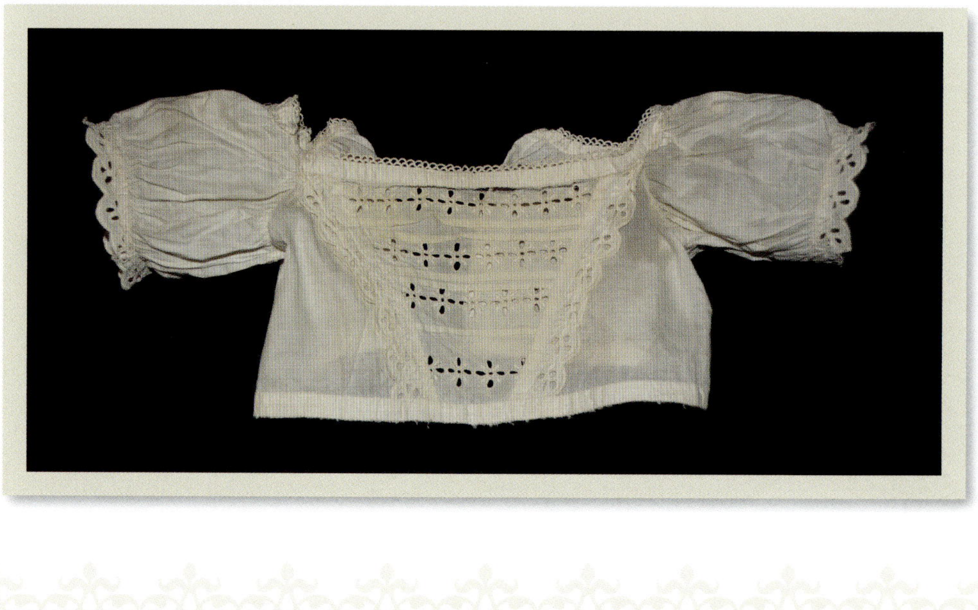

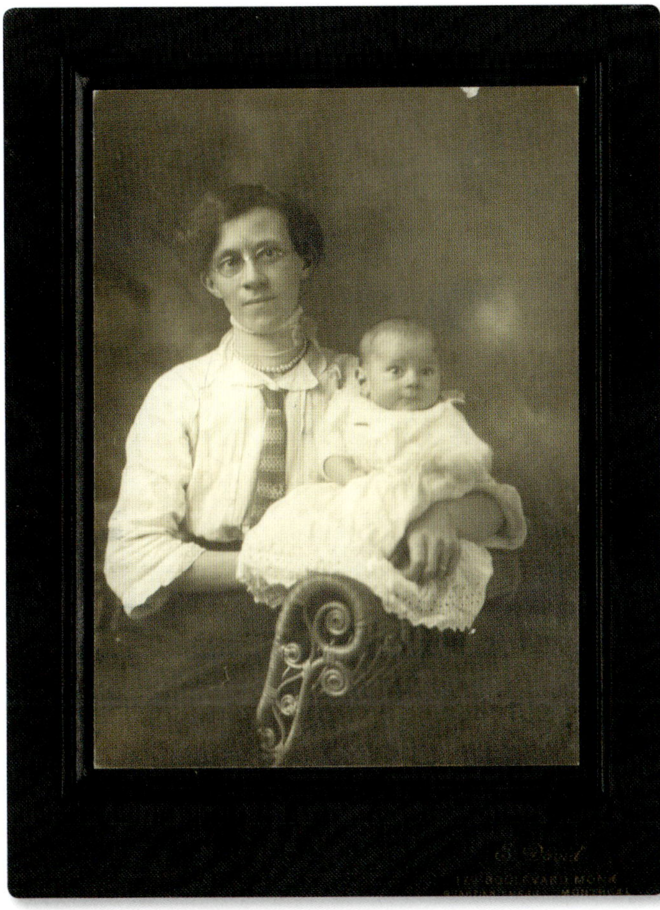

A 1914 cabinet card photo of infant Norman Hillyer in the arms of his mother. His lace-trimmed dress appears to be supported by multiple petticoats.

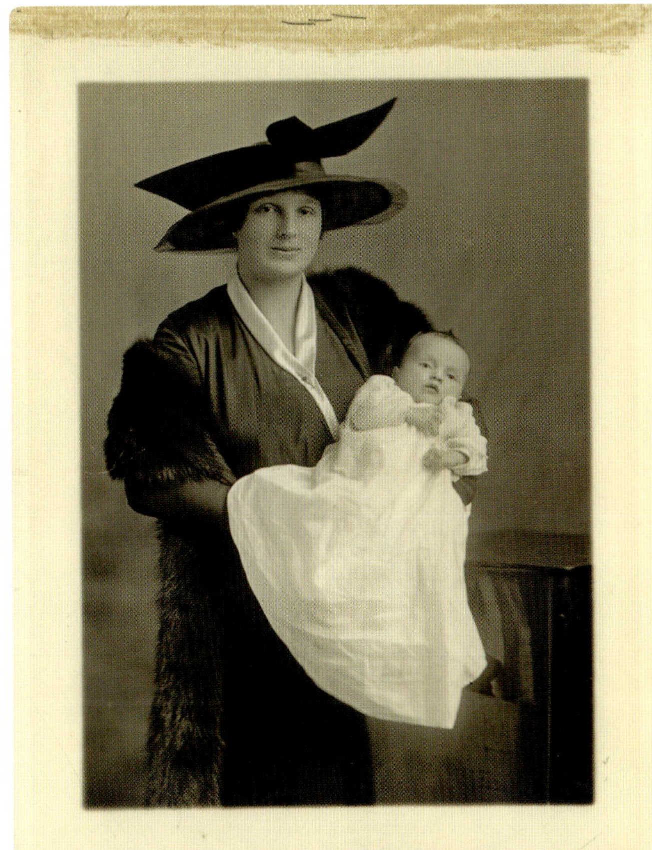

C.1914: This baby wears a long white dress typical for infants' wear at the time.

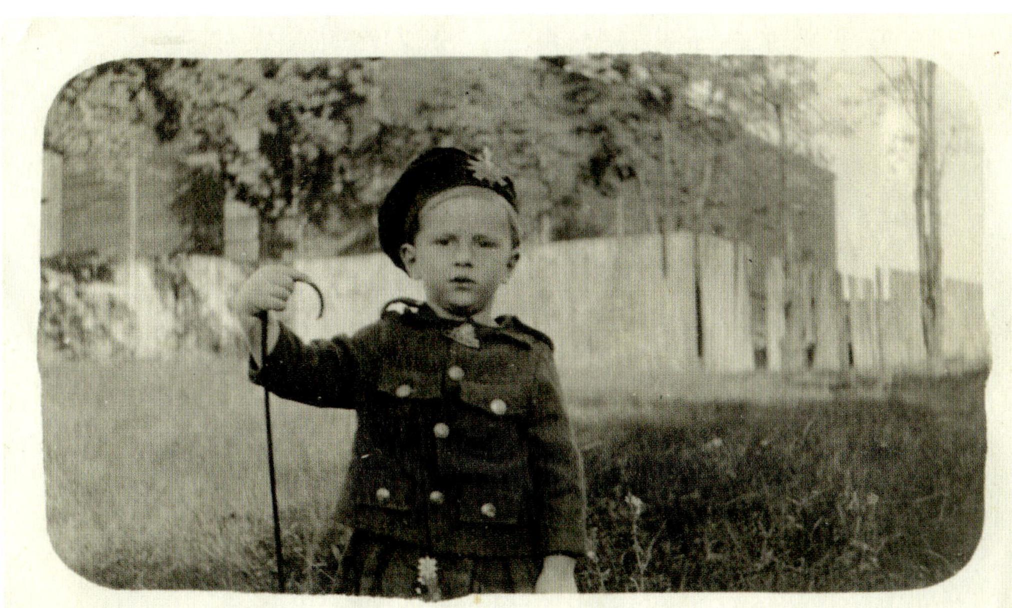

During the Great War many a young boy was proud to emulate the military by dressing in uniform.

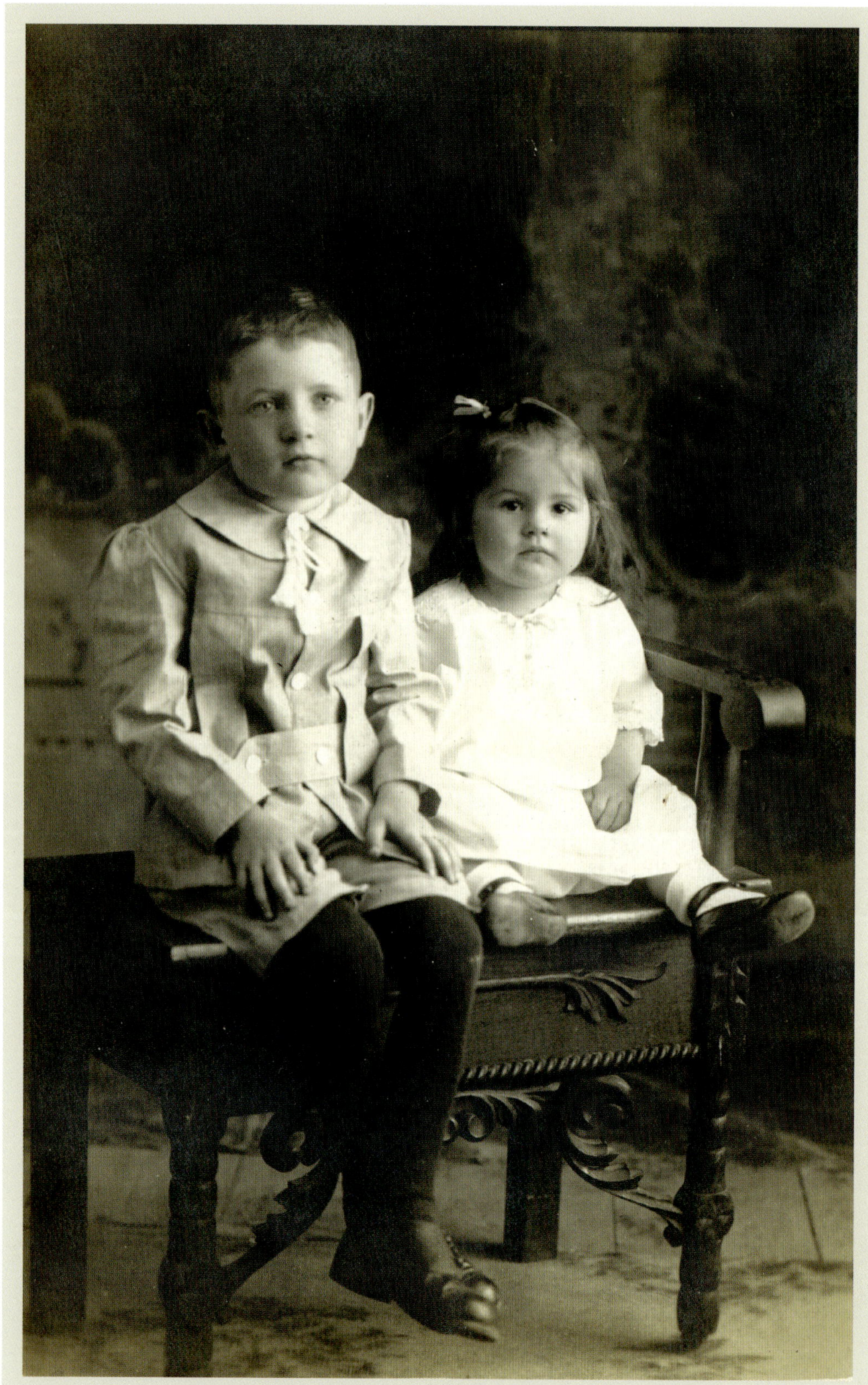

C.1919: Lorne and Kathleen O'Brien are dressed in the latest children's fashion for their brother-and-sister postcard portrait. The boy's crisp, belted and box-pleated short pant suit is particularly interesting.

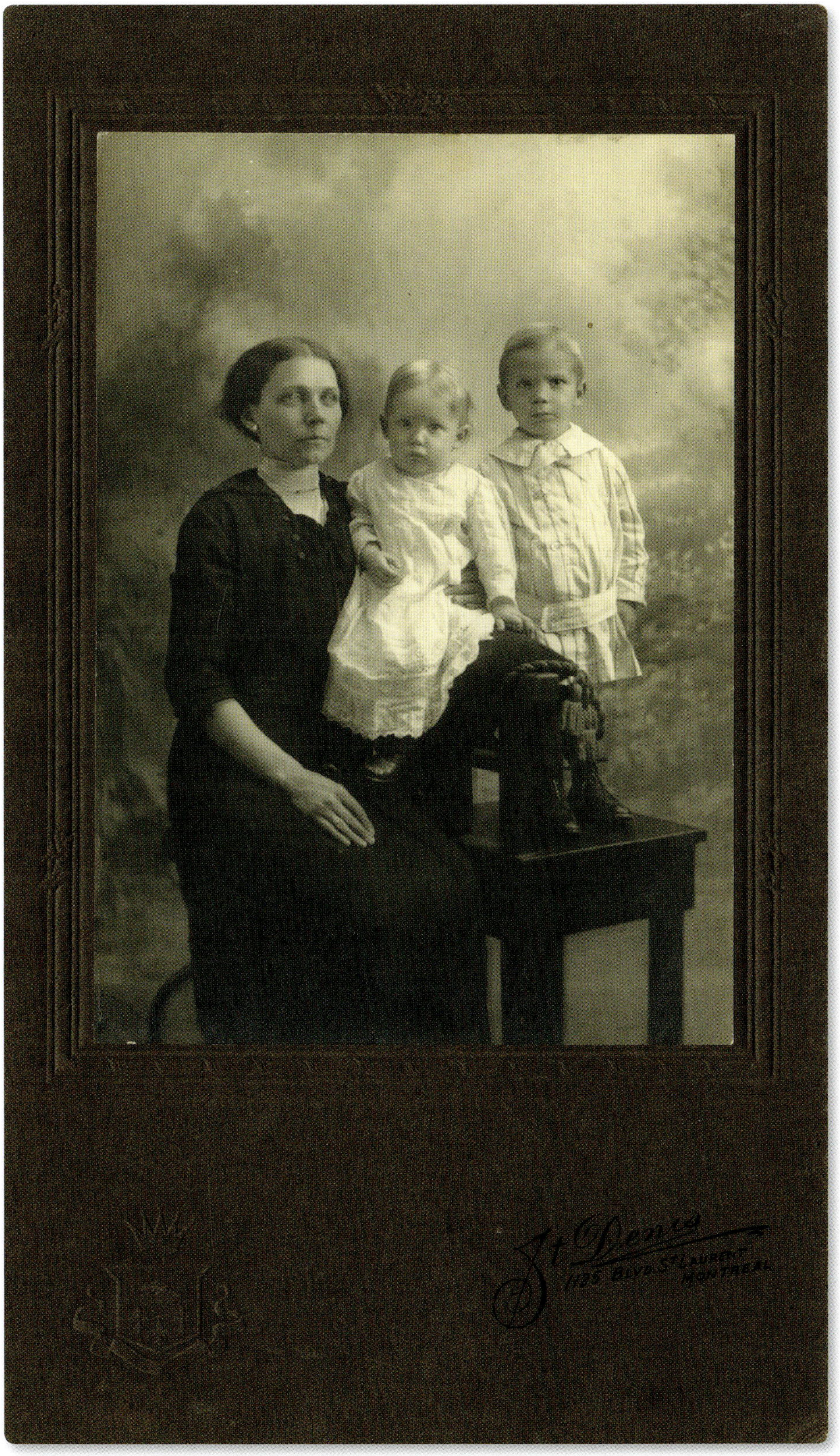

Studio portrait of Christie and Kenny Bethune taken in the early teens. Christie wears a lingerie dress of white eyelet with lace trim at the hem, while her older brother Kenny wears a Russian suit, pleated for fullness and belted low with a self-fabric band. What appears to be a silk bow adorns the neck. Mother-of-pearl buttons can be seen on the belt and placket, which is fashionably styled to the right of center. Cabinet card portrait by St. Denis, 1125 Blvd., St. Laurent, Montreal.

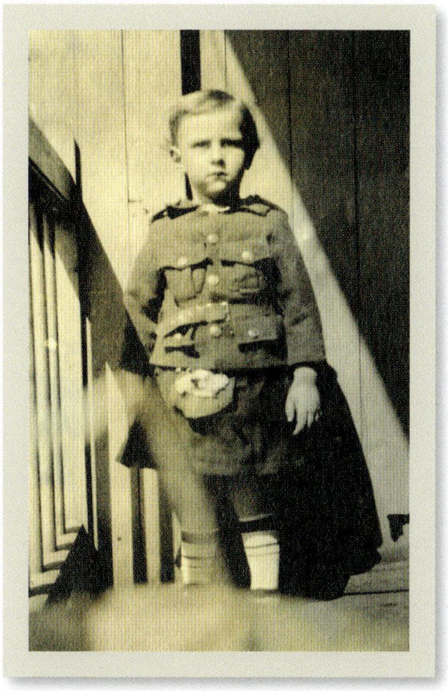

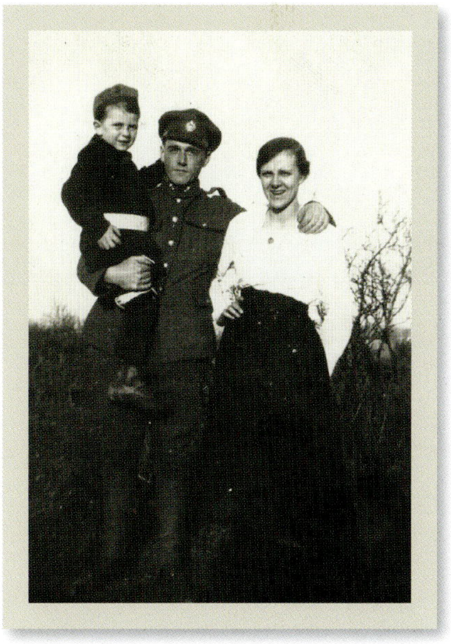

Top: Norman Hillyer c. 1917 in a military kilt suit, complete with sporran. Above: three-year-old Norman Hillyer in a child's belted military uniform.

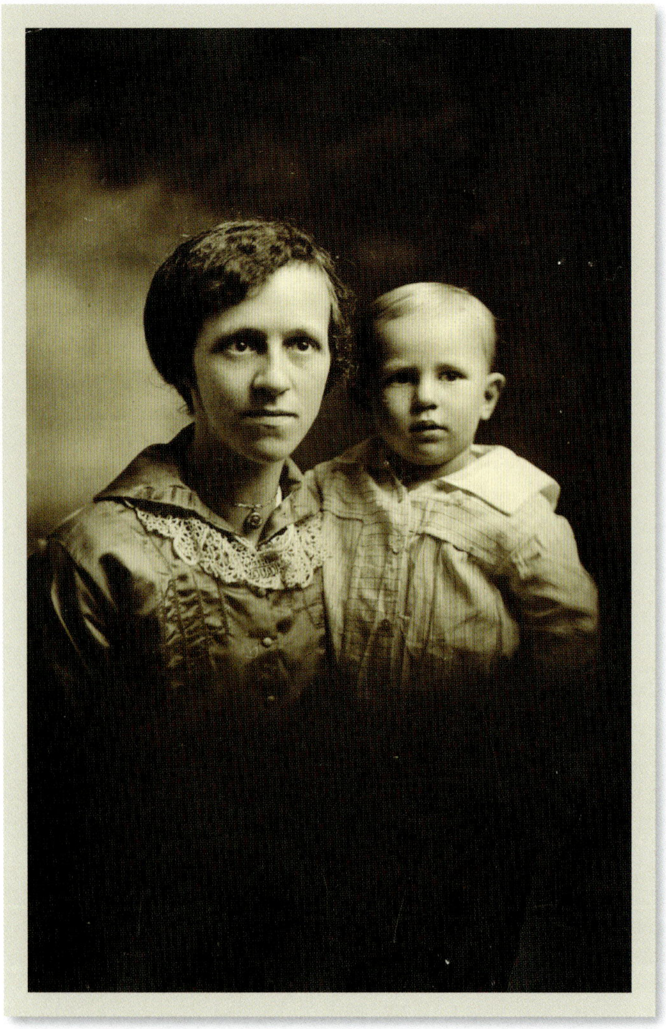

C. 1916: Formal portrait of two-year-old Norman Hillyer in a boy's suit with yoked bodice and broad collar.

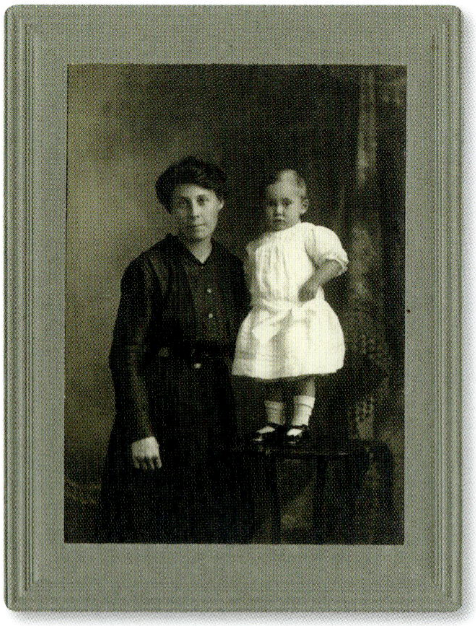

Though the dress is gender-neutral, the bow-trimmed ankle strap shoes suggest this smartly attired Edwardian model is a girl. Photo by Moore, Simcoe, Ontario.

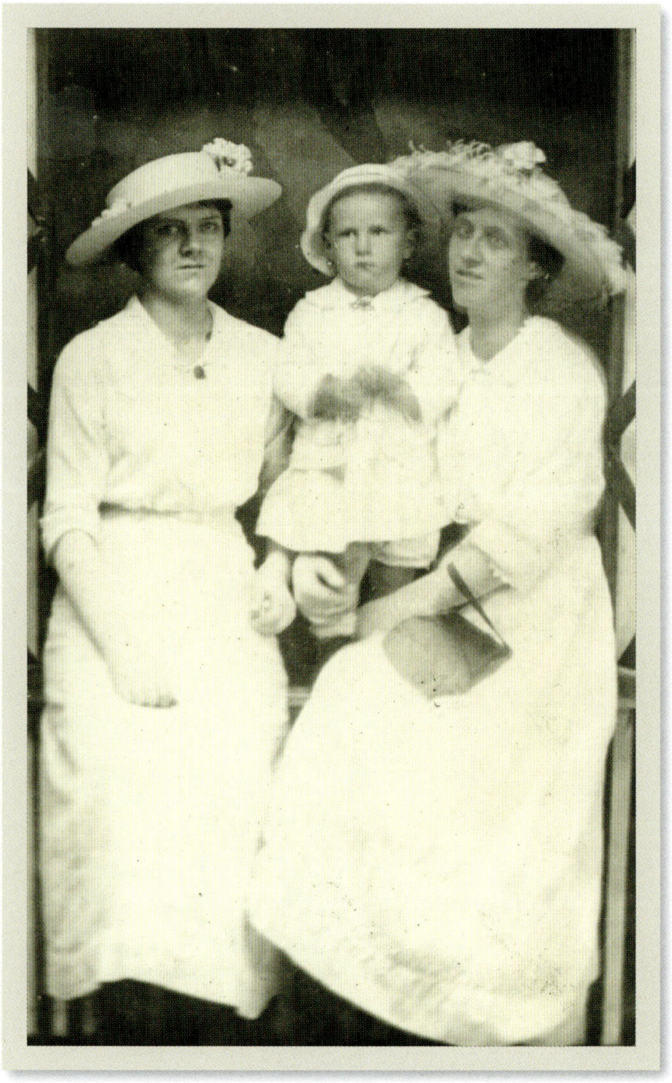

C.1916: The author's father poses for a postcard photo with his mother and aunt in a white knickers suit and summer hat.

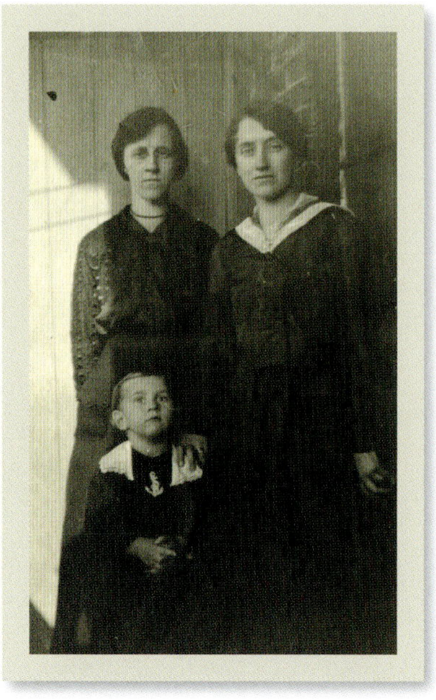

C.1917: The author's father, Norman Hillyer, in a sailor suit with large anchor appliqué. The photo was taken around the time of his father's death.

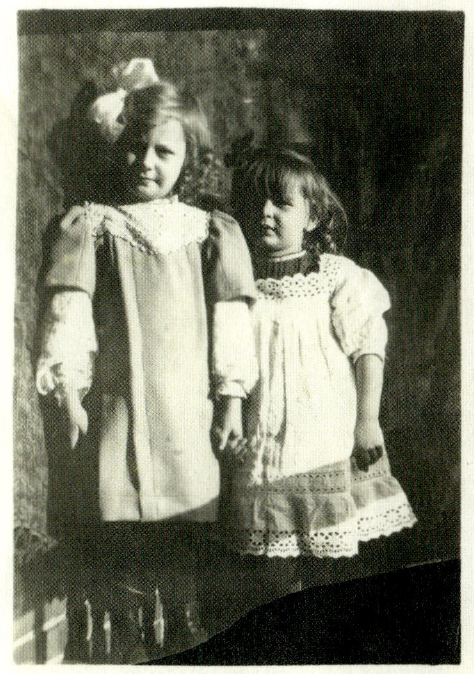

C.1916: Young sisters model loose-fitting frocks with exaggerated shoulders.

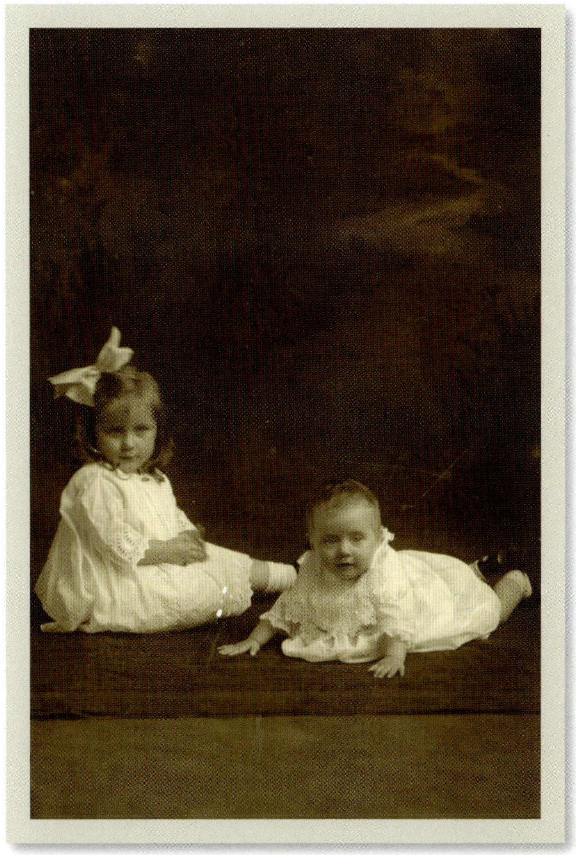

Photographic postcard image of sisters Muriel and Myrtle Hillyer in delicate white dresses with eyelet trim. Note the three-quarter-length sleeves typical of women's wear during the teen years. Muriel's hair is adorned with a fabric butterfly bow.

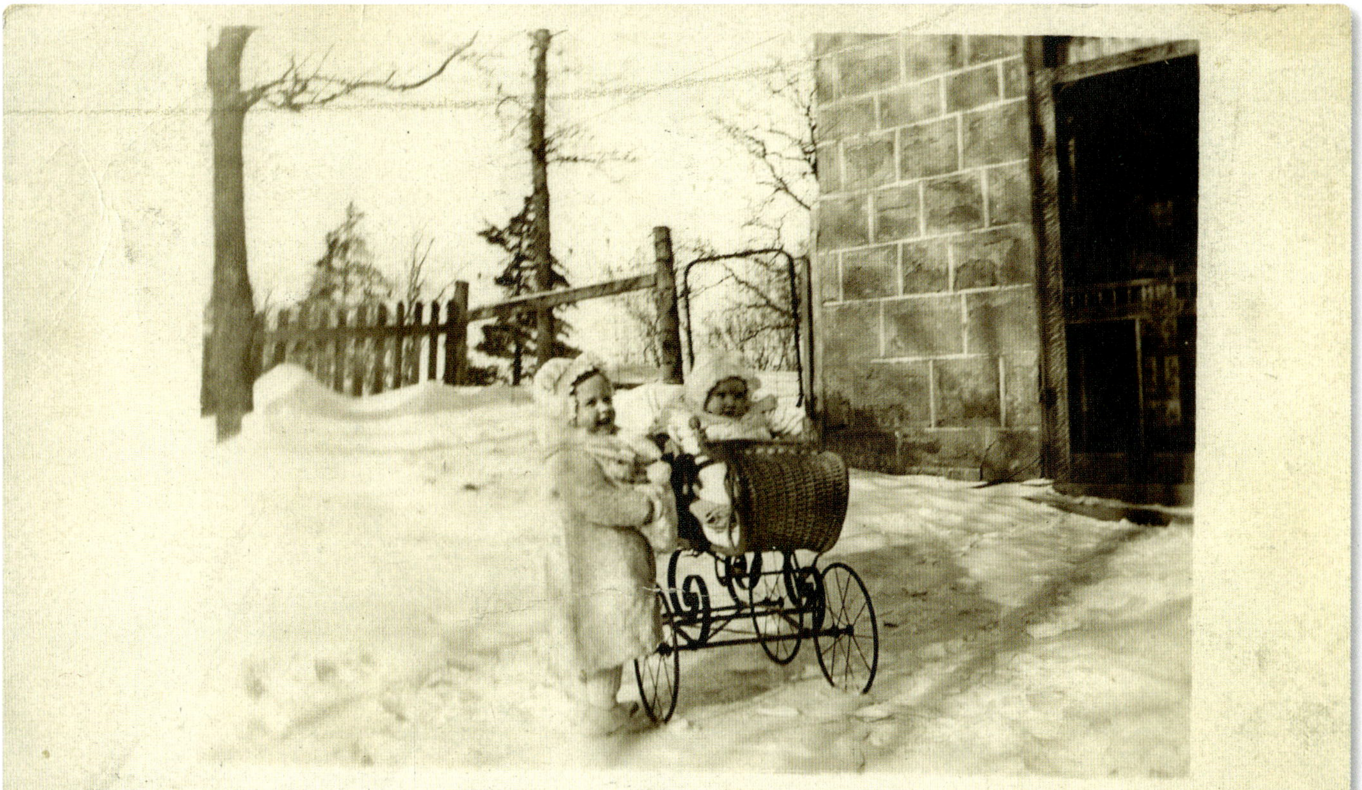

Picture postcard of Louise and Lillian Spence taken in March 1912. The girls are bundled in fur and brimmed bonnets.

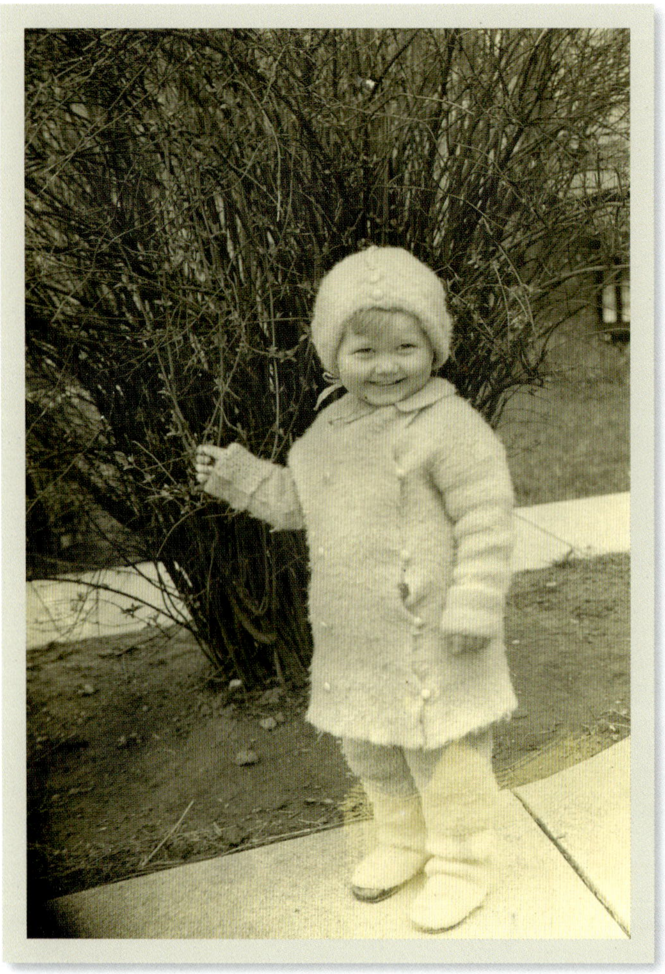

This little fellow's sweater attests to the knitting craze popularized during WWI.

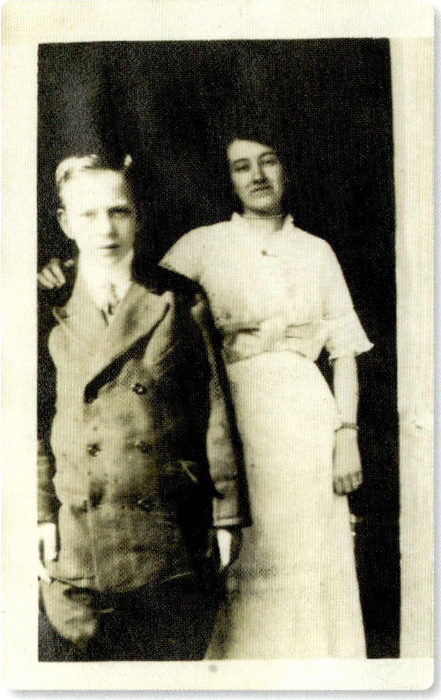

C.1912: Young teen Eddie Philip in a double-breasted woolen suit.

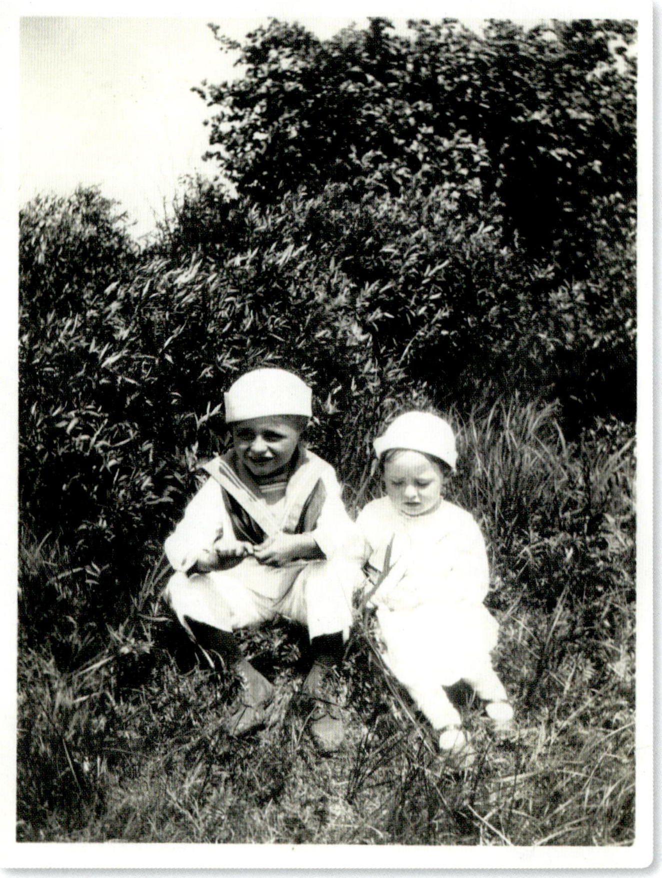

C.1919: His-and-hers sailor suits and caps.

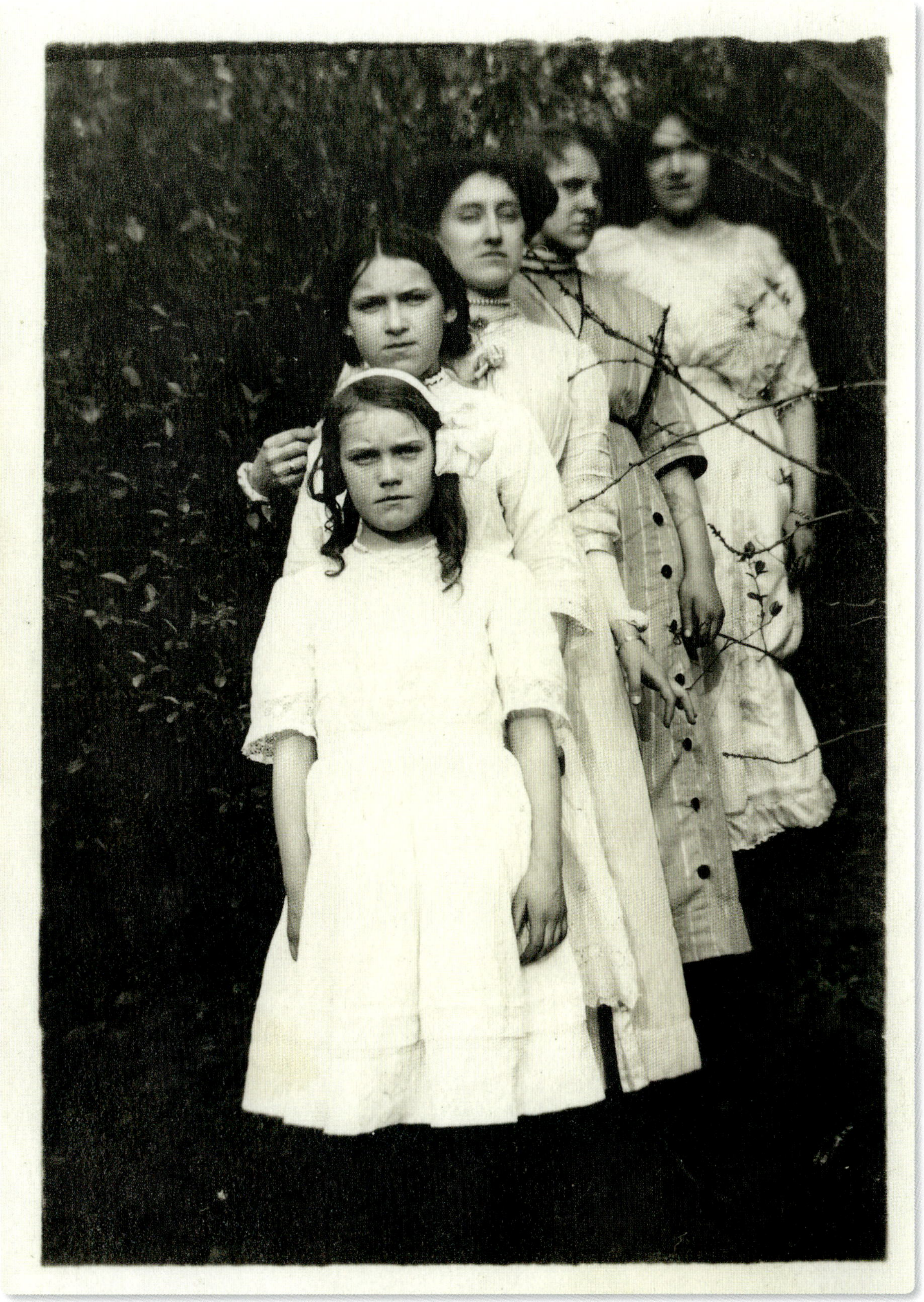

Who is hiding behind the shrubs (only a hand can be seen) beside five young ladies in ascending age and height? This charming photo illustrates typical casual summer wear for young girls, c.1914.

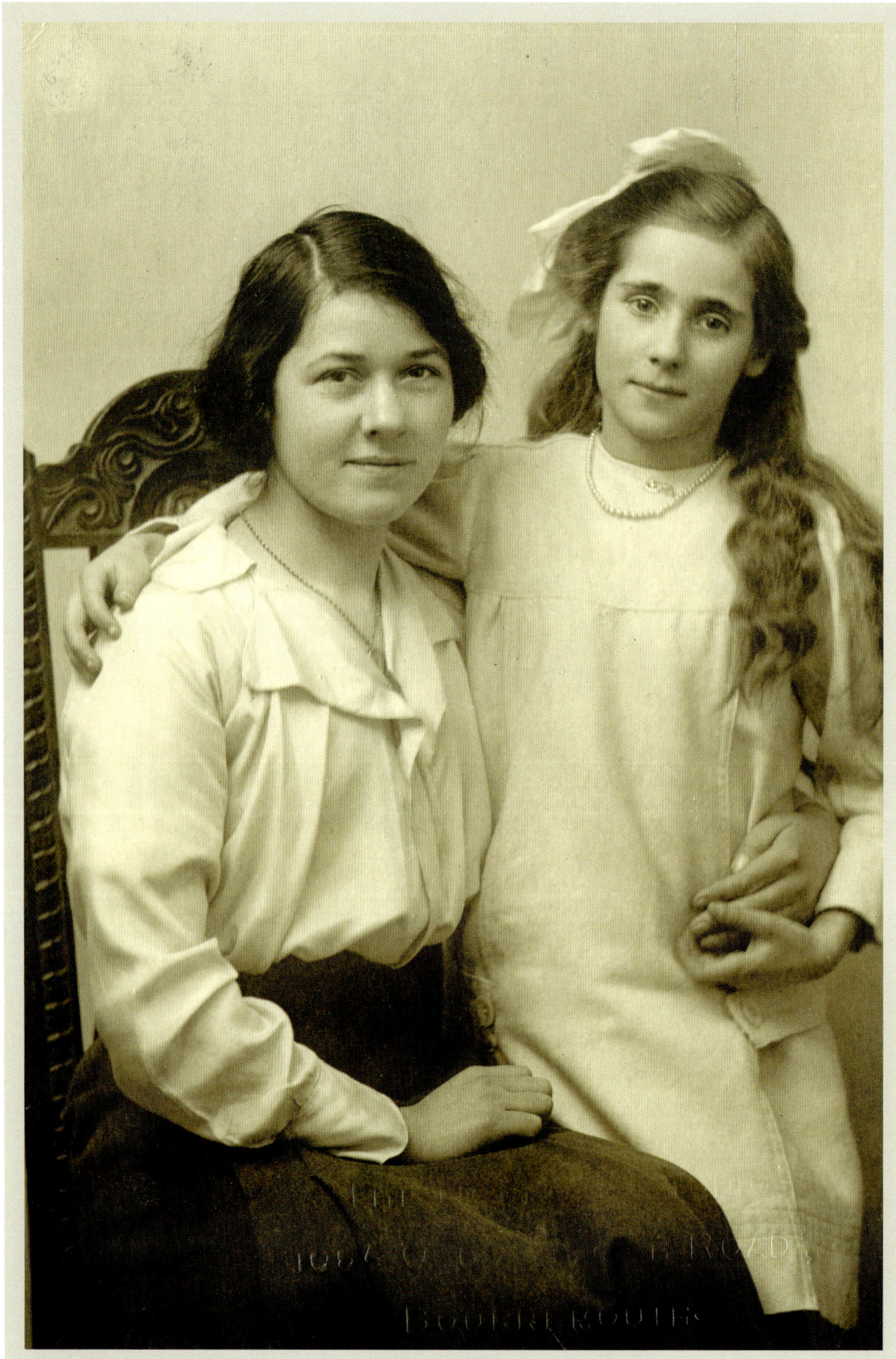

March 1917: Ten-year-old Miss Bracey poses with twenty-two-year-old Lucy Pearce in a long-sleeved, loose-fitting dress with square-cut yoke. Lucy's giant, flat bow is a cross between a hair adornment and a hat.

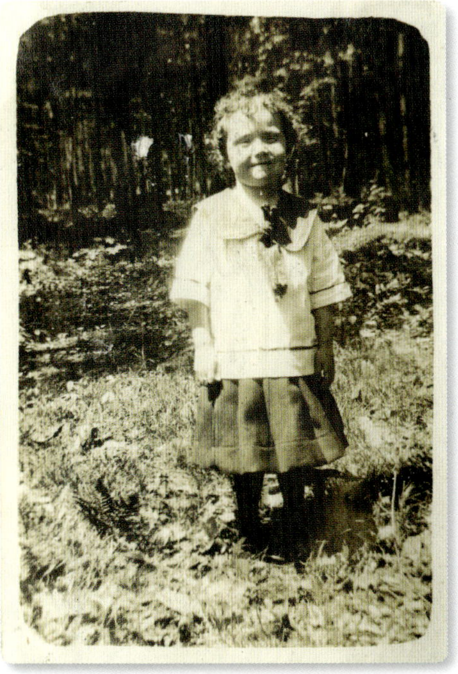

A smiley-faced girl in a square-cut middy blouse and skirt. Ella Philip collection.

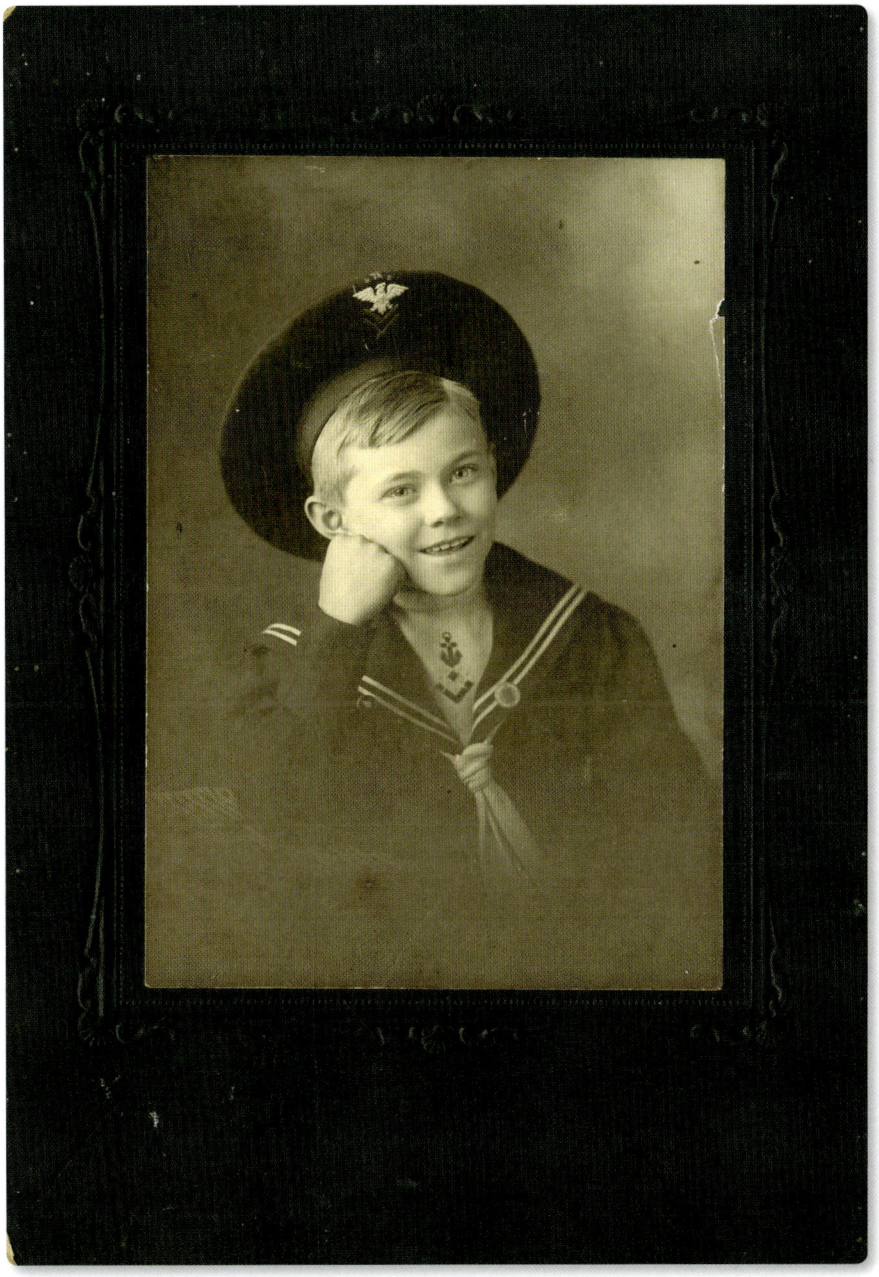

Lester Liddell strikes a nonchalant pose in a dark sailor suit. Note the anchor insignia on the vestee and American Eagle pin on the cap.

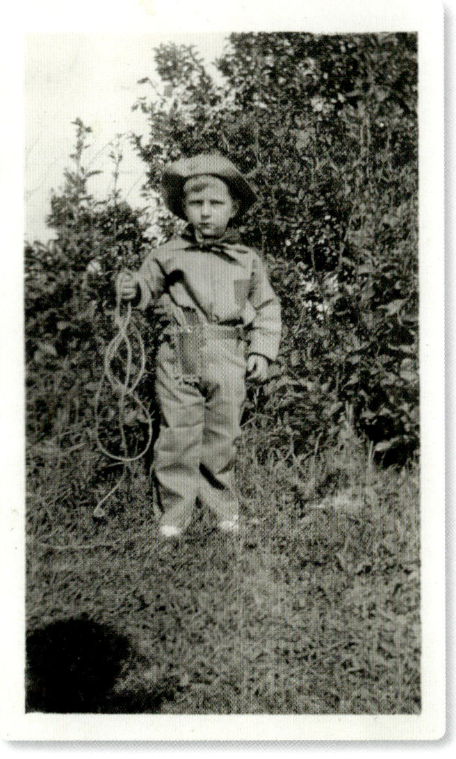

Learning to lasso? Young Norman Hillyer in a western inspired costume complete with neckerchief.

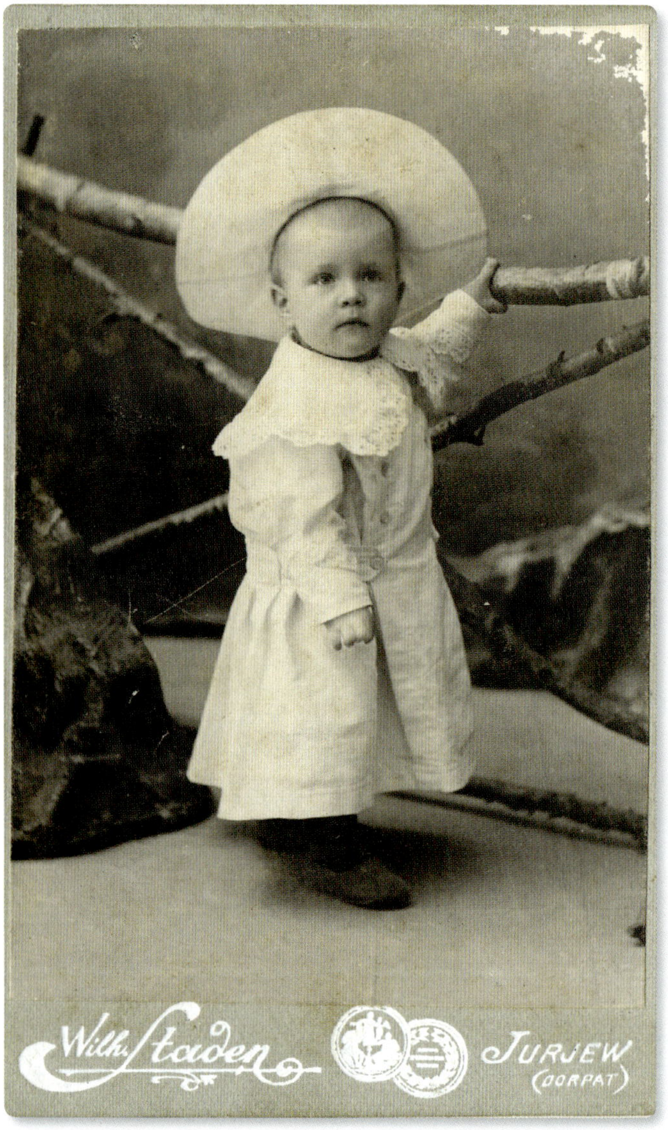

Summer dressing for a tiny tot. Note the puffed sleeves, enormous collar, and wide-brimmed hat. W. Staden studio photograph.

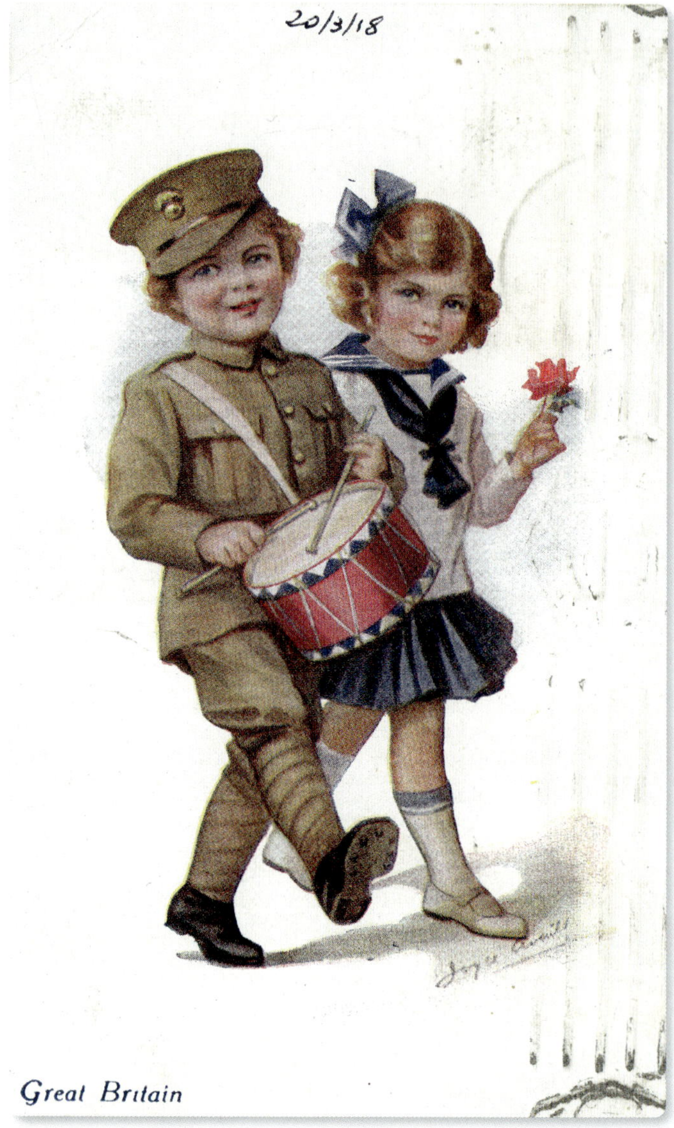

Spanish postcard c.1918 illustrating children's popular military and nautical dress.

Three tots in fashionable beachwear c.1919. For an amateur photograph, this is beautifully framed. The children's play clothes appear comfortable and stylish in keeping with early-twentieth-century dress reforms.

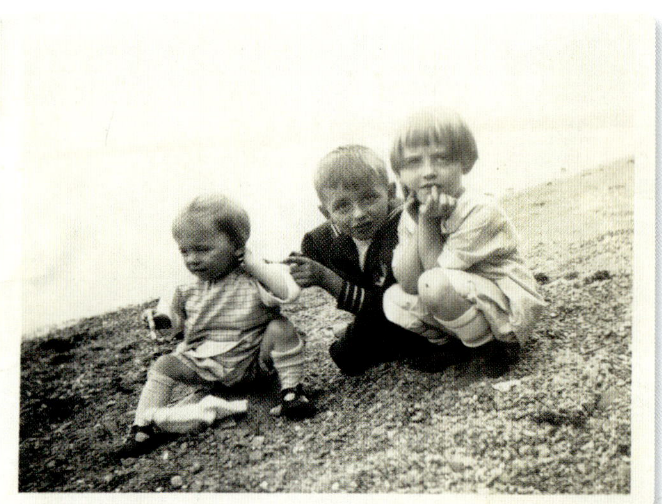

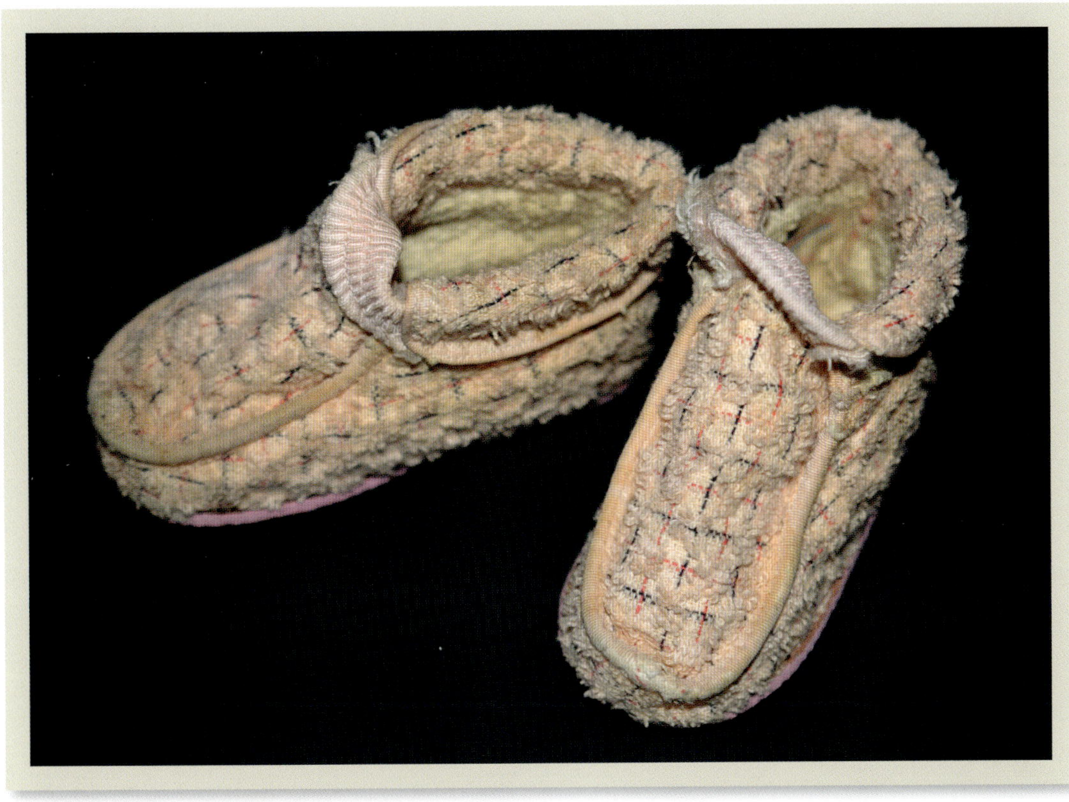

Soft chenille booties for a young child.

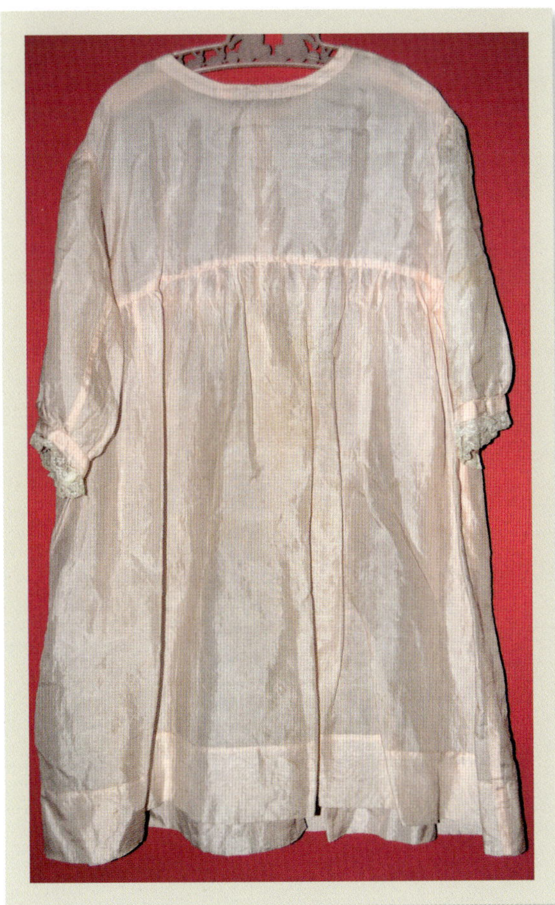

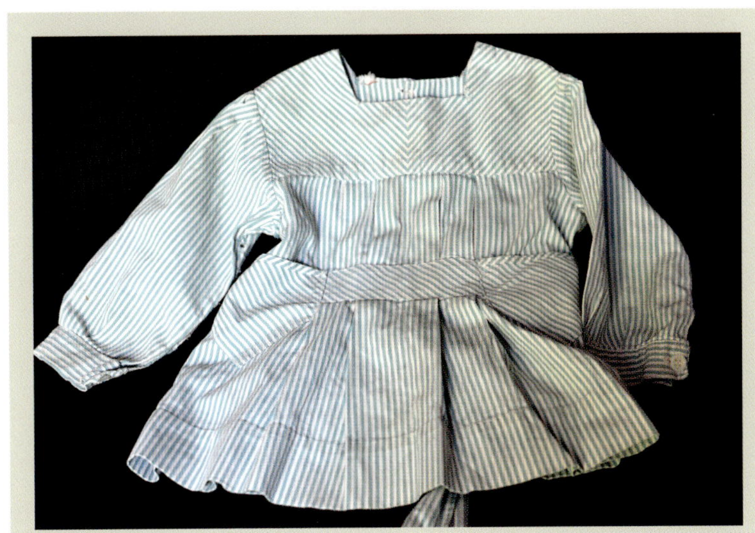

C. 1910: Young boy's blue stripe dress with three-quarter sleeves, box pleats, and self-fabric sash.

Young girl's pink silk loose-fitting dress.

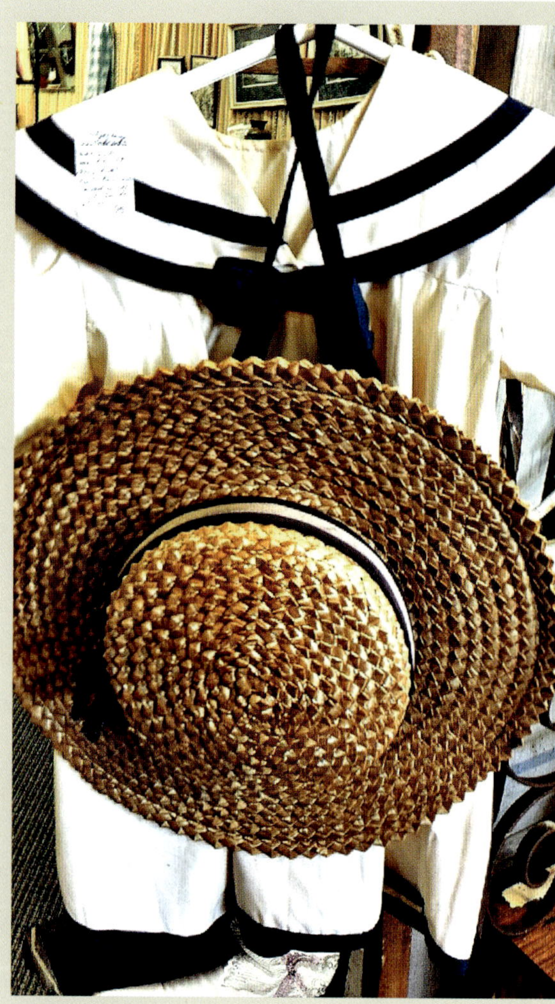

Fashioned from coarsely woven straw, this boy's sailor hat is the perfect accompaniment to the crisp blue-and-white sailor suit. They hang ready to tempt buyers at an Ontario antiques mall.

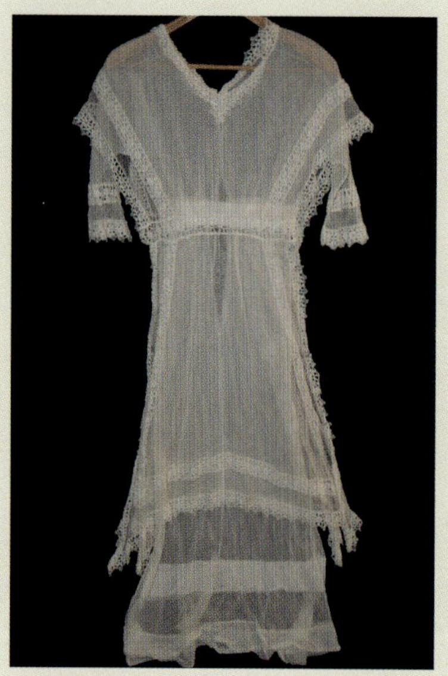

Teen girl's silk net lingerie dress with lace insertions.

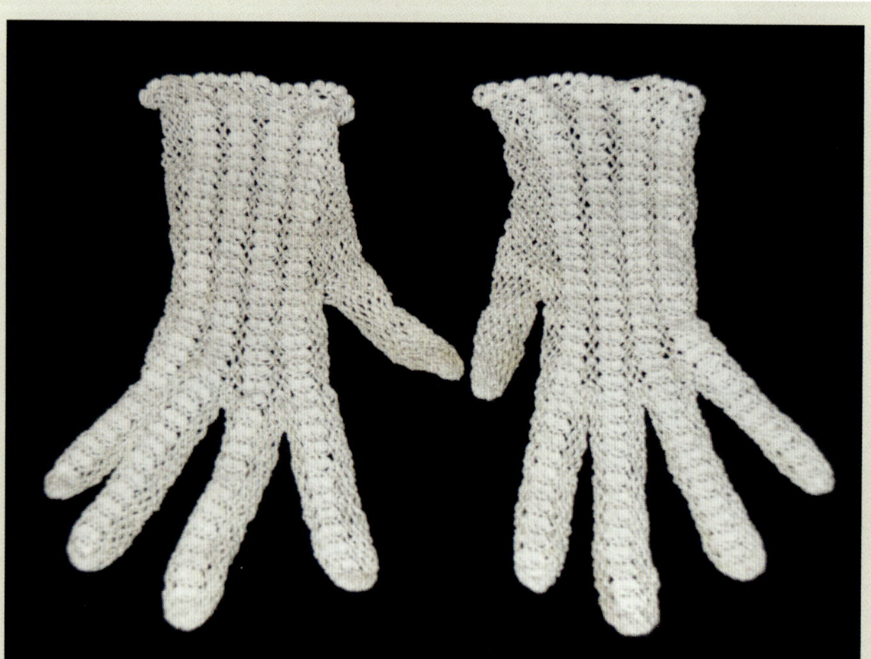

Teen girl's white lace gloves.

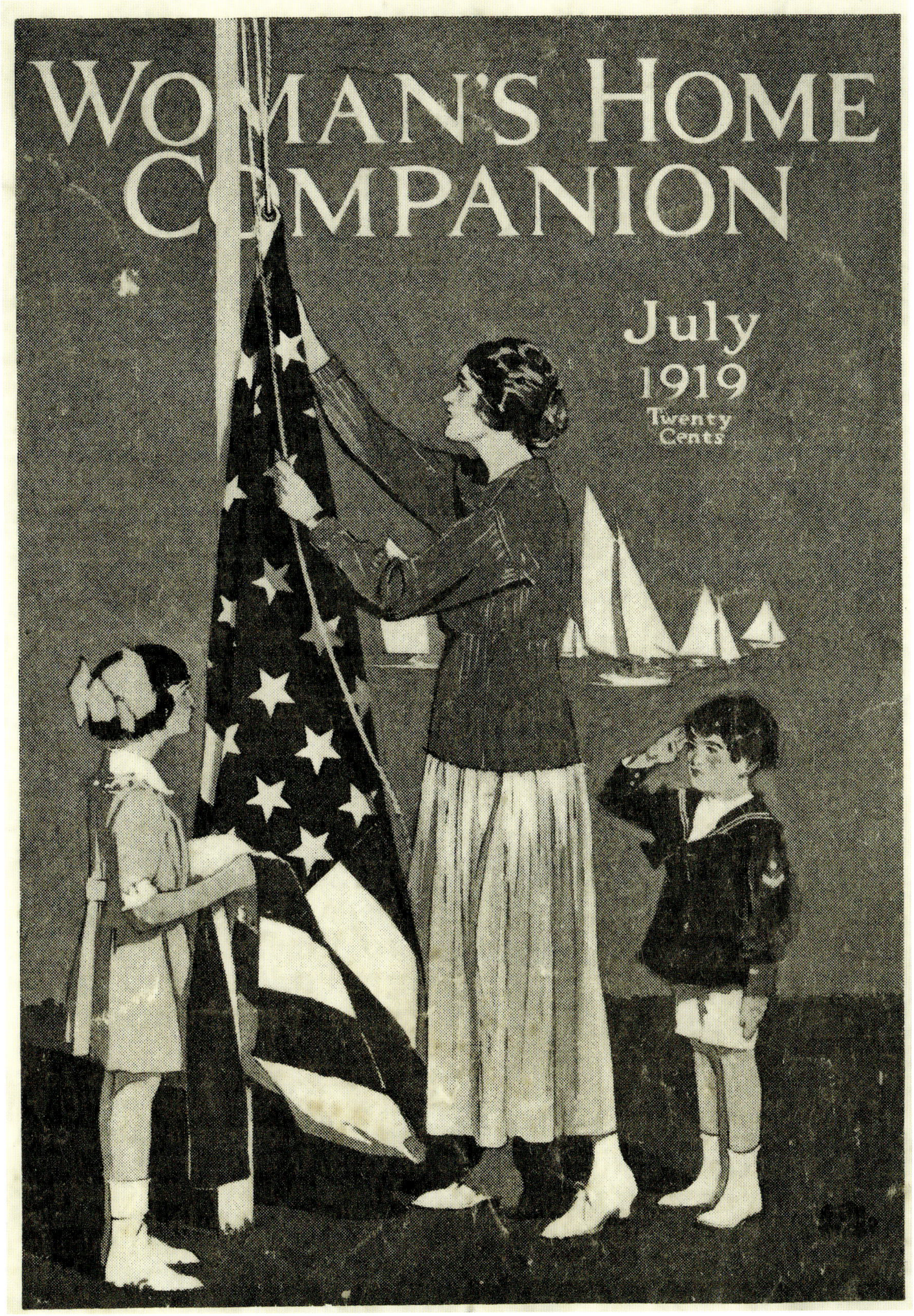

In this cover image for the July 1919 issue of *Woman's Home Companion*, artist Adolph Treidler portrayed this girl and boy in a strikingly modern-looking dress and sailor suit.

Glossary

Albatross: A fleecy cotton resembling the breast of the albatross bird.

Alizarin: An aniline dye producing a range of red hues.

Apron: A garment that ties at the waist and is worn to protect the front of one's clothing. Aprons are colorful reminders of twentieth-century homemaking when dishes were done by hand at the sink. At times, while mothers washed and daughters dried, husbands and sons playfully untied their aprons strings, causing shrieks and playful scolding. Commercially made examples exist, but many aprons were made at home on the sewing machine and represent a wide variety of tastes, patterns, and ingenuity.

Astrakhan: The soft, tightly coiled fleece harvested from Karakurl lambs three days old and younger.

Balmacaan: A single-breasted, knee-length, flared coat, loose-fitting with raglan sleeves and a Prussian collar.

Basque: A boned, close-fitting, hip-level jacket or bodice.

Bertha: A very large collar designed to complement the shoulders.

Bloomers: Originally described as a divided skirt, this invention of lecturer and dress reform proponent Amelia Bloomer is the precursor to modern-day underpants.

Blucher: A laced boot with rounded toe, the vamp and tongue of which are cut in one piece.

Bodice: The portion of a dress that covers the body from the shoulders to the waist.

Bohemian: An unconventional style; a description applied to certain hippie garments.

Box cloth: A felt-like woolen fabric.

Brandebourgs: Loup-and-toggle fasteners applied primarily to coats.

Breeching: A young boy's transition from dress to pants (breeches).

Bretelles: Shoulder straps attached to a waistband.

Briar-stitch: A hand embroidery stitch also called the feather stitch.

Brilliant: A glossy fabric made of cotton and mohair.

Cambric: A thin white fabric woven closely of cotton or linen fibres.

Challis: A thin silk-wool blend.

Chambray: A lightweight fabric of white fibers (usually cotton), woven against a colored warp.

Chambrette: A variation of chambray.

Chemise: A loose gown falling straight down from shoulders to hem.

Chemisette: A lacy insertion for an open neckline bodice or gown.

Cheviot: A coarse twill weave fabric derived from the Cheviot species of sheep, known for their medium-length heavy fleece.

Cloak: A loose-fitting, cape-like outer garment, usually devoid of fasteners.

Collarette: A small collar of beads, lace, fur, etc.

Combination: An all-in-one dress reform undergarment.

Crinoline: A stiff, nineteenth-century fabric comprised of horse hair strengthened with linen or cotton fibers; later used to describe a stiffened tulle half-slip.

Cutwork: An embroidery technique in which segments of the fabric are cut away.

Dagged: Cut into points or scallops.

Daguerreotype: An early type of photograph produced on a silver or silver-coated copper plate.

Débutante: French for female beginner. The word refers to an upper-class young lady being presented to society for the first time.

Dickie: A false blouse front that usually slips over the head.

Dimity: A lightweight cotton fabric with a corded effect.

Dolly Varden: During the late Victorian era, a number of products were named for this popular Dickens character including the revival polonaise dress and flat, forward-tilting beribboned straw hat.

Drawers: A Victorian undergarment for women, the legs of which extend to the knees.

Eton collar: This wide, stiff collar was a nineteenth-century style originally designed as part of the uniform for students of Eton College.

Ferrule: The metal ring or protective cap fitted to the tip of an umbrella or parasol handle.

Festoons: Textiles suspended in loops.

Flowers of sulphur: A bright yellow powder with antifungal and antibacterial properties, obtained from brimstone deposits.

Frieze: A curly-nap woolen fabric.

Galatea: A washable twill weave fabric with a lustrous finish.

Gingham: A cotton fabric usually woven in a check pattern of two colors.

Glengarry cap: A traditional Scots cap, made from wool and trimmed with a tassel and left-sided ribbon cockade.

Guimpe: A removable yoked insert for a low-necked dress.

Henrietta: Twilled fabric with a silk warp.

Kaftan: A long-sleeved ankle-length garment.

Kersey: A ribbed woolen textile popular for heavy stockings and outerwear.

Knickerbockers: Trousers for young boys that closed under the knee.

Krimmer: A pile fabric imitative of a certain type of fur.

Lansdowne: A botanical print in stony colors on soft cotton velvet.

Limerick lace: A net-based Irish lace.

Lisle: A fine, smooth knit produced from Eygptian yarn.

Mauveine: A synthetic aniline dye discovered in 1856; purplish in color.

Melton cloth: A heavy woolen fabric woven with a short nap.

Mercerization: A chemical process applied to cotton to strengthen the fibers, patented in 1850 by John Mercer.

Merino: A particularly soft wool, finely crimped, derived from Merino sheep.

Moire: A treatment applied to fabrics, primarily silks, which produces a wavy appearance (i.e, moiré and watered silk).

Mousquetaire: A style of glove.

Mousseline: A sheer, lightweight fabric often of silk.

Nainsook: A soft, plain-weave cotton fabric.

Ooze: An early name for suede, derived from the process of oozing chemicals through leather.

Palazzo pants: Women's pants with extremely wide legs.

Paletot: A jacket meant to cover a bodice.

Pantalettes: A leg covering popular in the 1860s, the lace or ruffled hems of which can be seen below the dress.

Parasol: A hand-held sunshade with a canopy made of cotton, silk, lace, paper, plastic, or nylon.

Pea jacket (i.e., reefer): A short, double-breasted woolen coat.

Peau de soie: A soft, satin-weave fabric with a dull finish.

Pelerine: A style of cape that tapers at the front, ending in long points.

Percale: A closely woven plain-weave cotton.

Persian lawn: A very fine plain-weave cotton fabric.

Petticoat: An underskirt with or without attached bodice.

Pilot jacket: An aviator-style leather jacket.

Piqué: A cotton, woven to produce raised parallel ribs.

Plaid: A tartan pattern.

Plumassier: A workshop for the creation of feather arrangements.

Pneumonia blouse: An Edwardian shirt waist with transparent yoke.

Poet's collar: A large collar with elongated points (i.e., Barrymore collar).

Polonaise: A gown with a swagged overskirt.

Poplin: A plain weave fabric or blend with corded appearance. Also known as Tabinet.

Quilling: An embellishment technique usually achieved by winding thread or yarn around a quill or rolled piece of fabric to create a decorative raised ridge; usually done in multiples.

Redingote: A coat with close-fitting bodice and flared skirt.

Rick rack: This decorative trim was first known as wave braid.

Rondelle: Circular decorative element.

Rosaniline: A reddish-brown synthetic dye.

Sacque: Loose-fitting coat or jacket.

Skimmer: A shallow-crowned circular straw hat with a flat brim.

Smock frock: A loose outer garment originally of cotton or linen.

Soutache: A narrow, flat decorative braid.

Spencer: A short jacket or coat that stops at the waistline of the garment it covers.

Stay: A length of whalebone, wood, or metal; multiples are incorporated into the design of a bodice or corset to support the back, midriff, or breasts.

Suspenders: Fabric or leather straps worn on the body and attached to stockings or trousers to keep them up.

Tabinet: See poplin.

Thibet: The white wool of the Tibetan lamb.

Trig: Neat and trim.

Ulster: A double breasted informal overcoat.

Ulster cloth: A high-quality linen.

Vest: A sleeveless garment covering the upper body.

Whitework: An embroidery technique worked in white thread on a white fabric.

Yoke: The fitted segment of a garment (usually at the neck and shoulders) to which an unfitted segment of the garment is gathered and attached.

Zephyr: A durable, lightweight cotton fabric.

Zibeline: A thick, soft, long-nap fabric made from wool or animal hair.

Zouave: A suit comprised of baggy trousers and a short, open fronted jacket. The jacket style, popular during the 1860s, was patterned after the military uniform of French Zouave troops during the Crimean War (1853–1856).

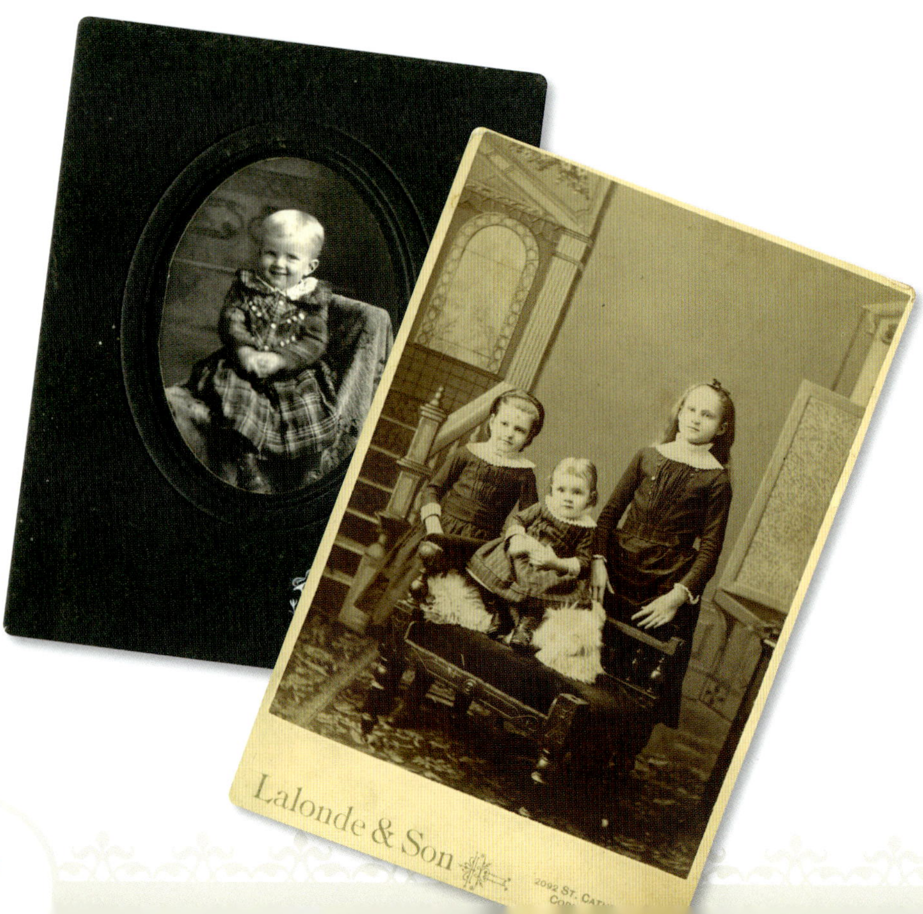

Bibliography

Bajorek, Lagretta. *America's Early Advertising Paper Dolls.* Atlgen, PA: Schiffer, 1999.

Ball, Jopanne Dubbs & Caroline Torem-Craig. *Wedding Traditions*. Atlgen, PA: Schiffer, 2001.

Bateman, Mildred, E. "Pretty Things for the Wee Folk," *Needlecraft Magazine*, April 1916.

Blackman, Cally. *100 Years of Fashion*. London: Laurence King Publishing Limited, 2012.

Blum, Stella. *Victorian Fashions and Costumes from Harper's Bazaar, 1867–1898.* New York: Dover Publications, 1974.

Boucher, Francois. *Histoire Du Costume; En Occident De L'Antiquité A Nos Jours.* France: Flammarion et Cie., 1965.

Bremer, Debra. "Every Portrait Tells a Lie," *Portrait Society Essays*, October 2010. www.portraitsocietygallery.com.

Brett, K. B. *Women's Costume in Ontario (1867–1907).* Toronto, Ontario: University of Toronto Press, 1966.

Burdett, Robert F., "The Mending Basket," *Ladies' Home Journal*, April 1898. Philadelphia: The Curtis Publishing Company.

Dolan, Maryanne. *Vintage Clothing 1880–1960.* Florence, AL: Books Americana, 1987.

Douglas, Dora. "The Art of Dressing," *Needlecraft Magazine*, March 1915.

Dubin, Tiffany. *Vintage Style: Buying and Wearing Classic Vintage Clothes*. New York: HarperCollins, 2000.

Florence, Judy. *Aprons of the Mid-20th Century*. Atglen, PA: Schiffer, 2001.

Fraser, Sylvia. *A Woman's Place: Seventy Years in the Lives of Canadian Women.* Toronto: Key Porter Books Ltd., 1997.

Fukai, Akido. *Fashion, The Collection of the Kyoto Costume Institute*. Tokyo: Taschen, 2002.

Godey, Louis A. & Sarah Buell Hale. *Godey's Lady's Book and Magazine*, January to June 1861, July to December 1864.

Grant, Neil. *History of Theatre*. London: Octopus Publishing Group Ltd., 2002.

Hand, Anna-Marie. *Clothes Tell Stories: Reuse and Recycle*. The Costume Collection at the Maryland Historical Society. www.mdhs.org/costumeblog.

Hemingway, Karen. *The Essential Guide to Embroidery*. London: Murdoch Books, 2002.

Luscomb, Sally C. *The Collector's Encyclopedia of Buttons*. Atglen, PA: Schiffer Publishing, 2007.

Mellor, C. M. & D. S. L. Cardwell. *Dyes and Dyeing 1775–1860*, Vol.1, No.3. The British Journal for the History of Science. Cambridge: Cambridge University Press.

nicDhuinnshleibhe, Lady Siobhan. "A Brief History of Dyestuffs & Dyeing." www.kws.atlantia.sca.org.

Polan, Brenda. *The Great Fashion Designers*. New York: Bloomsburg, 2009.

Vocelle, Kathleen, *Victorian Picture Buttons*. www.bnb.jewelrymakingmagazines.com.

To hear author Norma Shephard read an excerpt from "On the Habit of Being a Girl," a column by Helen C. Candee in the May 1991 issue of *Ladies Home Journal*, scan the QR code or listen to the audio recording at https://youtu.be/efquenGW5Dc.

Index